Cancer Treatment and Research

Volume 178

This book series provides detailed updates on the state of the art in the treatment of different forms of cancer and also covers a wide spectrum of topics of current research interest. Clinicians will benefit from expert analysis of both standard treatment options and the latest therapeutic innovations and from provision of clear guidance on the management of clinical challenges in daily practice. The research-oriented volumes focus on aspects ranging from advances in basic science through to new treatment tools and evaluation of treatment safety and efficacy. Each volume is edited and authored by leading authorities in the topic under consideration. In providing cutting-edge information on cancer treatment and research, the series will appeal to a wide and interdisciplinary readership. The series is listed in PubMed/Index Medicus.

More information about this series at http://www.springer.com/series/5808

Daniel D. Von Hoff · Haiyong Han
Editors

Precision Medicine in Cancer Therapy

Springer

Editors
Daniel D. Von Hoff
Molecular Medicine Division
Translational Genomics Research Institute
Phoenix, AZ, USA

Haiyong Han
Molecular Medicine Division
Translational Genomics Research Institute
Phoenix, AZ, USA

ISSN 0927-3042 ISSN 2509-8497 (electronic)
Cancer Treatment and Research
ISBN 978-3-030-16390-7 ISBN 978-3-030-16391-4 (eBook)
https://doi.org/10.1007/978-3-030-16391-4

Library of Congress Control Number: 2019935844

This Springer imprint is published by the registered company Springer Nature Switzerland AG
The registered company address is: Gewerbestrasse 11, 6330 Cham, Switzerland

Foreword

Alas, our fragility is the cause, not we!
For, such as we are made of, such we be.
Viola, in Shakespeare, *Twelfth Night*

The science of "precision medicine" is in many ways the delicate quest for gaining insights into the fashion *Nature* deals the cards of human variability across the >200+ different classes of cancer.

Most applications of genomic profiling can be roughly categorized into one of two paradigms on the basis of the anticipated or desired outcome for analysis:

- Research to Discover Generalized Knowledge
- Search to Recover Individualized Knowledge

In the past, our hope has largely been on the former—that by simply acquiring the knowledge of genetic, genomic, and immunologic changes across a massive enough number of cancers, it would allow us to anticipate the strategies, capriciousness, and fallibilities that are deployed against us in successful cancer treatment for an individual patient.

This volume on "precision medicine" captured by Von Hoff and Han takes the important step forward toward modifying the intellectual framework on which to hang "multi-omic data". As described across the chapters (and summarized in the chapter by Schork et al.), more precise medical management of an individual with cancer has to extend beyond discovery-based data analysis. Such data is likely to be cross-sectional and leverages scientific approaches that try and uncover patterns across populations to make new generalized discoveries, and although this approach has an incredible "greater good" potential, nonetheless it has only limited direct benefit for the individuals who participate. Most often the patient is left with the hope that with time more people will participate, more knowledge will be generated, and eventually, there will be additional indirect benefits for the individuals who participate today.

We lack an embracing of conceptual frameworks which process the rich individualized information more comprehensively, leverage previously available knowledge, and intelligently recovering clinical relevant meaning. The framework for "precision medicine" that is outlined in this volume is a collaborative strategy to provide such a "lingua franca" that can help improve our hand in the face of the often, hopeless odds we are dealt by cancer.

Precision medicine has changed options and outcomes for cancer patients—for a few, a transformative, durable response—but by no means a guarantee and we must strive to do better. The hope for the future of precision medicine is in our continued embracing of conceptual frameworks, which process both the rich individualized information more comprehensively, leverage previously available knowledge more completely, and intelligently recover clinical relevant meaning in near real time. We should be prepared for surprises!

Phoenix, Arizona, USA

Jeffrey M. Trent, Ph.D., F.A.C.M.G.
Founding Scientific Director of the National Human Genome Research Institute, NIH

President and Research Director
Translational Genomics Research Institute (TGen)

Professor, City of Hope
Comprehensive Cancer Center

Preface

The words of personalized medicine and indeed even the seemly more precise precision medicine are at the lips of many these days. They have become almost "catch phrases" used even in advertising campaigns to distinguish healthcare systems. Those of us engaged in the daily practice of oncology have felt there is no doubt that for an increasing number of patients with cancer, precision medicine has been a godsend for improving their individual clinical situation.

We are pleased to present for the readers what we feel is a valuable text on three aspects of precision medicine. The first aspect is how precision medicine is helping patients now. As you will see, these chapters provide an incredible update on the current status of precision medicine for day-to-day care. This is a must for the practicing clinicians.

The second aspect of precision medicine, which for some is a black hole of knowledge, is the technologies behind precision medicine. This is beautifully crafted by the chapters on basic technologies including the latest in precision medicine in immune-oncology.

The final aspect of this text is the future of precision medicine. This is provided to keep the readers well versed with knowledge they will be able to apply in the days ahead in their practice. This future will undoubtedly hold incredible new technologies and an increasing amount of artificial intelligence.

The assembly of this book has required the intelligence, skills, and devotion of many. We acknowledge our patients who have, with their sometimes insurmountable clinical situations, driven us to try to do better for them. We acknowledge the incredible contributors to this volume who have made these chapters exceptional readings. Finally, we acknowledge the tremendous effort of the editorial staff who have made this text possible.

Phoenix, Arizona, USA

Daniel D. Von Hoff, MD, FACP
Haiyong Han, Ph.D.

Contents

Part I
Individual Types of Cancer Precision Medicine

Targeted Therapies in Non-small-Cell Lung Cancer

1

Addie Hill, Rohan Gupta, Dan Zhao, Ritika Vankina, Idoroenyi Amanam and Ravi Salgia

Contents

A. Hill · R. Gupta · D. Zhao · I. Amanam · R. Salgia (✉)
Department of Medical Oncology, City of Hope Comprehensive Cancer Center, Duarte, CA, USA
e-mail: rsalgia@coh.org

R. Vankina
Department of Hematology-Oncology, Harbor-UCLA Medical Center, Torrance, CA, USA

D. D. Von Hoff and H. Han (eds.), *Precision Medicine in Cancer Therapy*,
Cancer Treatment and Research 178, https://doi.org/10.1007/978-3-030-16391-4_1

1.1 Introduction

Even though the incidence of lung cancer is decreasing, unfortunately over 160,000 people still die from the disease every year and it remains the leading cause of cancer death in the USA. Lung cancer has been traditionally classified as small-cell lung cancer and non-small-cell lung cancer. Non-small-cell lung cancer can further be classified into adenocarcinoma, squamous cell carcinoma, and large-cell carcinoma. Histologically, small-cell lung cancer and non-small-cell lung cancer have different natural histories and therapeutic approaches. Prior to 2004, there was no need of distinguishing various subtypes of non-small-cell lung cancer as the therapeutic management was similar within all subtypes.

However, management and treatment of lung cancer has transformed in the past decade. This changed particularly in 2004 when a small percentage of lung adenocarcinomas were identified with mutations in the EGFR gene that rendered those tumors sensitive to the EGFR tyrosine kinase inhibitors. Since then, there has been a surge of other actionable mutations in lung cancer. Up to 69% of the patients with advanced lung cancer have actionable mutations. The majority of them are KRAS (25%), EGFR sensitizing (17%), ALK (7%), MET (3%), HER-2 (2%), ROS1 (2%), BRAF (2%), RET (2%), NTRK1 (1%), PIK3CA (1%), and MEK1 (1%) [1]. In addition, 31% patients are found to have unknown oncogenic driver mutations for which we currently do not have any targets [1]. Because of these advances, the current guidelines such as American Society of Clinical Oncology (ASCO) or National Comprehensive Cancer Network (NCCN) guidelines recommend molecular profiling or next-generation sequencing to determine the best treatment options for the individual patients or small subsets of newly diagnosed lung cancer patients. There is also growing understanding that there are increased genomic alterations through treatment lines, and there is more emphasis on better understanding of mechanisms of resistance and clonal evolvement of tumor. Thus, precision or personalized medicine has become an emerging approach for treatment and research of lung cancer taking into account personalized genetic landscape, tumor microenvironment, and available therapeutics.

In this current chapter, we will review the available options for next-generation sequencing and the importance of value-based genomics. We will then attempt to define the molecular abnormalities in lung cancer with standards of care and also potential diagnostic platforms such as proteomics and genomics. Then, we will individually discuss the current actionable mutations, genomic alterations with emphasis on the underlying mechanism of abnormality with the potential to therapy and available therapeutic options with evidence of clinical trials.

1.2 Value-Based Genomic Profiling

In the past few years, there has been advancement in next-generation sequencing techniques which have led to the development of biomarker-driven cancer therapies. The NGS techniques have now become more commercialized and affordable with various different platforms. These sequencing data has not only impacted clinical decision making but also allocation of resources in research and development of therapeutics and lung cancer. However, the current challenge is the standardization of these recommended NGS across different academic and community practices in a more value-based approach to obtain a greater clinical benefit with minimizing cost and risk of genomic profiling in cancer care [2].

The human genome sequencing project was initially completed in 2003 and led to further investigations and understanding of the genomics of various mutations and alterations in development of cancer [1]. First-generation Sanger sequencing technique was used for sequencing of human genome which required a decade of multi-central collaboration, automated analysis, and roughly $3 billion [3]. However, there is an exponential decline in the sequencing cost since then. James Watson's genome was completed for less than $1 million. By 2009, the cost of genome sequencing dropped to $100,000 [4–6]. Since then, there has been development of several next-generation sequencers by different companies such as Roche, Life Technologies (SOLiD), Illumina, Pacific Biosciences, and Ion Torrent, all of which provide platform for faster and cheaper next-generation sequencing of cancer genome [4, 7–9]. The next-generation sequencing can be further subdivided into more affordable, interpretable, and commonly used targeted sequencing of a panel of recognized or putative cancer-associated genes versus whole-exome or whole-genome sequencing which provide comprehensive profiling of all protein-encoding genes of the genome giving more information and long-term cost-effectiveness [10–12].

In this rapidly progressing era, it is important to practice value-based medicine focusing not only on cancer drugs but also on value of genomic profiling in cancer clinic. Most of the next-generation sequencing platforms aim at detecting somatic mutations using formalin-fixed paraffin-embedded tissue tumor. Other rarely use samples include malignant fluid, blood samples, and salivary swabs. Common NGS platforms are FoundationOne that covers 315 genes costing $5800 with 14 day turnaround time; Caris Molecular Intelligence covering more than 600 genes with a cost of $6500 and similar 14 day turnaround; OncoDeep, 75 gene panel, costing $3500 with 7 day turnaround time; Paradigm cancer diagnostic with 186 genes and the cost of $4800 and 5-day return as well as Oncomine Dx Target Test (NSCLC only) with 23 genes and quick 4-day return [13–17].

There are multiple aspects of cost including sample collection, experimental design, sample sequencing, data management, and downstream analysis [18]. Even though the cost for the DNA sequencing may be reducing rapidly due to the advancements in NGS techniques, data management and downstream analysis costs still remain a challenge [19]. To date, no randomized controlled trials have investigated the cost-effectiveness of NGS and there is limited health economic evidence for genomic sequencing and a comprehensive calculation of genomic sequencing containing multiple aspects of the cost is needed.

Despite the high cost, it would be beneficial to use precision oncology if it shows clinical effectiveness. A large retrospective study of 143 single-agent phase II trials from Year 2000–2009 in over 7000 advanced non-small-cell lung cancer patients showed superior median overall response rate, progression-free survival, and overall survival in trials enriched for the presence of molecular targets compared to studies with non-selective patients [20]. Similarly another meta-analysis of 112 registration trials from 1998 to 2013 comparing efficacy outcomes between therapies employing a personalized treatment approach versus general non-selective treatment showed higher response rate, longer progression-free survival, and longer overall survival in patients treated based on precision medicine [21].

At the same time, it is important to keep in mind the treatment-related toxicity and financial burden for this personalized treatment approach. The same meta-analyses did not show any increased treatment-related mortality compared to the non-personalized treatment strategy [22]. Other meta-analyses have shown that cytotoxic agents have higher treatment-related or adverse effects compared to targeted therapies. In addition, a recent meta-analysis of 41 randomized clinical trials evaluating 28 targeted agents for solid tumors approved by the Food and Drug Administration (FDA) evaluating the rate of treatment discontinuation due to toxicity and grade 3–4 adverse effects showed that targeted therapies with companion diagnostic tests were associated with improved safety and tolerability [23].

The financial burden associated with the cancer care has increased rapidly with the cost of out-of-pocket expenses, copayments, and insurance premiums. Since most of these NGS diagnostic tests are associated with targeted therapies which are considered "experimental or investigational," insurance companies often do not reimburse for these agents which are considered "off label." Therefore, NGS has not yet become standard of care across most practices in USA.

However, undoubtedly precision medicine and value-based care may be the future of cancer medicine. There needs to be happy medium with guidelines or standardization in NGS so that insurance payers allow for coverage for appropriate and most cost-effective NGS testing which is in best interest of the patient.

1.3 Defining the Molecular Abnormalities in Lung Cancer

1.3.1 Molecular Abnormalities in Lung Cancer

In 2017, FDA approved immune checkpoint inhibitor pembrolizumab for treatment of cancer patients with high microsatellite instability or mismatch repair deficient markers, regardless of the tumor locations or tissue types. This is a milestone in the development of molecular profiling of cancer and its implications of cancer treatments. The future direction of precision medication in oncology will rely more on the molecular features of a tumor than the tissue types. Lung cancer has been histologically classified as small-cell lung cancer (SCLC) and non-small-cell lung cancer (NSCLC) which includes lung adenocarcinoma, large-cell carcinoma, and squamous cell carcinoma (SCC). With the advancement of technology especially next-generation sequencing, genetic and molecular profiling has identified different subtypes of lung cancer with specific molecular characteristics, which are associated with the clinical/pathological features, prognosis, and treatment responses. Molecular targeted therapy and immunotherapy based on specific somatic genetic mutations/alterations and molecular markers of lung cancer have been changing the paradigm of lung cancer management drastically.

The Cancer Genome Atlas Research Network analyzed 230 lung adenocarcinoma using messenger RNA, micro-RNA, and DNA sequencing integrated with copy number, methylation, and proteomic analyses [24]. The whole-exome sequencing had revealed high rates of somatic mutation (mean 8.9 mutations per mega base), and 18 genes were statistically significantly mutated. TP53 was the commonly mutated (46%), followed by mutations in KRAS (33%), EGFR (14%), BRAF (10%), as were PIK3CA (7%), MET (7%) and the small GTPase gene, RIT1 (2%). Mutations in tumor suppressor genes including STK11 (17%), KEAP1 (17%), NF1 (11%), RB1 (4%), and CDKN2A (4%) were observed. Mutations in chromatin modifying genes SETD2 (9%), ARID1A (7%), and SMARCA4 (6%) and the RNA splicing genes RBM10 (8%) and U2AF1 (3%) were also common. EGFR mutations were more frequent in female patients, whereas mutations in RBM10 were more common in males. Aberrations in NF1, MET, ERBB2, and RIT1 occurred in 13% of cases and were enriched in samples otherwise lacking an activated oncogene, suggesting a driver role for these events in certain tumors. By sequencing the DNA and mRNA sequence from the same sample, splicing alterations driven by somatic genomic changes such as exon 14 skipping in MET mRNA was found in 4% of cases.

When measured at the protein level, recurrent aberrations in multiple key pathways were characterized. Such as RTK/RAS/RAF pathway activation (76% of cases), PI3K-mTOR pathway activation (25%), p53 pathway alteration (63%), cell cycle regulation alteration (64%), and mutation of various chromatin and splicing factors (49%). There are mechanisms other than genetic mutations suggested for activations of signaling pathways. For example, the KRAS-mutated lung adenocarcinoma had higher levels of phosphorylated MAPK than KRAS wild-type tumors on average; however, a lot of KRAS wild-type tumors also have significant MAPK activation. MAPK and PI(3)K pathway activation can be explained by known mutations in only a fraction of cases. The somatic alterations involve key pathway components for RTK signaling, mTOR signaling, oxidative stress response, proliferation and cell cycle progression, nucleosome remodeling, histone methylation, and RNA splicing/processing [24].

Genetic analysis of lung adenocarcinoma is the standard of care for treatment selection nowadays. The Lung Cancer Mutation Consortium (LCMC) did a multi-institutional analysis of 10 potential oncogenic driver mutations in at least one of the 8 genes (EGFR, KRAS, ERBB2, AKT1, BRAF, MEK1, NRAS, and PIK3CA) in 1007 specimens and 733 specimens had all 10 markers tested (including ALK and MET) [25]. KRAS mutations are the most commonly found with a frequency of around 25% followed by EGFR mutations in 22% of the samples. In this cohort, EGFR mutations were highly associated with female sex, Asian race, and never-smoking status; and less strongly associated with stage IV disease, the presence of bone metastases, and absence of adrenal metastases. ALK rearrangements were strongly associated with never-smoking status and more weakly associated with the presence of liver metastases. ERBB2 mutations were strongly associated with Asian race and never-smoking status. Two mutations were seen in 2.7% of samples (27/1007), all but one of which involved one or more of PIK3CA,

ALK, or MET, including 14 with two small mutations and 13 with either a small mutation and ALK rearrangement (4); a small mutation and MET amplification (7); or concurrent ALK rearrangement and MET amplification (2). Of 14 cases with two small mutations, 13 (92%) had a PIK3CA mutation in addition to another mutation, including 9 with EGFR, 2 with BRAF, 1 with KRAS, and 1 with MEK1 mutation. One case had EGFR ex19del and AKT1 c.49G>A (p.E17K) mutations.

Unlike non-small-cell lung cancer (NSCLC), targeted therapy and molecular profiling are less utilized in small-cell lung cancer (SCLC) in clinical practice [26]. The most common genetic alterations in SCLC are inactivation of the tumor suppressor genes TP53 and RB1. In a study which sequenced 108 SCLC tumors without chromothripsis, TP53 and RB1 had bi-allelic losses in 100% and 93% of the cases, which included mutations, translocations, homozygous deletions, hemizygous losses, copy-neutral losses of heterozygosity (LOH), and LOH at higher ploidy [27]. The other common genetic alterations found in SCLC include copy-number gains of genes encoding MYC family members, mutations in enzymes involved in chromatin remodeling, receptor tyrosine kinases, and Notch pathway [27]. Around 98% of SCLC cases are associated with smoking and only 2% occur in non-smokers [28]. SCLCs have extremely high mutation rates (around 8.62 non-synonymous mutations per million base pairs), and C:G > A:T transversions were found in 28% of all mutations on average, a pattern indicative of heavy smoking [27]. The high mutational burden of SCLC might provide opportunities for immunotherapy.

According to the NCCN guidelines (Version 4.2018), molecular testing of EGFR mutation, ALK, ROS1, BRAF, and programmed death ligand 1 (PD-L1) is recommended in metastatic lung adenocarcinoma, large-cell lung cancer, and NSCLC not otherwise specified (NOS). For SCC, consider molecular testing of EGFR and ALK in never smokers or small biopsy or mixed histology, and consider ROS1, BRAF testing as part of broad molecular profiling. PD-L1 testing was also suggested for SCC. PD-L1 immunohistochemistry (IHC) testing is approved for formalin-fixed, paraffin-embedded (FFPE) surgical pathology specimens and helps select patients most likely to respond to immune checkpoint inhibitors. PD-L1 expression level $\geq 50\%$ is indicated for first-line pembrolizumab therapy of NSCLC.

Various methods have been utilized for molecular profiling of lung cancer. Mutations can be detected by next general sequencing as well as various methods including direct Sanger sequencing and pyrosequencing, mutation-specific PCR, multiplex PCR assay followed by single base extension sequencing (SNaPshot, Life Technologies, Grand Island, NY) or matrix-assisted laser desorption/ionization time-of-flight mass spectrometry (MassARRAY, Sequenom, San Diego, CA), high-performance liquid chromatography (HPLC), etc. [29]. Multiple commercial next-generation sequencing platforms are available now as summarized in a recent review [2]. Liquid biopsy which refers to testing mutations on circulating tumor DNA (ctDNA) in blood samples is a promising method to detect genomic alterations and can potentially be used a surrogate method for tissue biopsy testing and even complementary approach [30]. Due to the tumor heterogeneity, a single tissue biopsy may not reflect complete genomic mutations and there are discordance between tissue and ctDNA sequencing results, so both approaches are recommended to enhance mutation detection [31]. Fluorescence in situ hybridization (FISH) analysis is utilized for detecting copy number, amplification, and structural alterations such as gene arrangements. FISH is commonly used for ALK/ROS1 rearrangement and MET amplification.

1.4 Epidermal Growth Factor Receptor (EGFR)

1.4.1 EGFR Mutation in Lung Cancer

The epidermal growth factor receptor (EGFR) is a transmembrane signaling receptor that was discovered in the early 2000s [32]. Under normal conditions, once stimulated by epidermal growth factor, EGFR monomers on the cell surface dimerize to activate the intracellular tyrosine kinase. This activates the RAS, RAF, MEK, ERK pathway and the PI3K, AKT, mTOR pathway to increase expression of genes promoting cell growth and proliferation. In non-small-cell lung cancer (NSCLC), the EGFR gene can become mutated leading to constitutive activation of the EGFR tyrosine kinase. This permits increased tumor growth and proliferation uninhibited by extracellular or intracellular signals.

Approximately 15–20% of patients with NSCLC adenocarcinoma in the USA have mutations in the EGFR tyrosine kinase domain in their tumors [33]. The EGFR mutation frequency is highest in Asian populations. In a meta-analysis of 151 worldwide studies, the Asia-Pacific NSCLC subgroup had the highest EGFR mutation frequency at 47% but there was a wide range between studies from 20 to 76% [34]. The European subgroup in this meta-analysis had an overall EGFR mutation frequency of 15% [34]. EGFR mutations are also more prevalent in females and never smokers. However, EGFR mutations are not restricted to patients with Asian ethnicity, female gender, or never smoker status. The PIONEER study performed in Asia revealed that more than 50% of patients with EGFR mutations were not female non-smokers [35]. This highlights the need to test all patients with NSCLC adenocarcinoma for EGFR mutations regardless of clinical characteristics.

The two most common activating mutations in the tyrosine kinase domain of the EGFR are deletion of exon 19 (EGFR del19) and a point mutation in exon 21 (EGFR L858R) which substitutes an arginine for a leucine at position 858. Other possible mutations include T790M (substitution of a methionine for a threonine at position 790 in exon 20), S768I, L861Q, G719X, and many others. In a meta-analysis of studies from China, L858R accounted for 38.3% of all EGFR mutations and del19 accounted for 37% [36]. T790M occurred at a rate of 1.5% in treatment-naïve patients [36]. Of note, the T790M mutation rate increases with exposure to EGFR tyrosine kinase inhibitors, which will be discussed later. The rate of EGFR mutations sensitive to tyrosine kinase inhibitors was 88.5% [36].

The presence of an EGFR mutation is a key piece of clinical information because it is associated with a high response rate to therapy with EGFR tyrosine kinase inhibitors (TKIs). First-generation EGFR TKIs include erlotinib and gefitinib; these drugs compete with ATP to reversibly bind the intracellular catalytic domain of EGFR tyrosine kinase, thus blocking downstream signaling and reducing cell growth [37]. The second-generation EGFR TKIs include afatinib and dacomitinib; these drugs irreversibly inhibit the catalytic domain of the EGFR tyrosine kinase [37]. The third-generation EGFR TKI is osimertinib. Osimertinib is an irreversible EGFR TKI that inhibits both EGFR TKI sensitizing mutations and EGFR T790M resistance mutations. It is currently recommended for frontline treatment of advanced EGFR-mutant NSCLC based on the FLAURA trial [38].

In the FLAURA trial, 556 patients with previously untreated EGFR mutated advanced NSCLC were randomly assigned to either osimertinib 80 mg, PO, QD, or a standard EGFR TKI such as gefitinib 250 mg, PO, QD, or erlotinib 150 mg, PO, QD. The median PFS was longer with osimertinib at 18.9 months versus 10.2 months for the standard EGFR TKIs (HR 0.46; CI 0.37–0.57). The ORR was 80% with osimertinib and 76% with standard EGFR TKIs. The median duration of response was 17.2 months with osimertinib versus 8.5 months with standard EGFR TKIs. Data on OS is not yet mature. Grade 3 or higher adverse events were less common with osimertinib (34% vs. 45%). Osimertinib is now recommended in the first-line setting for EGFR mutated advanced NSCLC due to its improved PFS and lower rate of serious adverse events [38].

Prior to this trial, the standard of care was erlotinib, gefitinib, or afatinib in the frontline setting. After progression, the presence or absence of the resistance mechanism T790M was evaluated by liquid biopsy or tissue biopsy. This resistance mechanism develops in approximately 50% of cases [39]. If T790M is present, the patient is eligible for second-line therapy with osimertinib. This is based on the AURA3 trial; 419 patients with T790M-positive advanced NSCLC who had disease progression after standard EGFR TKI therapy received either osimertinib 80 mg PO QD or pemetrexed plus either carboplatin or cisplatin every 3 weeks for up to 6 cycles. Pemetrexed maintenance was permitted. The median PFS was significantly longer with osimertinib at 10.1 months versus 4.4 months (HR 0.30; CI 0.23–0.41). The ORR was 71% with osimertinib versus 31% with combination chemotherapy. Among patients with CNS disease, the median PFS was 8.5 months with osimertinib versus 4.2 months with chemotherapy. Furthermore, grade 3 or higher adverse events were lower with osimertinib (23% vs. 47%) [40]. As many patients have been on standard EGFR TKI therapy, this strategy for using second-line osimertinib remains relevant.

Erlotinib, gefitinib, and afatinib have all been evaluated by clinical trials comparing these agents to platinum-based chemotherapy doublets in patients with advanced NSCLC and EGFR activating mutations. One meta-analysis looked at 13 phase III trials including 2620 patients and concluded that the PFS was significantly prolonged with EGFR TKIs (HR 0.43; CI 0.38–0.49) compared to chemotherapy. Overall survival was not prolonged (HR 1.01; CI 0.87–1.18), but it was hypothesized that this is due to significant crossover between the treatment arms [41].

Three large trials assessed erlotinib versus chemotherapy. The OPTIMAL trial assigned 154 patients to erlotinib or gemcitabine plus carboplatin. Erlotinib increased PFS (13.1 vs. 4.6 months, HR 0.16; CI 0.10–0.26) and increased the ORR (83% vs. 36%) [42]. OS was not significantly different [43]. The EURTAC trial assigned 174 patients to erlotinib or a platinum-based chemotherapy doublet and found erlotinib increased PFS (9.7 vs. 5.2 months, HR 0.37; CI 0.25–0.54) but did not increase OS [44]. The ENSURE trial assigned 275 patients to erlotinib or gemcitabine plus cisplatin and found erlotinib increased PFS (11 vs. 5.5 months, HR 0.34; CI 0.22–0.51) but did not increase OS [45]. The most common side effects of erlotinib include rash, diarrhea, and less commonly interstitial pneumonitis and hepatic toxicity. The most common grade 3 or higher adverse event was rash (6.4–13%) in the erlotinib group, which had a favorable toxicity profile compared to chemotherapy [44, 45].

The IPASS trial assessed gefitinib versus chemotherapy. In this trial, 1217 Asian patients who were never or former light smokers with advanced NSCLC were assigned to gefitinib or carboplatin plus paclitaxel. Gefitinib improved PFS (12 month progression-free rate 25% vs. 7%, HR 0.74) but did not change overall survival in the cohort [46, 47]. Subgroup analysis revealed that patients with an EGFR mutation had a significantly improved PFS (9.5 vs. 6.3 months, HR 0.48). Patients without an EGFR mutation had a significantly shorter PFS (1.5 vs. 6.5 months, HR 2.85). This highlighted the importance of testing for the presence of EGFR mutation rather than relying on clinical characteristics to determine therapy [46, 47]. Further trials, such as the North East Japan Study Group 002 trial conducted in patients with known EGFR mutations, reported similar results to the IPASS trial [48]. The most common adverse events with gefitinib were rash (71%) and elevated liver function tests (55.3%). The rate of grade 3 or higher adverse events was approximately 41% in the gefitinib group and 71% in the chemotherapy group [48].

The LUX-Lung 3 and the LUX-Lung 6 trial assessed afatinib versus chemotherapy. The LUX-Lung 3 trial assigned 345 patients with EGFR mutated NSCLC to afatinib 40 mg PO QD or cisplatin plus pemetrexed for up to 6 cycles. Afatinib increased PFS compared with chemotherapy (11.1 months vs. 6.9 months, HR 0.58; CI 0.43–0.78). The ORR was increased with afatinib (56% vs. 23%), and time to symptom progression and quality of life were improved with afatinib [49, 50]. The most common side effects included diarrhea (95%), rash (89%), stomatitis (72%), nail changes (57%), and dry skin (29%) [49]. The LUX-Lung 6 trial assigned 364 Asian patients to afatinib or cisplatin plus gemcitabine. Afatinib increased PFS compared with chemotherapy (11 vs. 5.6 months) and afatinib increased the ORR (67% vs. 23%) [51]. When these two trials were combined, the median OS was not significantly different between the two therapy groups. However, there was a significant increase in OS in the subgroup of patients with the exon 19 deletion [52].

Of note, patients with NSCLC with uncommon EGFR mutations such as S768I, L861Q, or G719X can be treated with afatinib in the first-line setting based on analysis of the LUX-Lung trials, but afatinib is less active in other uncommon mutation types [53]. Dacomitinib is another second-generation EGFR TKI that was compared to gefitinib as first-line treatment for patients with EGFR mutation-positive NSCLC (ARCHER 1050). Dacomitinib did have a longer PFS, but it had greater toxicity and is not currently approved in the USA [54].

Erlotinib, gefitinib, and afatinib are considered to all have similar efficacy in EGFR mutated NSCLC and are all generally well tolerated. Some data suggests that afatinib may be slightly more efficacious but may also cause the most side effects, and many clinicians start at a lower dose than used in the LUX-Lung trials. Some data suggests gefitinib may be the best tolerated of the three agents, but the data is inconsistent. One study randomized 256 patients to either erlotinib 150 mg PO QD or gefitinib 250 mg PO QD and found no significant difference in PFS, ORR, OS, and grade 3 or 4 toxicities. The ORR was 56.3% versus 52.3% ($P = 0.53$), and the median OS was 22.9 versus 20.1 months ($P = 0.25$) [55]. The LUX-Lung 7 trial assessed afatinib 40 mg PO QD versus gefitinib 250 mg PO QD and found that median OS was 27.9 months with afatinib versus 24.5 months with gefitinib (HR 0.86, CI 0.62–1.36) [56]. In this trial, although there was no significant difference in OS with afatinib, PFS was improved with afatinib versus gefitinib [56].

The majority of patients who initially respond to an EGFR TKI eventually develop resistance to the drug and have progression of disease. We have already discussed using osimertinib in patients who develop T790M resistance after treatment with a first- or second-generation EFGR TKI. There are other mechanisms of resistance that can develop. One mechanism of resistance is the amplification of the MET oncogene. This has been linked to resistance in 5–20% of patients taking erlotinib or gefitinib [57]. This has been linked to resistance in up to 30% of patients taking osimertinib [58]. Another interesting but less common mechanism of resistance is histologic transformation of EGFR mutated NSCLC into small-cell lung cancer [59]. In one analysis of 37 tumor biopsies taken after progression on EGFR TKI therapy, 5 resistant tumors (14%) transformed from NSCLC into small-cell lung cancer; these tumors were sensitive to standard small-cell lung cancer chemotherapy regimens [59]. Although it is not standard of care, it may be reasonable to biopsy a site of progressive disease to determine if another targetable mutation is present or if there has been a transformation in histology.

There has been some investigation into whether or not continuing an EGFR TKI after progression has benefit. One retrospective analysis looked at Japanese patients with EGFR mutations who progressed on first- or second-line EGFR TKI and compared those who continued EGFR TKI beyond progression (39 patients) and those who were switched to cytotoxic chemotherapy alone (25 patients). The median OS was 32.2 months in the group receiving the EGFR TKI beyond progression and 23 months in the group receiving chemotherapy (HR 0.42, CI 0.21–0.83, $p = 0.013$) [60]. However, a prospective study is needed to confirm these results. Due to anecdotal evidence that EGFR-positive lung cancer can progress more rapidly even after progression when discontinuing EGFR TKI therapy, some clinicians elect to continue the EGFR TKI therapy until the next line of therapy can be initiated.

There has also been investigation into whether adding bevacizumab to EGFR TKI therapy adds benefit. During the JO25567 trial, 154 patients in Japan with EGFR mutations and no prior therapy were assigned to either erlotinib 150 mg PO QD alone or erlotinib plus bevacizumab 15 mg/kg every 3 weeks until disease progression or unacceptable toxicity. Median PFS with erlotinib plus bevacizumab was 16 months versus 9.7 months with erlotinib alone (HR 0.54, CI 0.36–0.79) [61]. Serious adverse events occurred at a similar frequency in both groups ($\sim$25%) [61]. The overall survival data is not yet mature. The combination of erlotinib plus bevacizumab is approved by the European Medicines Agency in Europe.

Finally, there has been investigation into whether adding chemotherapy to EGFR TKI therapy adds benefit. In the FASTACT-2 trial, 451 patients with were assigned to either chemotherapy (gemcitabine plus platinum) plus erlotinib or chemotherapy plus placebo. In the patients with an EGFR activating mutation, PFS was improved with chemotherapy plus erlotinib (7.6 vs. 6.0 months) and OS was improved with chemotherapy plus erlotinib (18.3 vs. 15.2 months) [62]. Another study evaluated gefitinib with and without pemetrexed in chemotherapy-naïve patients with EGFR-positive NSCLC. Median PFS was longer with gefitinib with pemetrexed (15.8 vs. 10.9 months, HR 0.68, CI 0.48–0.96) [63]. Overall survival data is immature.

Although these studies have shown a possible benefit of combining chemotherapy with EGFR TKI, four large randomized clinical trials using gefitinib or erlotinib all failed to show a survival benefit from the combination with chemotherapy [64–67]. However, these trials did not select patients based on the presence of an EGFR driver mutation so further investigation is needed in this area. In the IMPRESS trial, 265 patients with an EGFR mutation who had disease progression on gefitinib were assigned to cisplatin, pemetrexed, gefitinib or to cisplatin, pemetrexed, placebo. Patients completed 6 cycles of chemotherapy and then were continued on gefitinib or placebo for maintenance. There was no significant difference in median PFS (5.4 vs. 5.4 months, HR 0.86, CI 0.65–1.13) [68]. There was a decrease in median OS in those on chemotherapy plus gefitinib versus chemotherapy alone (13.4 vs. 19.5 months, HR 1.44, CI 1.07–1.94) [68]. At this time, patients with advanced EGFR-positive NSCLC generally do not receive combination chemotherapy with an EGFR TKI as initial therapy outside of a clinical trial.

1.5 Anaplastic Lymphoma Kinase (ALK)

Anaplastic lymphoma kinase (ALK) driver mutations are found in a variety of solid tumors. ALK receptor tyrosine kinase gene, located on chromosome 2p23, encodes a receptor that belongs to the insulin receptor superfamily. The protein is made up of an extracellular, transmembrane, and intracellular domain. It is believed that ALK plays a role in the development of neurons in the central nervous system.

Activation of ALKs kinase catalytic domains has been implicated in the growth and development of cancer. Multiple pathways are involved, including phospholipase Cγ (PLCγ), Janus kinase (JAK)–signal transducer and activator of transcription (STAT), PI3K–AKT, mTOR, sonic hedgehog (SHH), JUNB, CRKL–C3G–RAP1 GTPase, and MAPK. The most common mechanisms that are involved in ALK mutations are chromosomal translocations or rearrangements. The resultant oncogenic ALK fusion gene results in constitutive ALK activity.

The FDA has approved testing to identify ALK rearrangements with immunohistochemistry (IHC) and fluorescent in situ hybridization (FISH). In addition, ALK rearrangements and their resultant fusion proteins can also be identified via reverse transcription polymerase chain reaction (RT-PCR).

EML4-ALK is identified in 2–7% of all non-small-cell lung cancers, most prevalent in non-smokers, light smokers, and adenocarcinomas. These patients with ALK fusion lung cancers are relatively younger than typical NSCLC patients. Histologically almost all ALK fusion oncogenes are adenocarcinoma. In addition, signet ring cells, which portend for a poor prognosis and are associated with a more aggressive clinical course, have been identified to be more common.

The optimal approach to treat advanced NSCLC with an ALK fusion variant first line is an ALK inhibitor. The first ALK inhibitor approved by the FDA to treat metastatic NSCLC with an ALK rearrangement was crizotinib in 2011 under the accelerated approval process.

1.5.1 Crizotinib

Crizotinib, a first-generation ALK inhibitor, is a small-molecule tyrosine kinase inhibitor. Crizotinib was approved by the FDA after a phase I trial [69] with confirmatory trials in phases II [70] and III [71]. PROFILE 1014 compared crizotinib to a platinum doublet with pemetrexed for first-line treatment in advanced ALK rearranged NSCLC. Crizotinib had improved PFS, RR, and duration of response compared to traditional cytotoxic therapy. Crizotinib unfortunately has poor CSF penetration with the second- and next-generation ALK inhibitors shown to have better response rates intracranially [72].

1.5.2 Ceritinib

Ceritinib, a second-generation ALK inhibitor, initially received accelerated approval in 2014 for advanced NSCLC patients who progressed or who were intolerant to crizotinib based on the phase I study ASCEND-1 [73]. The phase III study ASCEND-4 compared ceritinib to front doublet platinum therapy and was found to be superior. Ceritinib has proven in preclinical studies to have activity against crizotinib-resistant cells including gatekeeper mutation L1196M. ASCEND-5 has also been evaluated in those who progressed on crizotinib to either ceritinib or single-agent chemotherapy with improvements in PFS and RR [74].

Ceritinib is currently approved to be used in either treatment-naïve ALK rearranged advanced NSCLC patients or those who have progressed on crizotinib.

1.5.3 Alectinib

Alectinib, also a second-generation ALK inhibitor, received accelerated approval in 2015 for ALK-positive metastatic NSCLC who progressed or who are intolerant to crizotinib after two single-arm clinical trials [75–77]. Alectinib is active against gatekeeper mutation L1196M and other crizotinib-resistant mutations such as C1156Y and F1174L. ALEX, an open-label phase III trial, compared alectinib and crizotinib in treatment-naïve advanced NSCLC. The primary end point, PFS, was superior in alectinib (25.7 months) compared to 10.4 months with crizotinib (HR 0.53; $p < 0.0001$) [78]. For CNS progression, a secondary end point in this study, alectinib showed superior aversion to progression in CNS in comparison with crizotinib (12% vs. 45%, respectively) [78]. The results of this study led to the approval of alectinib for use in treatment-naïve, ALK rearranged advanced NSCLC and is the treatment of choice in this setting.

1.5.4 Brigatinib

Brigatinib is a second-generation tyrosine kinase inhibitor, with potent activity against active ALK, developed to treat advanced NSCLC for those patient who have progressed or intolerant to crizotinib with activity against active ALK, and mutant L1196M. In 2017, the drug received accelerated approval based on the randomized, open-label, non-comparative, phase II ALTA study designed to evaluate anti-tumor activity of brigatinib in patients with metastatic ALK-positive NSCLC who have previously received crizotinib demonstrated improved PFS compared to historical data for patients who progressed on crizotinib (9.2 mo 90 mg/d vs. 12.9 mo 180 mg/d) [79]. Further investigation in the frontline setting is currently taking place with ALTA-1L. Brigatinib is approved to be used in crizotinib refractory or intolerant, advanced ALK rearranged NSCLC setting.

1.5.5 Lorlatinib

Lorlatinib is a novel third-generation, ALK inhibitor designed to overcome ALK-resistant mutations including G1202R, and improved CNS penetration was granted FDA breakthrough designation in 2017. It has shown promise (46% ORR, 9.6 mo PFS) in its first in human open-label phase I study in advanced ALK-positive NSCLC [80]. It is unclear in the sequence of available therapies where lorlatinib will lie but currently considered to be used in patients' refractory to second-generation inhibitors or multiple TKIs. An investigation for its efficacy in the first-line setting is being investigated currently (NCT03052608).

1.6 ROS Proto-oncogene 1 (ROS-1)

1.6.1 ROS-1 (Reactive Oxygen Species-1)

ROS-1 was initially discovered as the cellular homolog of the chicken c-ros gene. This gene is the proto-oncogene for v-ros which is the transforming sequence of UR2 sarcoma virus [81]. It is located at chromosome 6q22 and encodes for a receptor tyrosine kinase belonging to the insulin receptor family closely related to anaplastic lymphoma kinase (ALK) and leukocyte receptor tyrosine kinase (LTK) [82]. ROS1 protein expression in adult humans appears to be the highest in kidney but is also found in cerebellum, peripheral neural tissue, stomach, small intestine, and colon, with lower expression in several other tissues and absent in lungs. In mouse model studies, mice that lack the receptor appear to be healthy. No ligands for the receptor have been found.

Constitutive activation of ROS1 signaling leads to the phosphorylation of SHP-2 (tyrosine phosphatase, non-receptor type 11) and activation of downstream signaling pathways such as MEK/ERK, JAK/STAT, or PI3K/AKT [83]. Chromosomal rearrangements involving the *ROS1* gene were originally described in glioblastomas, where *ROS1* (chromosome 6q22) is fused to the *FIG* gene located on chromosome 6q22 immediately adjacent to *ROS1*. Known *ROS1* fusion partners in lung cancer include *FIG*, *CD74*, *SLC34A2,* and *SDC*. Expression of the *FIG-ROS1* and *SDC4-ROS1* fusions in murine Ba/F3 cells has been demonstrated to result in IL3 independent proliferation, and this proliferation was sensitive to treatment of small-molecule ROS1 inhibitors [84].

Crizotinib is approved as the first-line therapy for advanced *ROS1* fusion-positive NSCLC. *ROS1*-positive NSCLC demonstrated a 72% response rate and 19.2-month median progression-free survival in a phase I expansion cohort [73]. To date, acquired resistance to crizotinib has been reported in clinical studies because of the secondary S1986Y/F, G2032R, and D2033N mutations in *ROS1*. Preclinical data has suggested that missense mutations within the ROS1 kinase domain can drive acquired resistance to crizotinib. A patient with a crizotinib-sensitive NSCLC harboring a CD74-ROS1 fusion was found to have an acquired ROS1 G2032R mutation at the time of progression. However, preclinical data suggests that the next-generation ALK/MET/ROS1 inhibitors cabozantinib, foretinib, and PF-06463922 are capable of overcoming this resistance mutation [85].

1.7 V-Raf Murine Sarcoma Viral Oncogene Homolog B1 (BRAF)

1.7.1 BRAF in Non-small-Cell Lung Cancer

Mutations in the BRAF proto-oncogene were first described in 2002 with an incidence of 8% across all cancers and 3% in lung cancer [86]. The BRAF proto-oncogene encodes the intracellular B-Raf protein. The B-Raf protein phosphorylates and activates downstream MEK, which in turn phosphorylates and activates downstream ERK. This signaling pathway leads to the upregulation of genes promoting cell proliferation and survival. In healthy cells, this signaling pathway is modulated by extracellular signals such as growth factors transmitting information to the cell via transmembrane receptors. However, in cancer cells with a BRAF mutation, this regulation is lost due to constitutive activation of the B-Raf protein. This leads to increased cell proliferation and survival independent of extracellular factors [87].

BRAF mutations occur in 1–3% of patients with NSCLC [88–90]. The most common mutation is V600E, which is an amino acid substitution at position 600 from a valine to a glutamic acid. Other described mutations include G469A, D594G, K601E, G464E, G596R, A598T, G606R, and G469V [88, 89]. The BRAF V600E mutation is generally cited to be approximately 50% of all BRAF mutations in NSCLC, although various studies have documented rates from 30 to 80% [88, 91]. Compared to BRAF V600E mutations in melanoma, BRAF V600E mutations in NSCLC are less common.

To date, NSCLC patients with BRAF mutations are not statistically more likely to belong to a particular gender, sex, or race [91]. There is no unique histologic subtype that is more likely to harbor a BRAF mutation [89, 91]. There is no association of BRAF mutations with stage of disease at diagnosis [91]. Only smoking history consistently correlates with BRAF mutation status [89, 91, 92]. The majority of patients with BRAF mutations are former or current smokers. This signal is particularly strong with non-V600E mutations since patients with V600E mutations are more likely to be light/never smokers [92].

In general, concurrent mutations with other driver mutations in patients with BRAF mutations are rare. However, concurrent mutations have been reported with BRAF V600E or BRAF non-V600E mutations and mutations in other genes including EGFR, KRAS, ALK, and PIK3CA [88, 89, 91, 92].

Multiple studies have evaluated the prognosis and overall survival of patients with a BRAF mutation in NSCLC. Compared to patients with NSCLC with other driver mutations, patients with BRAF mutations had no statistically different overall survival [89]. In a study with 63 patients with BRAF mutations, their overall survival was intermediate between patients with EGFR and KRAS mutations but this was not statistically different [92]. In early-stage disease, there is no difference in overall survival between mutation types [92]. Overall survival may be slightly better with BRAF V600E mutations compared to non-V600E mutations, which may reflect the lighter smoking history of the former [92]. Finally, patients with concurrent driver mutations do have shorter overall survival compared to those with a single driver mutation [91].

Two BRAF inhibitors, vemurafenib and dabrafenib, have shown clinical activity in metastatic BRAF V600E mutated lung cancers. Vemurafenib works by inhibiting the active form of the B-Raf kinase by attaching to the ATP-binding site. In 2015, Hyman et al. evaluated vemurafenib in multiple non-melanoma cancers with BRAF

V600 mutations in a histology-independent phase II "basket" trial. A total of 122 patients with BRAF V600E mutations with various histologies received vemurafenib (960 mg, PO, BID) until progression of disease or unacceptable toxicity. In the 19 patients with NSCLC, there was a response rate (RR) of 42% (95% CI 20–67) with 8 patients having a partial response. Tumor regression was observed in most patients (14 of 19 patients). The median progression-free survival (PFS) was 7.3 months (95% CI 3.5–10.8). The 12-month overall survival (OS) was 66%. The majority of these patients received prior platinum-based chemotherapy. Common side effects included rash (68%), fatigue (56%), and arthralgia (40%) [93].

In 2016, Planchard et al. evaluated another BRAF inhibitor dabrafenib in patients with BRAF V600E mutations in advanced NSCLC in a phase II trial. Dabrafenib is an adenosine-triphosphate competitive inhibitor of B-Raf kinase that is selective for the V600E mutant. In this study, 84 patients with metastatic BRAF V600E NSCLC received dabrafenib (150 mg, PO, BID). Out of 6 patients who had no prior treatment, 4 (66%) had a partial response. Out of the remaining 78 patients who had prior treatment, 26 (33% [95% CI 23–45]) had an overall response (CR + PR). There was disease control in 58% of patients. The response was quick with 73% of responses occurring at 6 weeks. The side effects were mostly skin related with 42% of patients experiencing some adverse events. Grade 3 or 4 adverse reactions included cutaneous squamous cell carcinoma (12%), basal cell carcinoma (5%), and asthenia (5%). One patient died from an intracranial hemorrhage while concurrently taking a factor Xa inhibitor [94].

Unfortunately, treatment with a BRAF inhibitor alone can lead to resistance within 6–7 months in other tumor types. The BRAF inhibitor dabrafenib plus the MEK inhibitor trametinib has shown synergistic anti-tumor activity in BRAF mutant human cancer cell lines. Planchard et al. evaluated dabrafenib (150 mg, PO, BID) plus trametinib (2 mg, PO, QD) in patients with previously treated BRAF V600E mutant metastatic NSCLC. Out of 57 patients, 36 patients responded (63% [95% CI 49.3–75.6]). Approximately 79% of patients obtained disease control (CR + PR + stable disease). The median PFS was 9.7 months (95% CI 6.9–19.6). The median duration of treatment was 10.6 months with 30% of patients receiving treatment for more than 12 months. Common adverse events included fever, nausea, vomiting, diarrhea, asthenia, and anorexia. Grade 3–4 toxicity included neutropenia (9%), hyponatremia (7%), and anemia (5%). The combination of dabrafenib and trametinib had a high overall response rate, often a prolonged duration of response and manageable toxicity [95].

Planchard et al. also evaluated dabrafenib and trametinib in patients with previously untreated BRAF V600E mutant NSCLC. The study included 36 patients with an overall response rate of 64% (95% CI 46–79) and PFS of 10.9 months (95% CI 7.0–16.6). The median duration of response was 10.4 months, and the median overall survival was 24.6 months. The 2-year overall survival was 51%. Of note, there were similar response rates between patients who had been previously treated and those who had not (63% vs. 64%). Furthermore, PFS was similar between the previously treated and untreated groups (9.7 vs. 10.9 months). This suggests that treating clinicians have flexibility to treat patients with dabrafenib and trametinib in either the first-line metastatic setting or in the second line following chemotherapy [96].

1.8 MET Proto-oncogene (MET)

1.8.1 MET in Lung Cancer

MET proto-oncogene, located on chromosome 7q31, was identified in early 1980s. Its protein product is a transmembrane tyrosine kinase, which binds to the ligand scatter factor/hepatocyte growth factor (HGF). The downstream signaling activates the mitogen-activated protein kinase (MAPK), phosphoinositide-3-kinase (PI3K)/ AKT, signal transducer and activator of transcription proteins (STATs), and nuclear factor kappa B (NF-kB) pathways, thus promoting proliferation, escaping apoptosis, and increasing cell motility [97–100].

MET pathway abnormality is commonly found in lung cancer. The mechanisms include protein phosphorylation (p-MET), overexpression, amplification, rearrangement, and mutations [101]. Mutations in the splicing sites that cause MET exon 14 skipping are the most studied MET abnormality which occurs in around 3–4% of lung adenocarcinoma and 2% of SCC [102, 103]. Exon 14 of MET encodes the juxtamembrane domain of the protein, which is the binding site for E3 ubiquitin ligase for protein degradation; thus, skipping of exon 14 causes prolonged signal transduction of the MET pathway, which leads to cell proliferation and migration, and subsequently facilitates oncogenesis, cancer invasion, and metastasis [104, 105]. MET gene rearrangement is less reported, but the kinase fusion KIF5B-MET has been reported in lung adenocarcinoma [106]. Overexpression of MET is found in around 35–72% of the NSCLC, and p-MET can be found in 67% of the NSCLC, while amplification of MET is around 2–5% of newly diagnosed adenocarcinoma [107, 108]. The MET gene copy number (GCN) is associated with worse prognosis in surgically resected NSCLC, with overall survival (OS) of 25.5 months for patients with MET ≥ 5 copies/cell compared with 47.5 months for patients with MET < 5 copies/cell ($P = 0.0045$) [109].

Studies of targeting MET pathway in cancer have been ongoing for decades. The available agents and clinical trials have been summarized in recent reviews [108, 110]. There are small molecular tyrosine kinase inhibitors such as selective inhibitor tivantinib (targets MET), capmatinib (targets MET), savolitinib (targets MET), tepotinib (targets MET), SAR125844 (targets MET), sitravatinib (targets MET), AMG 337 (targets MET), non-selective inhibitor crizotinib (targets ALK/ROS/MET), cabozantinib (targets MET/RET/others), glesatinib (targets MET/AXL/others), merestinib (targets MET/ROS1/AXL/FLTs/others), S49076 (targets MET/AXL/FGFR1-3), as well as monoclonal antibodies including emibetuzumab (anti-MET), onartuzumab (anti-MET), rilotumumab (anti-HGF), and ficlatuzumab (anti-HGF) [108, 110].

Various clinical trials have investigated the efficacy of MET inhibition in lung cancer. Responses to non-selective MET inhibitors crizotinib and cabozantinib were reported in lung adenocarcinoma with MET abnormalities; however, cabozantinib also has activity against RET and had 28% overall response rate in a phase II clinical trial of 26 patients with RET-rearranged lung adenocarcinoma [111, 112]. So far the results of clinic trials for the selective MET inhibitors are not satisfactory, which may be partially due to lack of valid predictive biomarkers for patient selection as discussed previously [108, 110]. In the phase III OAM4971g (METLung) trial comparing erlotinib plus onartuzumab versus erlotinib plus placebo in patients with locally advanced or metastatic NSCLC with MET overexpressing defined by MET IHC staining, there is no difference in clinical outcomes (median OS was 6.8 vs. 9.1 months for onartuzumab vs. placebo, $P = 0.067$), with shorter OS in the onartuzumab arm, compared with erlotinib in patients with MET-positive non-small-cell lung cancer, and the median progression-free survival was 2.7 versus 2.6 months (stratified HR, 0.99; 95% CI 0.81–1.20; $P = 0.92$) with overall response rate of 8.4 and 9.6% for onartuzumab versus placebo, respectively [113]. A phase III trial of tivantinib (ARQ 197) plus erlotinib versus erlotinib alone in previously treated locally advance or metastatic non-squamous NSCLC reported by Scagliotti et al. in 2015 [114] showed OS did not improve, although PFS increased (median PFS, 3.6 vs. 1.9 months; HR, 0.74; 95% CI 0.62–0.89; $P < 0.001$). Subgroup analyses suggested OS improvement in patients with high MET expression (HR, 0.70; 95% CI 0.49–1.01). Most common adverse events occurring were rash (33.1% vs. 37.3%, respectively), diarrhea (34.6% vs. 41.0%), asthenia or fatigue (43.5% vs. 38.1%), and neutropenia (grade 3–4; 8.5% vs. 0.8%). It has been reported that MET amplification can increase to 5–22% after treatment with EGFR TKI erlotinib or gefitinib [115]. A phase II study of erlotinib plus tivantinib in 45 patients with locally advanced or metastatic EGFR mutation-positive non-small-cell lung cancer just after progression on EGFR TKI erlotinib or gefitinib did not prove clinical benefit of tivantinib in patients with acquired resistance to EGFR TKIs; however, the patients having high activated MET signaling have longer survival by tivantinib/erlotinib (c-Met high vs. low: median PFS 4.1 vs. 1.4 months; median OS 20.7 vs. 13.9 months) [116]. The ATTENTION study [117], a phase III trial of erlotinib plus tivantinib versus erlotinib in stage IIIB/IV Asian non-squamous NSCLC with wild-type EGFR, was prematurely terminated due to the increased interstitial lung disease (ILD) incidence in the tivantinib group. ILD developed in 14 patients (3 deaths) and 6 patients (0 deaths) in the tivantinib and the placebo groups, respectively, in total of 307 patients enrolled. Median OS was 12.7 and 11.1 months in the tivantinib and the placebo groups, respectively [hazard ratio (HR) = 0.891, $P = 0.427$]. Median PFS was 2.9 and 2.0 months in the tivantinib and the placebo groups, respectively (HR = 0.719, $P = 0.019$). Although this study lacked statistical power because of the premature termination and did not demonstrate an improvement in OS, the results suggest that tivantinib plus erlotinib might improve PFS compared to erlotinib alone in non-squamous NSCLC patients with WT-EGFR. The overexpression or phosphorylation of MET is less predictive for the response to MET inhibitors; according to the above-mentioned negative data and correlations between MET germline mutations, MET amplification, somatic mutation, overexpression, and activation with treatment responses have not been confirmed yet [113]. Targeting MET pathway is promising; however, we need better strategies to select the patients who are going to benefit from it [108].

MET mutations are frequently associated with other gene mutations (around 44%), and there are cross talks between MET pathway and other pathways such as mTOR, PI3K/AKT, STATs, MEK pathways, which may blunt the clinical benefit of MET inhibition [118]. Based on the synthetic lethality [119], combination of MET inhibitor and other pathway inhibitors could be an effective strategy. In a phase I study of tivantinib plus the mTOR inhibitor temsirolimus, the pharmacokinetic analysis showed no interaction in the plasma concentrations of the two drugs and the combination appears to be well tolerated with clinical activity [120]. MET abnormality is also common in NSCLC patients with brain metastases [121]. MET-amplified recurrent glioblastoma have been shown to respond to crizotinib treatment [122]. Intracranial activity of cabozantinib has also been shown in MET exon 14 skipping NSCLC patient with brain metastasis [123]. MET inhibitors penetrate the blood–brain barrier and could be effective for brain metastasis, especially for patients who failed the EGFR inhibitors due to brain metastasis.

1.9 Tropomyosin-Related Kinase (TRK) and (Rearranged During Transfection Kinase) RET

1.9.1 TRK

Tropomyosin receptor kinase (Trk) receptor family comprises 3 transmembrane proteins referred to as Trk A, B, and C receptors (TrkA, TrkB, and TrkC) that are encoded by the NTRK1, NTRK2, and NTRK3 genes [124]. These receptor tyrosine kinases are expressed in human neuronal tissue, activate neurotrophin (NTs), and play an role in nervous system. The NTRK1 gene is located on chromosome 1q21-q22, and mutation of which disrupts the function of the TrkA protein which can cause congenital insensitivity to pain with anhidrosis. The NTRK2 gene is on chromosome 9q22.1 (codes for TrkB receptor). The NTRK3 gene is located on chromosome 15q25 (TrkC) expressed in the human hippocampus, in the cerebral cortex, and in the granular cell layer of the cerebellum. Reported gene fusion SQSTM1-NTRK1, NTRK1-SQSTM1, CD74-NTRK 1, MPRIP-NTRK1, TRIM24-NTRK2, RFWD2-NTRK1. Gene fusions involving NTRK genes lead to the transcription of chimeric Trk proteins which elevates kinase function, resulting in oncogenic potential. Entrectinib is an orally bioavailable inhibitor of the tyrosine kinase TrkA, TrkB, and TrkC as well as of c-ros oncogene 1 (ROS1) and anaplastic lymphoma kinase (ALK). Entrectinib can cross the blood–brain barrier and could thus potentially be effective in the treatment of brain metastases and GBM with activating gene fusions of NTRK, ROS1, or ALK. In the subgroup of *NTRK-*

rearranged cancers, 100% of patients ($n = 5$) with various tumor histologies and fusion types responded to entrectinib treatment and had a good intracranial activity [125].

There are phase I trials investigating Altiratinib (DCC-2701) and sitravatinib (MGCD516) which are multi-kinase inhibitors with reported in vitro inhibitory activity against TrkA and TrkB. Other Trk inhibitors that are being investigated in phase I/II trial include TSR-011, PLX7486, DS-6051b, F17752, and cabozantinib (XL184). Larotrectinib is a selective small-molecule pan-TRK inhibitor currently being investigated in an adult/adolescent phase II trial. Primary objective of the trial was investigator-assessed overall response rate which was 78%, and duration of response has not reached [126]. NTRK gene fusions are emerging as novel target; however, due to the low incidence of Trk alterations across multiple histologies, it is challenging to study the various targets.

1.9.2 RET

RET (rearranged during transfection) is a proto-oncogene which through cytogenetic rearrangement and activating point mutations can undergo oncogenic activation. *RET* is localized to human chromosome 10q11.2. The expression of RET is the highest during development and the lowest in normal adult tissues. It is predominately expressed in neural crest-derived cells and urogenital cells. RET is required for the development of the enteric nervous system, kidney morphogenesis, and spermatogenesis [127]. Distinct chromosomal translocations produce different RET fusions which occur in 1–2% of NSCLCs and are mutually exclusive of mutations in *EGFR*, *KRAS*, *ALK*, *HER2*, and *BRAF*.

RET-rearranged lung adenocarcinomas (LUADs) are often found in never smokers (82%) and overall younger patients (≤ 60 years; 73%), more poorly differentiated (64%), solid subtype (64%), have a smaller size (≤ 3 cm) with N2 disease (54%). *RET* has been shown to form fusions with eight different genes in NSCLC: *KIF5B (most common)*, *CCDC6*, *NCOA*, *TRIMM33*, *CUX1*, *KIAA1468*, *KIAA1217*, and *FRMD4A*. Reverse transcriptase polymerase chain reaction (RT-PCR) is both sensitive and specific for the detection of known fusions, but it is not reliable for the detection of new fusion partners or isoforms. Currently, a few drugs have been investigated in phase II studies for RET-positive lung adenocarcinoma. Cabozantinib, an oral multi-kinase inhibitor of RET, was investigated in a phase II study ($n = 25$) which showed an objective response rate (ORR) of 28%. The median progression-free survival (PFS) was 5.5 months (95% CI [3.8, 8.4]), and the median overall survival (OS) was 9.9 months (95% CI [8.1, not reached]). Vandetanib, an oral RET, VEGFR-2, and EGFR kinase inhibitor, demonstrated an ORR of 18%, and a disease control rate (DCR) of 65% in patients with advanced/refractory *RET*-rearranged NSCLC. The PFS was 4.5 months, and the OS was 11.6 months. The 1-year OS rate was 33%. Ten out of 18 patients (56%) had died at the data cutoff. Lenvatinib, a multi-kinase inhibitor, achieved an ORR of 16% (four patients with partial responses), and a DCR of 76% with 48% of patients showed a durable response. Other multi-kinase inhibitors currently being investigated include Alectinib, a tyrosine kinase inhibitor of ALK that is also active against *RET* in vitro, and ponatinib. Studies showed that different multi-kinase inhibitors may produce variable responses depending on the type of *RET* fusion. RET inhibitor resistance was also found and investigated. Huang et al. recently identified cabozantinib-resistant *KIF5B-RETV804L* and the vandetanib-resistant *KIF5B-RETG810A* mutations in lung adenocarcinoma cells. Interestingly, vandetanib-resistant *KIF5B-RETG810A* mutant cells displayed gain of sensitivity to ponatinib and lenvatinib, suggesting that the different RET inhibitors can overcome vandetanib-induced mechanisms of resistance. A recent study of lung cancer cells that had *CCDC6-RET* genes suggested that activation of EGFR signaling may allow the cells to become resistant to *RET* inhibition via a bypass survival signaling through *ERK* and *AKT*. The combination of vandetanib and the mTOR inhibitor everolimus has demonstrated higher anti-tumor activity than either single agent alone. The combination is being further studied. At present, RET-mutated patients are a very small subgroup, which poses a challenge to develop a targeted therapy; however, identifying biomarkers in patients with NSCLC may result in clinical benefit from RET inhibitors and continues to be an active area of investigation [128].

1.10 Checkpoint Inhibitors

Immunotherapy has had drastic impacts on the treatment of some types of tumors including melanoma, renal cell cancer, and non-small-cell lung cancer. Immunotherapy in lung cancer has been used either as a single-agent or in combination with chemotherapy in a first- or second-line treatment setting in the recent times. Our own immune system consisting of the adaptive and innate immunity is one of the mechanisms of defense against tumor cells. Specifically, the immune response is initiated when T cell receptor recognizes and binds to major histocompatibility complex (MHC) on the surface off the antigen presenting cell (APC) or the tumor cells, which leads to the interaction between cytokines and stimulatory signals causing T lymphocyte activation, proliferation, and differentiation (Fig. 1.1).

However, the activation and proliferation of T cells are affected by inhibitory immune checkpoint molecules such as the cytotoxic T lymphocyte-associated protein 4 (CTLA-4), programmed cell death 1 (PD1), and programmed death ligand 1 and 2 (PD-L1, PDL2). For example, the interaction between CD28 on T cells and B7 on the APCs is a key step in activation of T cells; however, CTLA-4 competes with CD28 for binding to B7 and transmits an inhibitory signal that suppresses T cell activation. PD-L1/2 is expressed on the surface of multiple cell types including tumor cells and helps evade anti-tumor immune response. The interaction between PD-L1 with APC and PD1 on T cells inhibits apoptosis in tumor cells, promotes

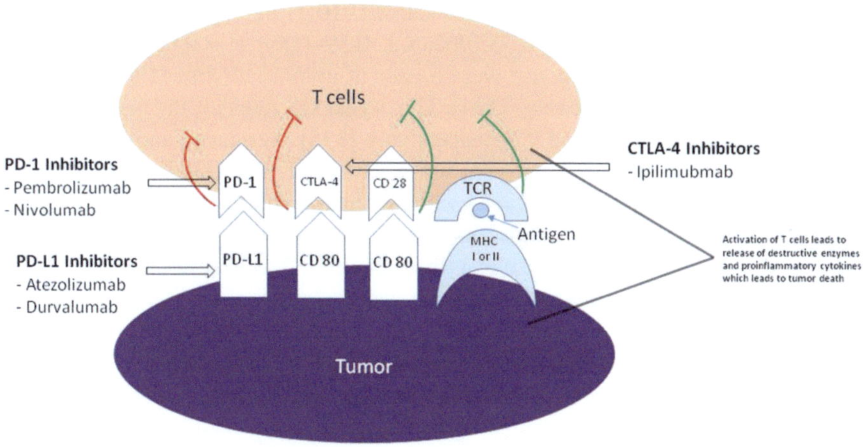

Fig. 1.1 Mechanism of action of checkpoint inhibitors

peripheral T effector cell exhaustion, and promotes the conversion of T effector cells to Treg cells [129, 130]. Other checkpoints which act as inhibitory receptors expressed by T cells or NK cells such as T cell Ig and T cell immunoglobulin mucin domain 3 (TIM3) and lymphocyte activation gene 3 (LAG3) and killer cell immunoglobulin-like receptor (KIR) have been discovered as well [131, 132]. Therefore, targeted treatments that inhibit these checkpoint proteins could restore and augment cytotoxic T cell responses, leading to potentially resilient responses and prolonged overall survival (OS) with tolerable toxicity.

1.10.1 PD1/PD-L1/2 Inhibitors

1.10.1.1 Nivolumab

Nivolumab is a fully humanized IgG4-blocking antibody against PD-1 checkpoint protein that disrupts interactions with PDL1/2. In an early phase I study of 39 patients with advanced metastatic melanoma, colon cancer, castrate resistant prostate cancer, renal cell cancer, and non-small-cell lung cancer (NSCLC), nivolumab was well tolerated with no dose-limiting toxicity. There was evidence of anti-tumor activity in 6/39 patients in the dose escalating and expansion phase up to the dose of 10 mg/kg [133].

Several phase II and III clinical trials have been performed with nivolumab to improve the outcomes of patients with NSCLC. Currently, nivolumab is FDA approved for the treatment of patients with advanced NSCLC who experience progression of disease on or after standard platinum-based chemotherapy. CheckMate 057, a phase III randomized control trial compared nivolumab versus docetaxel in a second-line treatment of advanced non-squamous NSCLC, showed a median OS of 12.2 months (95% CI: 9.7–15.0) among 292 patients in the nivolumab group and 9.4 months (95% CI: 8.1–10.7) among 290 patients in the docetaxel group (hazard ratio: 0.73; 96% CI: 0.59–0.89; $P = 0.002$) [134]. ORR and median durations of response were higher in nivolumab arm (19 vs. 12% and 18.3 vs. 5.6 months, respectively) [134]. The 3-year OS rates for the nivolumab and docetaxel arms were 18% and 9%, respectively [135]. Similarly, another phase III trial (CheckMate 017) compared nivolumab (3 mg/kg, IV, Q2W) with docetaxel (75 mg/m^2, IV, Q3W) in 272 patients with advanced, squamous NSCLC who had progressive disease on platinum-based doublet chemotherapy. OS was prolonged with nivolumab compared to docetaxel (median OS: 9.2 vs. 6.0 months) [136]. The two- and three-year OS rates for nivolumab versus docetaxel were 23% versus 8%, and 16% versus 6%, respectively [135, 137]. ORR was higher with nivolumab (20% vs. 9%), as was the duration of response (25.2 vs. 8 months) [136]. In terms of toxicity, when compared to docetaxel, nivolumab had fever severe grade 3–4 treatment-related adverse effects (7–10% vs. 54%) [134, 136]. In the subgroup analysis, OS benefit was only seen in non-squamous patients with increased tumor PD-L1 expression. There was no OS improvement in PD-L1-negative tumors in the non-squamous cohort and PD-L1 expressing tumors in the squamous cohort. However, better side effect and toxicity profile of nivolumab makes it a better choice than docetaxel [134, 136].

Currently, nivolumab as a single agent is not approved by FDA for the frontline setting in treatment-naïve patients regardless of PD-L1 level. The CheckMate 026 trial which sought to compare the activity of nivolumab versus platinum doublet chemotherapy in 541 treatment-naïve, PD-L1 positive (at least 1% of tumor cells with PD-L1 staining) NSCLC patients did not show any prolongation of OS or PFS with nivolumab [138] (Table 1.1). The combination of nivolumab plus ipilimumab in lung cancer is currently being tested in the CheckMate 227 trial (Table 1.1). In this trial, patients with PD-L1 expression level of at least 1% were randomly assigned in 1:1:1 ratio to receive nivolumab plus ipilimumab, nivolumab monotherapy, or chemotherapy. Additionally, patients with tumor PD-L1 expression less than 1% were randomly assigned in 1:1:1 ratio to receive nivolumab plus ipilimumab, nivolumab plus chemotherapy or chemotherapy alone. In the recently reported part 1 data ($n = 299$) of this trial, there was improvement in median PFS with frontline nivolumab plus ipilimumab compared to chemotherapy among patients with high tumor mutational burden (defined as >10 mutations per megabase) irrespective of PD-L1 expression level (7.2 months (95% CI: 5.5–13.2) vs. 5.5 months (95% CI: 4.4–5.8) [139]. The objective response rate was 45.3% with nivolumab plus ipilimumab and 26.9% with chemotherapy [139]. The OS data is not mature, but it is likely that after completion of this clinical trial, nivolumab will gain FDA approval in certain patients with lung cancer in the first-line setting.

Nivolumab has also been studied in untreated patients with surgically resectable early stage (stage I, II, or IIIA) NSCLC. In a phase I study with primary end point of safety and feasibility, nivolumab (at a dose of 3 mg/kg) was given IV every 2 weeks, with surgery planned approximately 4 weeks after the first dose. The study showed that neoadjuvant nivolumab was associated with few side effects, did not delay surgery, and induced a major pathological response in 45% of resected

Table 1.1 Key phase III checkpoint inhibitor trails in chemotherapy-naïve NSCLC patients

Study trial/agent	Trial description	Results timing	PFS (months)	RR (%)	Median OS (months)	AEs ≥ 3 (%)
KEYNOTE-407/pembrolizumab	Platinum doublet chemotherapy with pembrolizumab or placebo in squamous NSCLC	Median follow-up 87.8 months	6.4 versus 4.8	58 versus 38	15.9 versus 11.3	70 versus 68
KEYNOTE-189/pembrolizumab	Platinum doublet chemotherapy with pembrolizumab or placebo in non-squamous NSCLC	Median follow-up 10.5 months	8.8 versus 4.9	48 versus 19	69% versus 49%	67 versus 66
KEYNOTE-042/pembrolizumab (ongoing)	Pembrolizumab versus platinum doublet chemotherapy with ≥1% PD-L1 staining	Prelim at 12.8 months	PD-L1 ≥ 50%: 7.4 versus 6.4 PD-L1 ≥ 20%: 6.2 versus 6.6 PD-L1 ≥ 1%: 5.4 versus 6.5	NA	PD-L1 ≥ 50%: 20 versus 12 PD-L1 ≥ 20%: 18 versus 13 PD-L1 ≥ 1%: 17 versus 12	18 versus 41
KEYNOTE-024/pembrolizumab	Pembrolizumab versus platinum doublet chemotherapy with ≥50% PD-L1 staining	Prelim: at 25 months	10.3 versus 6	45 versus 28	30 versus 14.2	27 versus 53
CheckMate 227/nivolumab + ipilimumab (ongoing)	Platinum doublet chemotherapy versus nivolumab (N) + ipilimumab (I) versus nivolumab monotherapy (PD-L1 > 1%) versus nivolumab + chemotherapy (PD-L1 < 1%)	Part 1 with N + I versus chemo with known tumor mutation burden (TMB)	7.2 versus 5.4	For high TMB 45 versus 27	NA	Prelim: N + I: 25 N + chemo: 52 Chemo: 35
CheckMate 026/nivolumab	Nivolumab versus chemotherapy with PD-L1 > 1%	Study conclusion	4.2 versus 5.9		14.4 versus 13.2 (HR 1.02)	71 versus 92

(continued)

Table 1.1 (continued)

Study trial/agent	Trial description	Results timing	PFS (months)	RR (%)	Median OS (months)	AEs $\geq$ 3 (%)
IMpower 150/atezolizumab + bevacizumab (ongoing)	Platinum doublet chemotherapy with atezolizumab (ACP) or atezolizumab + bevacizumab (ABCP) or bevacizumab (BCP)	ABCP versus BCP	8.3 versus 6.8		19.2 versus 14.7	
IMpower 131/atezolizumab	Platinum doublet chemotherapy with atezolizumab or placebo	Median follow-up 17 months	6.3 versus 5.6		14 versus 14	68 versus 57

tumors. The tumor mutational burden was predictive of the pathological response to PD1 blockade [140].

1.10.1.2 Pembrolizumab

Pembrolizumab is another IgG monoclonal antibody that targets PD1 on T cells and inhibits the interaction between PD1 and PD-L1 on the tumor cells. Currently, it is approved by FDA for the frontline treatment of EGFR/ALK wild-type NSCLC with at least 50% of tumor cells expressing PD-L1. This approval came after completion of the phase III KEYNOTE024 trial which compared pembrolizumab monotherapy to standard platinum-based chemotherapy in EGFR/ALK wild-type NSCLC with at least 50% of tumor cells expressing PD-L1. There were both OS (6 month OS rate of 80.2% vs. 72.4% with HR: 0.60; 95% CI: 0.41–0.89; $P = 0.005$) and PFS (10.3 months vs. 6 months; HR: 0.50; 95% CI: 0.37–0.68; $P < 0.001$) benefit in the pembrolizumab arm [141].

Recently, pembrolizumab in combination with pemetrexed and carboplatin also received accelerated FDA approval for treatment of metastatic non-squamous NSCLC, irrespective of the PD-L1 expression. This approval was based on the KEYNOTE 021 phase II trial which compared chemotherapy alone or with pembrolizumab in 123 patients with advanced untreated non-squamous NSCLC without any EGFR or ALK alterations. This study showed that patients who receive progressive map had better ORR (55 vs. 29%, 95% CI 8–42) and PFS (13 vs. 6 months; HR 0.53, 95% CI 0.31–0.91) [142]. These findings were later confirmed in a larger phase III trial (KEYNOTE-189) which was reported this year and also showed improvement in OS (12 month OS rate: 69% vs. 49%; HR: 0.49; 95% CI: 0.38–0.64), PFS (8.8 month vs. 4.9 months; HR: 0.52; 95% CI: 0.43–0.64) and ORR (48% vs. 19%) in the platinum doublet plus pembrolizumab arm compared to the chemotherapy plus placebo arm [143] (Table 1.1).

Pembrolizumab has also been approved for treatment of advanced NSCLC as a second-line therapy after disease progression on platinum-based chemotherapy. This approval was based on the phase II/III KEYNOTE-010 study in which patients with disease progression on or after platinum-containing chemotherapy and had >1% tumor cell PD-L1 expression as determined by the 22C3 pharmDx test received either pembrolizumab (2 mg/kg or 10 mg/kg via IV) or docetaxel (75 mg/m^2) every 3 weeks. The HR and p value for OS was 0.71 (95% CI: 0.58–0.88) and <0.001 comparing pembrolizumab (2 mg/kg) with chemotherapy and 0.61 (95% CI: 0.49–0.75) and <0.001 comparing pembrolizumab (10 mg/kg) with chemotherapy [144].

1.10.1.3 Atezolizumab

Unlike nivolumab and pembrolizumab, atezolizumab is an antibody against PD-L1, the ligand for PD-1. By binding to the PD-L1 receptor present on tumor cells atezolizumab activates antibody depended cell mediated toxicity which enhances immune system to fight tumor cells. Currently, it is approved for the management of patients with metastatic NSCLC who are EGFR- or ALK-negative and have disease progression on platinum-containing chemotherapy. This approval was based on a phase III randomized controlled trial (the OAK trial) comparing atezolizumab at 1200 mg, IV, every three weeks (n = 425) to docetaxel at 75 mg/m^2, every 3 weeks (n = 425). OS was significantly better in the atezolizumab arm than the docetaxel arm (13.8 months [95% CI: 11.8–15.7] vs. 9.6 months [95% CI: 8.6–11.2]; HR: 0.73; 95% CI: 0.62–0.87; p = 0.0003). Patients with low PD-L1 or undetectable expression levels also benefited with improvement in survival in the atezolizumab arm [145].

Although atezolizumab has not been approved by FDA for the treatment of NSCLC in a frontline setting, there are ongoing clinical trials that show promising results. Specifically interim results of the phase III IMpower 131 trial showed improvement in PFS (6.3 vs. 5.6 months; HR: 0.7; 95% CI: 0.60–0.85) when patients were given platinum-based chemotherapy combined with atezolizumab versus chemotherapy alone. The improvement in PFS was the most significant in PD-L1-high (expression in $\geq$50% of tumor cells) group (10.1 vs. 5.5 months; HR: 0.44; 95% CI: 0.27–0.71), but benefits were seen in all PD-L1-positive subgroups and not in the PD-L1-negative subgroup [146] (Table 1.1). Final OS data is still pending.

Recently another phase III trial, IMpower150, showed that addition of atezolizumab to bevacizumab plus platinum-based chemotherapy can lead to improved PFS (8.3 vs. 6.8 months; HR: 0.62; 95% CI: 0.52–0.74) and OS (19.2 vs. 14.7 months; HR: 0.78; 95% CI: 0.64–0.96) in patients with metastatic non-squamous NSCLC, regardless of PD-L1 expression and EGFR or other genetic alterations [147] (Table 1.1).

Overall, pembrolizumab currently remains the drug of choice in the frontline setting for patients with NSCLC until other checkpoint inhibitors are approved by FDA.

1.10.1.4 Durvalumab

Durvalumab, a humanized immunoglobulin G1 kappa monoclonal antibody that blocks the binding of programmed cell death ligand 1 (PD-L1) to PD-1 and CD80 (B7.1), has been approved for treatment of unresectable stage III NSCLC that has not progressed following concurrent platinum-based chemotherapy and radiation therapy. This approval came on the basis of a large phase III trial (the PACIFIC trial) in which patients with unresectable stage III NSCLC without any progression after at least 2 lines of platinum-based chemotherapy were randomly assigned to the PD-L1 antibody or placebo. The immunotherapy group had improved PFS (16.8 vs. 5.6 months; HR: 0.52; 95% CI: 0.42–0.65), response rate (28% vs. 16%; relative risk [RR]: 1.78; 95% CI: 1.27–2.51), and median time to death or distant metastasis (23.2 vs. 14.6 months; HR: 0.52: 95% CI: 0.39–0.69) [148]. However, OS data of the study is still pending and therefore some investigators recommend against using immunotherapy in patients with stage III lung cancer at this point.

1.10.2 CTLA-4 Antagonists

The combination of a CTLA 4 inhibitor (ipilimumab) and a PD-1 blocker (nivolumab) has shown promising results in chemotherapy-naïve patients with metastatic NSCLC. However, without PD-1 blockade ipilimumab may not be as effective. There was one phase II randomized control trial that compared ipilimumab plus paclitaxel and carboplatin with paclitaxel and carboplatin alone as first-line treatment. However, there was no statistical difference in primary end point of progression-free survival between the two arms. In addition, there was no OS benefit in the ipilimumab arm [149].

1.10.3 Toxicity Associated with Immune Checkpoint Inhibitors

Although the immune checkpoint inhibitors are in general less toxic than chemotherapies, there have been several reports of immune-related adverse events that can occur occasionally. These immune-related adverse events include inflammatory reactions against normal cells apart from the tumor cells. Common side effects include rash (33%), colitis (14%), endocrinopathies (8%), hepatitis (4%), pneumonitis (2%), and acute kidney injury (2%) [150]. Other rare ones including pancreatitis, Guillain-Barré syndrome or myasthenia gravis, myocarditis or venous thromboembolism, thrombocytopenias or neutropenia, ocular inflammation, and inflammatory arthritis. Management of grade 1 toxicities includes close monitoring of patients and continuation of immune checkpoint inhibitors with the exception of some toxicities such as neurotoxicity, cardiotoxicity, and hematological toxicity. For grade 2 toxicities, immune checkpoint inhibitor treatment should be suspended with resumption when symptoms revert to grade 1 or less. Corticosteroids may be administered to help in reducing the inflammation. For grade 3 toxicities, high-dose steroids should be initiated along with suspension of immunotherapy. Corticosteroids should be tapered slowly over the course of at least 4–6 weeks. If patients are refractory to corticosteroids, then other forms of immunosuppressive agents such as infliximab could be used. For any grade 4-related toxicity permanent discontinuation of checkpoint inhibitors is recommended with the exception of endocrinopathies which can be controlled with hormone replacement therapy. Specific recommendations for the management of adverse events with checkpoint inhibitors have been published by American Society of Clinical Oncology [151].

1.10.4 Immunotherapy Biomarkers in Lung Cancer

With the approval of multiple checkpoint inhibitors, it is important to select the appropriate patients who might benefit from this class of therapies. In majority of the trials that led to the approval of these agents, it was noted that patients with tumors expressing high levels of PD-L1 benefit the most. For example in the

KEYNOTE 189 trial with chemotherapy-naïve patients, pembrolizumab showed the highest OS benefit in patients with PD-L1 expression in $\geq 50\%$ of tumor cells (12-month OS rate: 73.0% vs. 48.1%; HR: 0.42; 95% CI: 0.26–0.68) [143]. The clinical trial CheckMate 227 showed improved PFS in patients with higher tumor mutational burden which may be a new biomarker for immunotherapy.

One of the challenges facing these biomarkers is that PD-L1 and tumor mutational burden in tumor samples may be heterogeneous and repetitive tumor biopsies may be needed but is not always feasible [152]. Additionally, companion tests for evaluating PD-L1 expression as a biomarker of response use a variety of detection platforms for different forms (protein or mRNA), employ diverse biopsy and surgical samples, and have disparate positivity cutoff points and scoring systems, all of which complicate the standardization of clinical decision-making process [153]. Currently, four immunohistochemistry (IHC)-based assays using diagnostic monoclonal antibodies, 22C3 (pembrolizumab), 28-8 (nivolumab), SP142 (atezolizumab), or SP263 (durvalumab), to detect PD-L1 expression have been approved by FDA. Finally, the expression levels of PD-L1 may change after treatment with chemotherapy or immunotherapy and the patterns of resistance need to be better studied. In case of clear progressive disease upon immunotherapy, chemotherapy should be offered to the patients. However, if there are only 1 or 2 sites of progressive disease local modalities such as radiation or surgery with continuation of immunotherapy may be considered. It is important to develop a feasible, predictive, and reproducible biomarker which can predict patient response and help improve the overall survival among all these immunotherapies.

1.11 Other Potential Immune Therapy Targets

1.11.1 HER2

ERBB2 gene, a proto-oncogene on chromosome 17q12, encodes the ERBB2 protein which is also known as human epidermal growth factor receptor 2 (Her2), a tyrosine kinase receptor of the EGFR family. Her2 alterations have been detected in 1–4% of NSCLC tumors by multiplex testing and next-generation sequencing [154, 155]. These tumors are most commonly found in never smokers, adenocarcinomas, and women. Aberrations on exon 20 lead to phosphorylation of Her2 and activation of downstream pathways including RAS/RAF/MEK/ERK and PI3K/AKT/mTOR. These pathways have been implicated in the cancer cell proliferation, survival, growth, and tumor angiogenesis. The mutations most frequently found in Her2 gene are in-frame insertions in exon 20. There are currently no approved targeted agents for these patients. Her-2 targeted agents studied include: dacomitinib, neratinib, neratinib in combination with temsirolimus, afatinib, trastuzumab in combination with pertuzumab, and ado-trastuzumab emtansine. Response rates for these regimens have been meager at best (0–19%) [156–158] with ado-trastuzumab emtansine showing some of the most promise with a response rate up to 44% [159].

Another drug under investigation, poziotinib has been shown to have robust responses in preclinical models, and currently, there is a phase II study evaluating Her2 exon 20 insertion mutant advanced NSCLC with poziotinib as a treatment (NCT 03318939). Her2 amplification and Her2 exon 20 mutated advanced NSCLC represent two distinct subsets of disease in an ever-expanding field of potential clinically relevant targets.

1.11.2 Kirsten Rat Sarcoma Viral Oncogene Homolog (KRAS)

The KRAS gene (located on chromosome 12p12.1) is primarily involved in regulating cell division. It is a member of the RAS family of genes that encodes four proteins that are highly related mediators of the mitogen-activated protein kinase (MAPK) pathway: HRAS, KRAS4a, KRAS4b, and NRAS. These proteins function as guanosine triphosphatases (GTPases) binary switches that turn on or turn off multiple pathways involved in cancer cell survival, proliferation, angiogenesis, and differentiation via effector proteins. KRAS mutations have been found to be one of the most common oncogenic drivers in NSCLC (20–30%). The most common KRAS mutations are G12C with KRAS transversions typical for smokers and transitions typical for never smokers. Targeting RAS mutations remains elusive with most of the research focusing on RAF/MAPK pathway or novel approaches to RAS inhibition. MEK inhibitors such as trametinib and selumetinib have yet to show any survival benefit in patients with KRAS mutations compared to non-mutated patients [160–164]. Prior to activation of downstream effectors of RAS, RAS attaches to the cell membrane via farnesyl transferase. Investigations on utilizing farnesyl transferase inhibition have also failed to yield any promising results [165, 166]. The RAF/MEK inhibitor, RO5126766 (CH5127566), has shown some promising results in a basket trial with KRAS mutant NSCLC showing a 60% response rate [167].

1.11.3 Phosphatidylinositol-4,5-Bisphosphate 3-Kinase Catalytic Subunit Alpha (PIK3CA)

PI3K/AKT signaling promotes carcinogenesis and development of NSCLC. PIK3CA encodes for PI3K which promotes cell survival. Its activation triggers downstream AKT. Mutations in the pathway include gain of function mutations in PIK3CA and AKT1 or loss of function mutations in the negative regulator protein PTEN, which occur in 16% of cancer cases. These mutations are found predominantly in SCC and smokers. Investigation is ongoing to determine if these are passenger or driver mutations. A variety of small molecules have been or currently being investigated as single agents or in combination with others but thus far failed to show improved efficacy over standard approaches [168–171]. Pictilisib in combination with standard of care did show some encouraging anti-tumor activity as a first-line treatment in a phase IB dose-escalation study [172], but this activity did not translate into improved PFS in the phase II FIGARO study [173].

1.11.4 Ephrin Type-B Receptor 4 (EPHB4)

EphB4 is a receptor found on venous endothelial cells, while its companion ligand Ephrin B2 is often expressed on arterial endothelial cells. EphB4 is overexpressed in epithelial tumors, which has been shown to be associated with poor prognosis in a variety of tumor types. This induces bidirectional signaling between EphB4 and EphB2 incudes the activation of PI3K/AKT/mTOR, Rho, Ras, Abl, Src, and MAPK signaling pathways, leading to increased cancer cell migration, proliferation, and adhesion. A biologic drug, sEphB4-HSA, which interferes the interaction between EphB4 and its ligand, has shown promising results in a dose finding phase IA study [174]. sEphB4-HSA in combination with pembrolizumab is currently under investigation in a phase II clinical trial (NCT03049618).

1.11.5 Fibroblast Growth Factor Receptor (FGFR)

Fibroblast growth factor receptor (FGFR) and its associated pathway are important in cell cycle progression, survival, and proliferation and can activate RAS and MAPK signaling cascades. FGFR mutations have been detected in 3–19% of non-small-cell lung cancer cases. These aberrations are mostly gene amplifications as well as nucleotide sequence alterations. FGFR inhibitors are mostly still investigational and their clinical significance remains to be seen [175–178].

1.12 Conclusions

In summary, the treatment of the lung cancer has advanced rapidly with the emergence of targeted therapy, immunotherapy, biomarker-based treatments, and availability of new clinical trials. Precision medicine may become increasingly important in the future of lung cancer treatment. Currently, testing for PD-L1 expression levels, EGFR mutations, ALK and ROS1 translocations are essential in selecting the best therapy for lung cancer patients, especially those with lung adenocarcinoma, large-cell histology, and non-small-cell lung cancer. Those tests can also be extended to patients who are never smokers or light smokers with squamous cell histology. Furthermore, broad genomic profiling to identify molecular alterations such as HER2 insertions, BRAF mutations, MET, TRK and RET alterations can help to identify investigational targeted agents that are in clinical trials.

For patients who are EGFR-positive, EGFR TKIs remain standard of care in the first-line metastatic setting. Patients with a ROS1 fusions should consider crizotinib as the initial treatment. For patients with ALK mutations, recent trials have shown that the next-generation ALK inhibitor such as alectinib may be superior to crizotinib in the first-line setting. Patients whose tumors have high PD-L1 expression ($\geq 50\%$) should receive pembrolizumab as the first-line therapy. Ongoing clinical trials are evaluating the benefits of combining immunotherapy or targeted therapy with chemotherapy. Patients whose tumors harbor other mutations should be encouraged to participate in clinical trials for corresponding targeted agents.

Acknowledgements Special thanks to Sam Garcia, Library Assistant, and Andrea Lynch, Scholarly Communications Librarian at the City of Hope Graff Library in Duarte, California.

References

1. Wheeler DA, Wang L (2013) From human genome to cancer genome: the first decade. Genome Res 23(7):1054–1062
2. Gong J et al (2018) Value-based genomics. Oncotarget 9(21):15792–15815
3. National Human Genome Research Institute (NHGRI) (2003) Human genome project completion: frequently asked questions. In: National Human Genome Research Institute (ed) 2003 release: international consortium completes HGP
4. El-Metwally S, Ouda OM, Helmy M (2014) Next generation sequencing technologies and challenges in sequence assembly. SpringerBriefs in Systems Biology, vol 7. XII, 118 11 b/w illustrations, 1 illustrations in colour. Springer-Verlag, New York
5. Mardis ER (2011) A decade's perspective on DNA sequencing technology. Nature 470 (7333):198–203
6. Wheeler DA et al (2008) The complete genome of an individual by massively parallel DNA sequencing. Nature 452(7189):872–876
7. Goodwin S, McPherson JD, McCombie WR (2016) Coming of age: ten years of next-generation sequencing technologies. Nat Rev Genet 17(6):333–351
8. Heather JM, Chain B (2016) The sequence of sequencers: the history of sequencing DNA. Genomics 107(1):1–8
9. Quail MA et al (2012) A tale of three next generation sequencing platforms: comparison of Ion Torrent, Pacific Biosciences and Illumina MiSeq sequencers. BMC Genom 13:341
10. Feliubadalo L et al (2017) Benchmarking of whole exome sequencing and ad hoc designed panels for genetic testing of hereditary cancer. Sci Rep 7:37984
11. Khotskaya YB, Mills GB, Mills Shaw KR (2017) Next-generation sequencing and result interpretation in clinical oncology: challenges of personalized cancer therapy. Annu Rev Med 68:113–125
12. Schram AM, Berger MF, Hyman DM (2017) Precision oncology: charting a path forward to broader deployment of genomic profiling. PLoS Med 14(2):e1002242
13. Cubiella J et al (1999) Prognostic factors in nonresectable pancreatic adenocarcinoma: a rationale to design therapeutic trials. Am J Gastroenterol 94(5):1271–1278
14. Frampton GM et al (2013) Development and validation of a clinical cancer genomic profiling test based on massively parallel DNA sequencing. Nat Biotechnol 31(11):1023–1031
15. Herzog TJ et al (2016) Impact of molecular profiling on overall survival of patients with advanced ovarian cancer. Oncotarget 7(15):19840–19849

16. Radovich M et al (2016) Clinical benefit of a precision medicine based approach for guiding treatment of refractory cancers. Oncotarget 7(35):56491–56500
17. Weiss GJ et al (2015) Evaluation and comparison of two commercially available targeted next-generation sequencing platforms to assist oncology decision making. Onco Targets Ther 8:959–967
18. Sboner A et al (2011) The real cost of sequencing: higher than you think! Genome Biol 12 (8):125
19. Frank M et al (2013) Genome sequencing: a systematic review of health economic evidence. Health Econ Rev 3(1):29
20. Jardim DL et al (2015) Impact of a biomarker-based strategy on oncology drug development: a meta-analysis of clinical trials leading to FDA approval. J Natl Cancer Inst 107(11)
21. Schwaederle M et al (2015) Impact of precision medicine in diverse cancers: a meta-analysis of phase II clinical trials. J Clin Oncol 33(32):3817–3825
22. Schwaederle M et al (2016) Association of biomarker-based treatment strategies with response rates and progression-free survival in refractory malignant neoplasms: a meta-analysis. JAMA Oncol 2(11):1452–1459
23. Ocana A et al (2015) Influence of companion diagnostics on efficacy and safety of targeted anti-cancer drugs: systematic review and meta-analyses. Oncotarget 6(37):39538–39549
24. Cancer Genome Atlas Research Network (2014) Comprehensive molecular profiling of lung adenocarcinoma. Nature 511(7511):543–550
25. Sholl LM et al (2015) Multi-institutional oncogenic driver mutation analysis in lung adenocarcinoma: the Lung Cancer Mutation Consortium experience. J Thorac Oncol 10 (5):768–777
26. Sabari JK et al (2017) Unravelling the biology of SCLC: implications for therapy. Nat Rev Clin Oncol 14(9):549–561
27. George J et al (2015) Comprehensive genomic profiles of small cell lung cancer. Nature 524 (7563):47–53
28. Pesch B et al (2012) Cigarette smoking and lung cancer—relative risk estimates for the major histological types from a pooled analysis of case-control studies. Int J Cancer 131 (5):1210–1219
29. Ellison G et al (2013) EGFR mutation testing in lung cancer: a review of available methods and their use for analysis of tumour tissue and cytology samples. J Clin Pathol 66(2):79–89
30. Mayo-de-Las-Casas C et al (2017) Large scale, prospective screening of EGFR mutations in the blood of advanced NSCLC patients to guide treatment decisions. Ann Oncol 28 (9):2248–2255
31. Toor OM et al (2018) Correlation of somatic genomic alterations between tissue genomics and ctDNA employing next-generation sequencing: analysis of lung and gastrointestinal cancers. Mol Cancer Ther 17(5):1123–1132
32. Yarden Y, Sliwkowski MX (2001) Untangling the ErbB signalling network. Nat Rev Mol Cell Biol 2(2):127–137
33. Rosell R et al (2009) Screening for epidermal growth factor receptor mutations in lung cancer. N Engl J Med 361(10):958–967
34. Midha A, Dearden S, McCormack R (2015) EGFR mutation incidence in non-small-cell lung cancer of adenocarcinoma histology: a systematic review and global map by ethnicity (mutMapII). Am J Cancer Res 5(9):2892–2911
35. Shi Y et al (2014) A prospective, molecular epidemiology study of EGFR mutations in Asian patients with advanced non-small-cell lung cancer of adenocarcinoma histology (PIONEER). J Thorac Oncol 9(2):154–162
36. Wang S, Wang Z (2014) EGFR mutations in patients with non-small cell lung cancer from mainland China and their relationships with clinicopathological features: a meta-analysis. Int J Clin Exp Med 7(8):1967–1978
37. Information NCfB, NIH. PubChem. NIH

38. Soria JC et al (2018) Osimertinib in untreated EGFR-mutated advanced non-small-cell lung cancer. N Engl J Med 378(2):113–125
39. Xu J, Wang J, Zhang S (2017) Mechanisms of resistance to irreversible epidermal growth factor receptor tyrosine kinase inhibitors and therapeutic strategies in non-small cell lung cancer. Oncotarget 8(52):90557–90578
40. Mok TS et al (2017) Osimertinib or platinum-pemetrexed in EGFR T790M-positive lung cancer. N Engl J Med 376(7):629–640
41. Lee CK et al (2013) Impact of EGFR inhibitor in non-small cell lung cancer on progression-free and overall survival: a meta-analysis. J Natl Cancer Inst 105(9):595–605
42. Zhou C et al (2011) Erlotinib versus chemotherapy as first-line treatment for patients with advanced EGFR mutation-positive non-small-cell lung cancer (OPTIMAL, CTONG-0802): a multicentre, open-label, randomised, phase 3 study. Lancet Oncol 12(8):735–742
43. Zhou C et al (2015) Final overall survival results from a randomised, phase III study of erlotinib versus chemotherapy as first-line treatment of EGFR mutation-positive advanced non-small-cell lung cancer (OPTIMAL, CTONG-0802). Ann Oncol 26(9):1877–1883
44. Rosell R et al (2012) Erlotinib versus standard chemotherapy as first-line treatment for European patients with advanced EGFR mutation-positive non-small-cell lung cancer (EURTAC): a multicentre, open-label, randomised phase 3 trial. Lancet Oncol 13(3): 239–246
45. Wu YL et al (2015) First-line erlotinib versus gemcitabine/cisplatin in patients with advanced EGFR mutation-positive non-small-cell lung cancer: analyses from the phase III, randomized, open-label, ENSURE study. Ann Oncol 26(9):1883–1889
46. Fukuoka M et al (2011) Biomarker analyses and final overall survival results from a phase III, randomized, open-label, first-line study of gefitinib versus carboplatin/paclitaxel in clinically selected patients with advanced non-small-cell lung cancer in Asia (IPASS). J Clin Oncol 29(21):2866–2874
47. Mok TS et al (2009) Gefitinib or carboplatin-paclitaxel in pulmonary adenocarcinoma. N Engl J Med 361(10):947–957
48. Maemondo M et al (2010) Gefitinib or chemotherapy for non-small-cell lung cancer with mutated EGFR. N Engl J Med 362(25):2380–2388
49. Sequist LV et al (2013) Phase III study of afatinib or cisplatin plus pemetrexed in patients with metastatic lung adenocarcinoma with EGFR mutations. J Clin Oncol 31(27):3327–3334
50. Yang JC et al (2013) Symptom control and quality of life in LUX-Lung 3: a phase III study of afatinib or cisplatin/pemetrexed in patients with advanced lung adenocarcinoma with EGFR mutations. J Clin Oncol 31(27):3342–3350
51. Wu YL et al (2014) Afatinib versus cisplatin plus gemcitabine for first-line treatment of Asian patients with advanced non-small-cell lung cancer harbouring EGFR mutations (LUX-Lung 6): an open-label, randomised phase 3 trial. Lancet Oncol 15(2):213–222
52. Yang JC et al (2015) Afatinib versus cisplatin-based chemotherapy for EGFR mutation-positive lung adenocarcinoma (LUX-Lung 3 and LUX-Lung 6): analysis of overall survival data from two randomised, phase 3 trials. Lancet Oncol 16(2):141–151
53. Yang JC et al (2015) Clinical activity of afatinib in patients with advanced non-small-cell lung cancer harbouring uncommon EGFR mutations: a combined post-hoc analysis of LUX-Lung 2, LUX-Lung 3, and LUX-Lung 6. Lancet Oncol 16(7):830–838
54. Wu YL et al (2017) Dacomitinib versus gefitinib as first-line treatment for patients with EGFR-mutation-positive non-small-cell lung cancer (ARCHER 1050): a randomised, open-label, phase 3 trial. Lancet Oncol 18(11):1454–1466
55. Yang JJ et al (2017) A phase III randomised controlled trial of erlotinib vs gefitinib in advanced non-small cell lung cancer with EGFR mutations. Br J Cancer 116(5):568–574
56. Paz-Ares L et al (2017) Afatinib versus gefitinib in patients with EGFR mutation-positive advanced non-small-cell lung cancer: overall survival data from the phase IIb LUX-Lung 7 trial. Ann Oncol 28(2):270–277

57. Chabon JJ et al (2016) Circulating tumour DNA profiling reveals heterogeneity of EGFR inhibitor resistance mechanisms in lung cancer patients. Nat Commun 7:11815
58. Piotrowska Z et al (2017) MET amplification (amp) as a resistance mechanism to osimertinib. J Clin Oncol 35:6
59. Sequist LV et al (2011) Genotypic and histological evolution of lung cancers acquiring resistance to EGFR inhibitors. Sci Transl Med 3(75):75ra26
60. Nishie K et al (2012) Epidermal growth factor receptor tyrosine kinase inhibitors beyond progressive disease: a retrospective analysis for Japanese patients with activating EGFR mutations. J Thorac Oncol 7(11):1722–1727
61. Seto T et al (2014) Erlotinib alone or with bevacizumab as first-line therapy in patients with advanced non-squamous non-small-cell lung cancer harbouring EGFR mutations (JO25567): an open-label, randomised, multicentre, phase 2 study. Lancet Oncol 15 (11):1236–1244
62. Wu YL et al (2013) Intercalated combination of chemotherapy and erlotinib for patients with advanced stage non-small-cell lung cancer (FASTACT-2): a randomised, double-blind trial. Lancet Oncol 14(8):777–786
63. Cheng Y et al (2016) Randomized phase II trial of gefitinib with and without pemetrexed as first-line therapy in patients with advanced nonsquamous non-small-cell lung cancer with activating epidermal growth factor receptor mutations. J Clin Oncol 34(27):3258–3266
64. Gatzemeier U et al (2007) Phase III study of erlotinib in combination with cisplatin and gemcitabine in advanced non-small-cell lung cancer: the Tarceva Lung Cancer Investigation Trial. J Clin Oncol 25(12):1545–1552
65. Giaccone G et al (2004) Gefitinib in combination with gemcitabine and cisplatin in advanced non-small-cell lung cancer: a phase III trial—INTACT 1. J Clin Oncol 22(5):777–784
66. Herbst RS et al (2004) Gefitinib in combination with paclitaxel and carboplatin in advanced non-small-cell lung cancer: a phase III trial—INTACT 2. J Clin Oncol 22(5):785–794
67. Herbst RS et al (2005) TRIBUTE: a phase III trial of erlotinib hydrochloride (OSI-774) combined with carboplatin and paclitaxel chemotherapy in advanced non-small-cell lung cancer. J Clin Oncol 23(25):5892–5899
68. Mok TSK et al (2017) Gefitinib plus chemotherapy versus chemotherapy in epidermal growth factor receptor mutation-positive non-small-cell lung cancer resistant to first-line gefitinib (IMPRESS): overall survival and biomarker analyses. J Clin Oncol 35(36):4027–4034
69. Kwak EL et al (2010) Anaplastic lymphoma kinase inhibition in non-small-cell lung cancer. N Engl J Med 363(18):1693–1703
70. Crino L et al (2011) Initial phase II results with crizotinib in advanced ALK-positive non-small cell lung cancer (NSCLC): PROFILE 1005. J Clin Oncol 29(15):1
71. Solomon BJ et al (2014) First-line crizotinib versus chemotherapy in ALK-positive lung cancer. N Engl J Med 371(23):2167–2177
72. Awad MM, Shaw AT (2014) ALK inhibitors in non-small cell lung cancer: crizotinib and beyond. Clin Adv Hematol Oncol 12(7):429–439
73. Shaw AT et al (2014) Crizotinib in ROS1-rearranged non-small-cell lung cancer. N Engl J Med 371(21):1963–1971
74. Shaw AT et al (2017) Ceritinib versus chemotherapy in patients with ALK-rearranged non-small-cell lung cancer previously given chemotherapy and crizotinib (ASCEND-5): a randomised, controlled, open-label, phase 3 trial. Lancet Oncol 18(7):874–886
75. Yang JC et al (2017) Pooled systemic efficacy and safety data from the pivotal phase II studies (NP28673 and NP28761) of alectinib in ALK-positive non-small cell lung cancer. J Thorac Oncol 12(10):1552–1560
76. Shaw AT et al (2016) Alectinib in ALK-positive, crizotinib-resistant, non-small-cell lung cancer: a single-group, multicentre, phase 2 trial. Lancet Oncol 17(2):234–242
77. Bendell JC et al (2016) Clinical activity and safety of cobimetinib (cobi) and atezolizumab in colorectal cancer (CRC). J Clin Oncol 34(15):2

78. Peters S et al (2017) Alectinib versus crizotinib in untreated ALK-positive non-small-cell lung cancer. N Engl J Med 377(9):829–838
79. Kim DW et al (2017) Brigatinib in patients with crizotinib-refractory anaplastic lymphoma kinase-positive non-small-cell lung cancer: a randomized, multicenter phase II trial. J Clin Oncol 35(22):2490–2498
80. Shaw AT et al (2017) Lorlatinib in non-small-cell lung cancer with ALK or ROS1 rearrangement: an international, multicentre, open-label, single-arm first-in-man phase 1 trial. Lancet Oncol 18(12):1590–1599
81. Davies KD, Doebele RC (2013) Molecular pathways: ROS1 fusion proteins in cancer. Clin Cancer Res 19(15):4040–4045
82. Rossi G et al (2017) Detection of ROS1 rearrangement in non-small cell lung cancer: current and future perspectives. Lung Cancer (Auckl) 8:45–55
83. Ogura H et al (2017) TKI-addicted ROS1-rearranged cells are destined to survival or death by the intensity of ROS1 kinase activity. Sci Rep 7(1):5519
84. Bergethon K et al (2012) ROS1 rearrangements define a unique molecular class of lung cancers. J Clin Oncol 30(8):863–870
85. Sporn JR (1999) Practical recommendations for the management of adenocarcinoma of the pancreas. Drugs 57(1):69–79
86. Davies H et al (2002) Mutations of the BRAF gene in human cancer. Nature 417(6892):949–954
87. Ascierto PA et al (2012) The role of BRAF V600 mutation in melanoma. J Transl Med 10:85
88. Kinno T et al (2014) Clinicopathological features of nonsmall cell lung carcinomas with BRAF mutations. Ann Oncol 25(1):138–142
89. Paik PK et al (2011) Clinical characteristics of patients with lung adenocarcinomas harboring BRAF mutations. J Clin Oncol 29(15):2046–2051
90. Sequist LV et al (2011) Implementing multiplexed genotyping of non-small-cell lung cancers into routine clinical practice. Ann Oncol 22(12):2616–2624
91. Villaruz LC et al (2015) Clinicopathologic features and outcomes of patients with lung adenocarcinomas harboring BRAF mutations in the Lung Cancer Mutation Consortium. Cancer 121(3):448–456
92. Litvak AM et al (2014) Clinical characteristics and course of 63 patients with BRAF mutant lung cancers. J Thorac Oncol 9(11):1669–1674
93. Hyman DM et al (2015) Vemurafenib in multiple nonmelanoma cancers with BRAF V600 mutations. N Engl J Med 373(8):726–736
94. Planchard D et al (2016) Dabrafenib in patients with BRAF(V600E)-positive advanced non-small-cell lung cancer: a single-arm, multicentre, open-label, phase 2 trial. Lancet Oncol 17(5):642–650
95. Planchard D et al (2016) Dabrafenib plus trametinib in patients with previously treated BRAF(V600E)-mutant metastatic non-small cell lung cancer: an open-label, multicentre phase 2 trial. Lancet Oncol 17(7):984–993
96. Planchard D et al (2017) Dabrafenib plus trametinib in patients with previously untreated BRAF(V600E)-mutant metastatic non-small-cell lung cancer: an open-label, phase 2 trial. Lancet Oncol 18(10):1307–1316
97. Giordano S et al (1989) Tyrosine kinase receptor indistinguishable from the c-met protein. Nature 339(6220):155–156
98. Bottaro DP et al (1991) Identification of the hepatocyte growth factor receptor as the c-met proto-oncogene product. Science 251(4995):802–804
99. Naldini L et al (1991) Scatter factor and hepatocyte growth factor are indistinguishable ligands for the MET receptor. EMBO J 10(10):2867–2878
100. Ponzetto C et al (1994) A multifunctional docking site mediates signaling and transformation by the hepatocyte growth factor/scatter factor receptor family. Cell 77(2):261–271

101. Sadiq AA, Salgia R (2013) MET as a possible target for non-small-cell lung cancer. J Clin Oncol 31(8):1089–1096
102. Ma PC et al (2008) Expression and mutational analysis of MET in human solid cancers. Genes Chromosomes Cancer 47(12):1025–1037
103. Sattler M, Salgia R (2016) MET in the driver's seat: exon 14 skipping mutations as actionable targets in lung cancer. J Thorac Oncol 11(9):1381–1383
104. Maulik G et al (2002) Role of the hepatocyte growth factor receptor, c-Met, in oncogenesis and potential for therapeutic inhibition. Cytokine Growth Factor Rev 13(1):41–59
105. Krishnaswamy S et al (2009) Ethnic differences and functional analysis of MET mutations in lung cancer. Clin Cancer Res 15(18):5714–5723
106. Stransky N et al (2014) The landscape of kinase fusions in cancer. Nat Commun 5:4846
107. Watermann I et al (2015) Improved diagnostics targeting c-MET in non-small cell lung cancer: expression, amplification and activation? Diagn Pathol 10:130
108. Salgia R (2017) MET in lung cancer: biomarker selection based on scientific rationale. Mol Cancer Ther 16(4):555–565
109. Cappuzzo F et al (2009) Increased MET gene copy number negatively affects survival of surgically resected non-small-cell lung cancer patients. J Clin Oncol 27(10):1667–1674
110. Raghav K et al (2018) Untying the gordion knot of targeting MET in cancer. Cancer Treat Rev 66:95–103
111. Waqar SN, Morgensztern D, Sehn J (2015) MET mutation associated with responsiveness to crizotinib. J Thorac Oncol 10(5):e29–e31
112. Drilon A et al (2016) Cabozantinib in patients with advanced RET-rearranged non-small-cell lung cancer: an open-label, single-centre, phase 2, single-arm trial. Lancet Oncol 17 (12):1653–1660
113. Spigel DR et al (2017) Results from the phase III randomized trial of onartuzumab plus erlotinib versus erlotinib in previously treated stage IIIB or IV non-small-cell lung cancer: METLung. J Clin Oncol 35(4):412–420
114. Scagliotti G et al (2015) Phase III multinational, randomized, double-blind, placebo-controlled study of tivantinib (ARQ 197) plus erlotinib versus erlotinib alone in previously treated patients with locally advanced or metastatic nonsquamous non-small-cell lung cancer. J Clin Oncol 33(24):2667–2674
115. Bean J et al (2007) MET amplification occurs with or without T790M mutations in EGFR mutant lung tumors with acquired resistance to gefitinib or erlotinib. Proc Natl Acad Sci U S A 104(52):20932–20937
116. Azuma K et al (2016) Phase II study of erlotinib plus tivantinib (ARQ 197) in patients with locally advanced or metastatic EGFR mutation-positive non-small-cell lung cancer just after progression on EGFR-TKI, gefitinib or erlotinib. ESMO Open 1(4):e000063
117. Yoshioka H et al (2015) A randomized, double-blind, placebo-controlled, phase III trial of erlotinib with or without a c-Met inhibitor tivantinib (ARQ 197) in Asian patients with previously treated stage IIIB/IV nonsquamous nonsmall-cell lung cancer harboring wild-type epidermal growth factor receptor (ATTENTION study). Ann Oncol 26(10):2066–2072
118. Zenali M et al (2015) Retrospective review of MET gene mutations. Oncoscience 2(5): 533–541
119. McLornan DP, List A, Mufti GJ (2014) Applying synthetic lethality for the selective targeting of cancer. N Engl J Med 371(18):1725–1735
120. Kyriakopoulos CE et al (2017) A phase I study of tivantinib in combination with temsirolimus in patients with advanced solid tumors. Invest New Drugs 35(3):290–297
121. Preusser M et al (2014) Amplification and overexpression of CMET is a common event in brain metastases of non-small cell lung cancer. Histopathology 65(5):684–692
122. Chi AS et al (2012) Rapid radiographic and clinical improvement after treatment of a MET-amplified recurrent glioblastoma with a mesenchymal-epithelial transition inhibitor. J Clin Oncol 30(3):e30–e33

123. Klempner SJ et al (2017) Intracranial activity of cabozantinib in MET exon 14-positive NSCLC with brain metastases. J Thorac Oncol 12(1):152–156
124. Amatu A, Sartore-Bianchi A, Siena S (2016) NTRK gene fusions as novel targets of cancer therapy across multiple tumour types. ESMO Open 1(2):e000023
125. Broderick JM (2017) Entrectinib granted breakthrough designation by FDA for NTRK + solid tumors. Targeted Oncology News article
126. Hyman DM et al (2017) The efficacy of larotrectinib (LOXO-101), a selective tropomyosin receptor kinase (TRK) inhibitor, in adult and pediatric TRK fusion cancers. J Clin Oncol 35 (18_suppl):LBA2501
127. Bagheri-Yarmand R et al (2015) A novel dual kinase function of the RET proto-oncogene negatively regulates activating transcription factor 4-mediated apoptosis. J Biol Chem 290 (18):11749–11761
128. Cascone T, Subbiah V, Heymach JV (2017) Targeting RET rearrangements in non-small cell lung cancer
129. Amarnath S et al (2011) The PDL1-PD1 axis converts human T H1 cells into regulatory T cells. Sci Transl Med 3(111)
130. Francisco LM et al (2009) PD-L1 regulates the development, maintenance, and function of induced regulatory T cells. J Exp Med 206(13):3015–3029
131. Shin DS, Ribas A (2015) The evolution of checkpoint blockade as a cancer therapy: what's here, what's next? Curr Opin Immunol 33:23–35
132. Kusnierczyk P (2013) Killer cell immunoglobulin-like receptor gene associations with autoimmune and allergic diseases, recurrent spontaneous abortion, and neoplasms. Front Immunol 4:8
133. Brahmer JR et al (2010) Phase I study of single-agent anti-programmed death-1 (MDX-1106) in refractory solid tumors: safety, clinical activity, pharmacodynamics, and immunologic correlates. J Clin Oncol 28(19):3167–3175
134. Borghaei H et al (2015) Nivolumab versus docetaxel in advanced nonsquamous non-small-cell lung cancer. N Engl J Med 373(17):1627–1639
135. Vokes EE et al (2018) Nivolumab versus docetaxel in previously treated advanced non-small-cell lung cancer (CheckMate 017 and CheckMate 057): 3-year update and outcomes in patients with liver metastases. Ann Oncol 29(4):959–965
136. Brahmer J et al (2015) Nivolumab versus docetaxel in advanced squamous-cell non-small-cell lung cancer. N Engl J Med 373(2):123–135
137. Horn L et al (2017) Nivolumab versus docetaxel in previously treated patients with advanced non-small-cell lung cancer: two-year outcomes from two randomized, open-label, phase III trials (CheckMate 017 and CheckMate 057). J Clin Oncol 35(35):3924–3933
138. Carbone DP et al (2017) First-line nivolumab in stage IV or recurrent non-small-cell lung cancer. N Engl J Med 376(25):2415–2426
139. Hellmann MD et al (2018) Nivolumab plus ipilimumab in lung cancer with a high tumor mutational burden. N Engl J Med 378(22):2093–2104
140. Forde PM et al (2018) Neoadjuvant PD-1 blockade in resectable lung cancer. N Engl J Med 378(21):1976–1986
141. Reck M et al (2016) Pembrolizumab versus chemotherapy for PD-L1-positive non-small-cell lung cancer. N Engl J Med 375(19):1823–1833
142. Langer CJ et al (2016) Carboplatin and pemetrexed with or without pembrolizumab for advanced, non-squamous non-small-cell lung cancer: a randomised, phase 2 cohort of the open-label KEYNOTE-021 study. Lancet Oncol 17(11):1497–1508
143. Gandhi L et al (2018) Pembrolizumab plus chemotherapy in metastatic non-small-cell lung cancer. N Engl J Med 378(22):2078–2092
144. Herbst RS et al (2016) Pembrolizumab versus docetaxel for previously treated, PD-L1-positive, advanced non-small-cell lung cancer (KEYNOTE-010): a randomised controlled trial. Lancet 387(10027):1540–1550

145. Rittmeyer A et al (2017) Atezolizumab versus docetaxel in patients with previously treated non-small-cell lung cancer (OAK): a phase 3, open-label, multicentre randomised controlled trial. Lancet 389(10066):255–265
146. Jotte RM et al (2018) IMpower131: primary PFS and safety analysis of a randomized phase III study of atezolizumab + carboplatin + paclitaxel or nab-paclitaxel vs carboplatin + nab-paclitaxel as 1L therapy in advanced squamous NSCLC. J Clin Oncol 36 (18_suppl):LBA9000
147. Socinski MA et al (2018) Atezolizumab for first-line treatment of metastatic nonsquamous NSCLC. N Engl J Med 378(24):2288–2301
148. Antonia SJ et al (2017) Durvalumab after chemoradiotherapy in stage III non-small-cell lung cancer. N Engl J Med 377(20):1919–1929
149. Lynch TJ et al (2012) Ipilimumab in combination with paclitaxel and carboplatin as first-line treatment in stage IIIB/IV non-small-cell lung cancer: results from a randomized, double-blind, multicenter phase II study. J Clin Oncol 30(17):2046–2054
150. Weber JS et al (2017) Safety profile of nivolumab monotherapy: a pooled analysis of patients with advanced melanoma. J Clin Oncol 35(7):785–792
151. Brahmer JR, Lacchetti C, Thompson JA (2018) Management of immune-related adverse events in patients treated with immune checkpoint inhibitor therapy: American society of clinical oncology clinical practice guideline summary. J Oncol Pract 14(4):247–249
152. The Lancet Respiratory Medicine (2018) Lung cancer immunotherapy biomarkers: refine not reject. Lancet Respir Med 6(6):403
153. Liu D, Wang S, Bindeman W (2017) Clinical applications of PD-L1 bioassays for cancer immunotherapy. J Hematol Oncol 10(1):110
154. Stephens P et al (2004) Lung cancer: intragenic ERBB2 kinase mutations in tumours. Nature 431(7008):525
155. Shigematsu H et al (2005) Somatic mutations of the HER2 kinase domain in lung adenocarcinomas. Can Res 65(5):1642–1646
156. Kris M et al (2015) Targeting HER2 aberrations as actionable drivers in lung cancers: phase II trial of the pan-HER tyrosine kinase inhibitor dacomitinib in patients with HER2-mutant or amplified tumors. Ann Oncol 26(7):1421–1427
157. Gandhi L et al (2017) MA04. 02 neratinib ± temsirolimus in HER2-mutant lung cancers: an international, randomized phase II study. J Thorac Oncol 12(1): S358–S359
158. Lai WCV et al (2017) Afatinib in patients with metastatic HER2-mutant lung cancers: an international multicenter study. Am Soc Clin Oncol
159. Li BT et al (2018) Ado-trastuzumab emtansine for patients with HER2-mutant lung cancers: results from a phase II basket trial. J Clin Oncol. https://doi.org/10.1200/JCO.2018.77.9777
160. Blumenschein G Jr et al (2015) A randomized phase II study of the MEK1/MEK2 inhibitor trametinib (GSK1120212) compared with docetaxel in KRAS-mutant advanced non-small-cell lung cancer (NSCLC). Ann Oncol 26(5):894–901
161. Gandara DR et al (2013) Oral MEK1/MEK2 inhibitor trametinib (GSK1120212) in combination with docetaxel in KRAS-mutant and wild-type (WT) advanced non-small cell lung cancer (NSCLC): a phase I/Ib trial. Am Soc Clin Oncol
162. Kelly K et al (2013) Oral MEK1/MEK2 inhibitor trametinib (GSK1120212) in combination with pemetrexed for KRAS-mutant and wild-type (WT) advanced non-small cell lung cancer (NSCLC): a phase I/Ib trial. Am Soc Clin Oncol
163. Jänne PA et al (2013) Selumetinib plus docetaxel for KRAS-mutant advanced non-small-cell lung cancer: a randomised, multicentre, placebo-controlled, phase 2 study. Lancet Oncol 14 (1):38–47
164. Jänne PA et al (2017) Selumetinib plus docetaxel compared with docetaxel alone and progression-free survival in patients with kras-mutant advanced non-small cell lung cancer: the select-1 randomized clinical trial. JAMA 317(18):1844–1853
165. Aviel-Ronen S et al (2006) K-ras mutations in non-small-cell lung carcinoma: a review. Clin Lung Cancer 8(1):30–38

166. Reuter CW, Morgan MA, Bergmann L (2000) Targeting the Ras signaling pathway: a rational, mechanism-based treatment for hematologic malignancies? Blood 96(5):1655–1669
167. Chenard-Poirier M et al (2017) Results from the biomarker-driven basket trial of RO5126766 (CH5127566), a potent RAF/MEK inhibitor, in RAS- or RAF-mutated malignancies including multiple myeloma. Am Soc Clin Oncol
168. Vansteenkiste JF et al (2015) Safety and efficacy of buparlisib (BKM120) in patients with PI3K pathway-activated non-small cell lung cancer: results from the phase II BASALT-1 study. J Thorac Oncol 10(9):1319–1327
169. Soria J-C et al (2015) Phase I dose-escalation study of pilaralisib (SAR245408, XL147), a pan-class I PI3K inhibitor, in combination with erlotinib in patients with solid tumors. Oncologist 20(3):245–246
170. Levy B et al (2014) A randomized, phase 2 trial of docetaxel with or without PX-866, an irreversible oral phosphatidylinositol 3-kinase inhibitor, in patients with relapsed or metastatic non-small-cell lung cancer. J Thorac Oncol 9(7):1031–1035
171. Wade JL et al (2017) A phase II study of GDC-0032 (taselisib) for previously treated PI3K positive patients with stage IV squamous cell lung cancer (SqNSCLC): LUNG-MAP sub-study SWOG S1400B. Am Soc Clin Oncol
172. Soria J-C et al (2017) A phase IB dose-escalation study of the safety and pharmacokinetics of pictilisib in combination with either paclitaxel and carboplatin (with or without bevacizumab) or pemetrexed and cisplatin (with or without bevacizumab) in patients with advanced non-small cell lung cancer. Eur J Cancer 86:186–196
173. Besse B et al (2015) A phase II trial of pictilisib with chemotherapy in first-line non-squamous NSCLC. J Thorac Oncol. Elsevier
174. Thomas JS et al (2018) A first-in-human phase I study of sEphB4-HSA (sEphB4) with expansion in hepatocellular (HCC) and cholangiocarcinoma (CCA). Am Soc Clin Oncol
175. Nogova L et al (2017) Evaluation of BGJ398, a fibroblast growth factor receptor 1-3 kinase inhibitor, in patients with advanced solid tumors harboring genetic alterations in fibroblast growth factor receptors: results of a global phase I, dose-escalation and dose-expansion study. J Clin Oncol 35(2):157–165
176. Tabernero J et al (2015) Phase I dose-escalation study of JNJ-42756493, an oral pan–fibroblast growth factor receptor inhibitor, in patients with advanced solid tumors. J Clin Oncol 33(30):3401–3408
177. Paik PK et al (2014) A phase 1b open-label multicenter study of AZD4547 in patients with advanced squamous cell lung cancers: preliminary antitumor activity and pharmacodynamic data. Am Soc Clin Oncol
178. Smyth EC et al (2015) Phase II multicenter proof of concept study of AZD4547 in FGFR amplified tumours. Am Soc Clin Oncol

Update on Precision Medicine in Breast Cancer

2

Jasgit C. Sachdev, Ana C. Sandoval and Mohammad Jahanzeb

Contents

J. C. Sachdev (✉)
HonorHealth Research Institute, Scottsdale, AZ, USA
e-mail: Jasgit.Sachdev@honorhealth.com

J. C. Sachdev
Translational Genomics Research Institute (TGen), Phoenix, AZ, USA

A. C. Sandoval · M. Jahanzeb
Sylvester Comprehensive Cancer Center, University of Miami, Miami, FL, USA

D. D. Von Hoff and H. Han (eds.), *Precision Medicine in Cancer Therapy*,
Cancer Treatment and Research 178, https://doi.org/10.1007/978-3-030-16391-4_2

2.1 Introduction

Breast cancer is a very heterogeneous disease; it has different molecular subtypes with distinct clinical implications. Inter-tumor heterogeneity refers to molecular differences in the tumors among different patients. Intra-tumor (spatial) heterogeneity refers to the difference within a single tumor mass, and temporal heterogeneity refers to the changes over time during tumor growth and under treatment pressure in an individual patient [1]. The overarching aim of precision medicine is to decipher and target this heterogeneity allowing physicians to tailor effective treatments based on the precise molecular makeup of a tumor.

In 2000, Perou et al. described the four basic molecular subtypes of breast cancer: Luminal A, Luminal B, HER2 enriched, and basal-like (Table 2.1) [2]. There are important biological differences that allowed the clustering of breast cancers into Luminal A or Luminal B subtypes, despite both of them being defined by expression of hormone-regulated pathways. For example, Luminal B cancers are often associated with higher expression of proliferation-related and HER2 signaling pathway genes. The basal-like tumors have higher expression of proliferation-related genes and of keratins commonly found in the basal layer of the epidermis. This classification gave us the first glimpse into the complexity that exists within tumors that share the same anatomic site of origin. This also allowed prognostication of patient outcomes with different subtypes of breast cancer and the evaluation of specific therapeutic vulnerabilities within these molecular subtypes. The development of multigene classifiers like the Oncotype Dx 21-gene recurrence score, the Mammaprint 70-gene signature, and the PAM50-based Prosigna assay has advanced the adjuvant treatment of breast cancer patients by identifying the subset of hormone-receptor-positive breast cancer patients that derive little benefit from adjuvant chemotherapy and can be treated safely with adjuvant endocrine therapy alone.

Since then, the subclassification of breast cancers has continued to evolve through the availability of high-throughput next-generation sequencing platforms and new subgroups have been identified [3]. We have also discovered that tumors can change longitudinally during treatment resulting in treatment failures and requiring different therapeutic approaches. There are ongoing trials looking at molecular mechanisms of resistance at progression and matching therapies to precisely target the aberration at an individual level.

Table 2.1 Major molecular differences in intrinsic subtypes of breast cancer

Intrinsic molecular subtype	Common Mutations (>5% frequency) [79]	IHC approx	Upregulation/amplification/copy number/methylation	Downregulated (decreased expression)	Potential therapeutic agents	Prevalence (%)
Luminal A	PIK3CA 45%, MAP3K1 13%, GATA3 14%, TP53 12%, CDH1 9%, MAP2K4 7%, MLL3 8%, CDH1 9%, RUNX1 5%, NCOR1 5%	ER+, PR+, HER2 −	Luminal expression signature: ESR1, GATA3, FOXA1, XBP1, MYB1 RB1signature: retained RB expression Cyclin D1 amp (29%) CDK4 gain (14%) Mostly Diploid No significant hypermethylation	Proliferation/cell cycle genes (MKI67 and AURKA)	Hormonal blockade CDK4/6 inhibitors PI3K/mTOR inhibitors	64.3
Luminal B	TP53 29%, PIK3CA 29%, MAP3K1 5%, GATA3 15%, MLL3 6%, CDH1 5%	ER+, PR+, HER2 +	High proliferation/cell cycle genes (MKI67 and AURKA) Cyclin-D1 amp (58%) CDK4 gain (25%) Mostly aneuploid Hypermethylated	ER cluster	Hormonal blockade, anti-HER2 CDK4/6 inhibitors PI3K/mTOR inhibitors	
HER2− enriched	TP53 75%, PIK3CA 42%, MLL3 7%, CDH1 5%, AFF2 5%, PTPN22 5%	ER−, PR−, HER2 +	HER2 amplicon Proliferation FGFR4, EGFR Cyclin D1 amp (38%) CDK4 gain (24%) MDM2 gain (30%) Mostly aneuploid	Luminal cluster	Anti-HER2, PI3K/mTOR inhibitors, FGFR inhibitors, CDK4/6 inhibitors	11.2
Basal-like	TP53 84%, PIK3CA 7%, PTEN mut/loss (39%) MLL3 5%,	ER− PR−	Proliferation-related genes (MKI67), basal signature	Luminal-related genes RB signature	Platinums and other	12.3

(continued)

Table 2.1 (continued)

Intrinsic molecular subtype	Common Mutations (>5% frequency) [79]	IHC approx	Upregulation/amplification/copy number/methylation	Downregulated (decreased expression)	Potential therapeutic agents	Prevalence (%)
	RB1 mut/loss (20%), BRCA mut/loss 20%	HER2 –	(keratins 5/6, 17), WNT pathway (CDKN2A) Cycle E1 amp (9%) MYC amp HIF1∞-ARNT pathway Mostly aneuploid Hypomethylated		DNA-damaging drugs DNA damage repair inhibitors: PARP inhibitors ATR inhibitors Angiogenesis inhibitors PI3K/mTOR inhibitors	

Recently, there have been promising advances in the treatment of many solid tumors through harnessing the patient's own immune system to recognize and eliminate established metastatic disease. The immune checkpoint inhibitor pembrolizumab is the first immunotherapy agent approved for tumors that share a common molecular abnormality, i.e., mismatch repair deficiency or microsatellite instability, irrespective of their site of origin. Though only a small proportion of breast cancers fall in this category, it has set a new precedence for drug development and getting effective therapies to patients in an expeditious manner in this era of precision medicine.

Herein, we discuss the current applications of precision medicine in breast cancer and the ongoing research in this field.

2.2 Single-Gene/Pathway Targeting Approaches

It has long been known that greater than two-thirds of all breast cancers express the estrogen receptor (ER). Abrogation of estrogenic stimulation of breast cancers by performing an oophorectomy was the earliest example of precision medicine in the treatment of breast cancer. ER expression in breast cancer is so prevalent that the first approval of tamoxifen, a selective ER modulator (SERM) in advanced breast cancer, was based on responses seen in multiple Phase II trials in unselected patient populations [4, 5]. Subsequently, the benefit of tamoxifen and other SERMs was shown to be restricted to ER- and/or PR-positive (collectively known as hormone-receptor-positive) tumors only, so that histological identification of hormone-receptor expression on breast cancer cells now guides the use of hormone-receptor-targeted therapies (alternatively known as endocrine therapy) both in the advanced and early-stage settings. For the treatment of metastatic hormone-receptor-positive breast cancer, sequential lines of endocrine therapy incorporating tamoxifen, an aromatase inhibitor (AI), and the selective estrogen receptor down-regulator (SERD) fulvestrant are currently recommended as single agents or in combination with other targeted agents such as CDK4/6 inhibitors and mTOR inhibitors, or with each other [6]. In the early-stage setting, the use of tamoxifen for at least 5 years has shown a 39 and 31% reduction in the annual odds of recurrence and death, respectively, for ER-positive tumors [7]. Furthermore, a meta-analysis comparing 5 years of tamoxifen to 5 years of AIs in postmenopausal women with early-stage breast cancer demonstrated that AIs were superior to tamoxifen in terms of 5-year recurrence rate (HR = 0.59) and 10-year breast cancer mortality (HR = 0.66) rate [7].

By the late 1990s, it was shown that a subset of breast cancers ($\sim$15–20%) overexpress the HER2 protein or have additional copies of the HER2 gene (HER2 amplification), an important regulator of cell proliferation. It was shown that targeting HER2 signaling provides an effective way of inhibiting cell proliferation and survival in HER2-positive breast cancer cells. Trastuzumab, an antagonistic HER2 monoclonal antibody, emerged as the pivotal agent to be approved for the treatment of HER2-positive metastatic breast cancer (mBC) based on improved OS when combined with standard chemotherapy versus the same chemotherapy alone [8]. This laid the path to the development of subsequent small molecule inhibitors (lapatinib, neratinib) and monoclonal antibodies (pertuzumab) as well as antibody-drug conjugates (e.g., TDM1-emtansine) targeting the HER2 pathway. Because receptor tyrosine kinases like HER2 exert their action through dimerization, pertuzumab, another monoclonal antibody, was developed to disrupt HER2 dimerization and resultant activation. Baselga et al. reported a Phase III clinical trial (the **CLEOPATRA** trial) that showed that the addition of pertuzumab to trastuzumab + chemotherapy increased OS for HER2+ mBC patients from 12.4 to 18.5 months with no increase in adverse events (Fig. 2.1) [9]. The combination therapy with two HER2 targeting antibodies + chemotherapy was approved for the first-line treatment of HER2-positive mBC later that year. As mentioned above, trastuzumab has also formed the basis for antibody-drug conjugates (ADCs) like trastuzumab–emtansine (T-DM1) that targets the delivery of the bound cytotoxic drug (emtansine) directly to tumor cells with high expression of HER2 (discussed in more detail later in this chapter).

Until the advent of molecular techniques, ER, PR, and HER2 represented the only validated targets in mBC with predictive utility for selecting therapies. It remains perplexing that a large percentage of patients harboring these targets do not respond to corresponding therapies, because few biomarkers exist that clearly

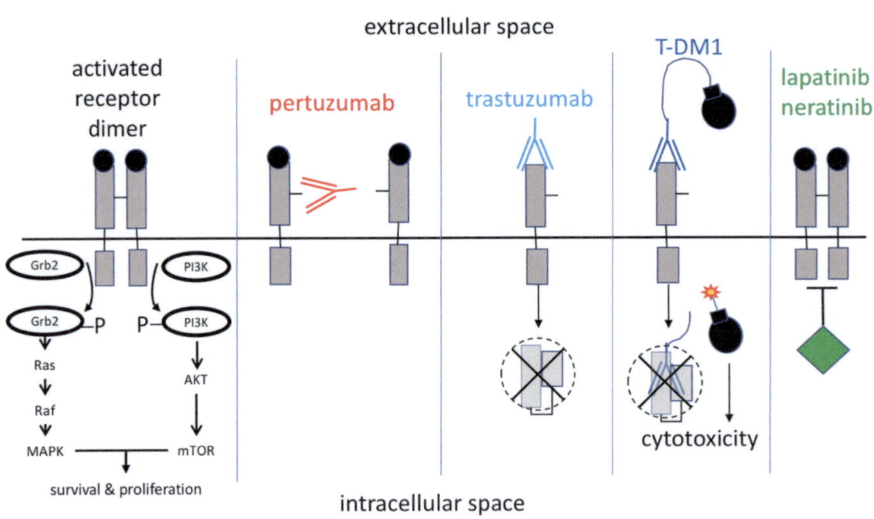

Fig. 2.1 Mechanism of action of HER2 targeted therapies. Increased expression and activation of the tyrosine receptor kinase HER2 leads to increased breast cancer cell proliferation as HER2 dimerizes and phosphorylates its downstream targets. HER2-targeted drugs act by: (1) blocking dimerization (pertuzumab), (2) competitive inhibition and proteolytic degradation (trastuzumab), (3) competitive inihibition and cytotoxicity (T-DM1), or (4) direct inhibition of HER2 kinase activity

differentiate responders from non-responders. Since both de novo (primary) resistance and acquired (secondary) resistance to endocrine and HER2 targeting therapies limit the magnitude and duration of benefit, there is immense interest in identifying biomarkers predictive of efficacy and resistance [10, 11].

Multiple putative mechanisms of resistance have been elucidated, some of which have only been identified through the use of next-generation sequencing technologies. For example, mutations in the gene ESR-1 that encodes the ERα receptor have recently been uncovered as a cause of secondary endocrine resistance. ESR-1 mutations result in the clonal selection of endocrine-resistant cell populations after prior treatment with aromatase inhibitors specifically, but not post-tamoxifen treatment [12, 13]. Tumors harboring ESR1 mutations in patients with prior treatment with non-steroidal AIs respond less well to subsequent single-agent AI like exemestane [14, 15]. However, in combination with other agents like CDK4/6 inhibitors, this resistance seems to be at least partially overcome. Thus, it is likely that other signaling pathways could function in conjunction with ESR1 mutations to confer therapeutic resistance. These often constitute products of compensatory changes that are triggered in other parts of the same or related signaling pathways. These compensatory changes provide an escape mechanism that results in tumor cell resistance to the targeted therapy. Molecular profiling of tumor tissues can potentially reveal such genetic alterations or compensatory transcriptional or proteomic changes that confer resistance to a therapy of interest.

2.3 Overcoming Cross Talk and Resistance Mechanisms

To tackle the problem of therapeutic resistance, dual-target inhibition strategies have been investigated and subsequently successfully applied in the treatment of hormone-receptor and HER2-positive mBC.

The biggest advance in the treatment of hormone-receptor-positive mBC has been the incorporation of CDK4/6 inhibitors in combination with endocrine agents in the first-line treatment and beyond. CDK4 and CDK6 kinases form complexes with D-type cyclins and promote cell proliferation by hyperphosphorylating the retinoblastoma (RB) protein leading to inactivation of cell cycle checkpoint and G1-S cell cycle progression. Alterations in the CDK-RB pathway like loss of function mutations in the RB gene, amplification of CDK encoding genes like CCND1 are implicated in endocrine resistance [16]. CDK4/6 inhibitors block the inactivation of the RB checkpoint and restore cell cycle control in endocrine-resistant cells. Three CDK4/6 inhibitors are currently approved for treatment of hormone-receptor-positive metastatic breast cancer. In the first-line setting, palbociclib, abemaciclib, and ribociclib in combination with an AI improve PFS by approximately 10 months when compared with an AI alone in postmenopausal women with very similar efficacy observed for all three agents across the trials (HR: 0.54–0.58) [17–19]. In the second-line setting, CDK4/6 inhibitors in combination with fulvestrant improve PFS by about 5–7 months in postmenopausal women or premenopausal women who get ovarian suppression [20, 21]. Abemaciclib is the only CDK4/6 inhibitor that is also approved by FDA as a single agent in heavily pretreated postmenopausal women at a higher dose of 200 mg BID instead of 150 mg BID in combination therapy [22]. Results recently reported from randomized trials that involved the three CDK4/6 inhibitors leading to regulatory approval are summarized in Table 2.2.

CDK4/6 inhibitors differ in their toxicity profiles. All of them cause some degree of neutropenia which is manageable with dose and schedule modification and unlike chemotherapy-induced neutropenia which is not amenable to or requisites G-CSF support due to daily administration and a short break. Ribociclib is known to cause elevation of the liver enzymes, and they need to be monitored during treatment. Prolongation of the QT interval, an electrophysiological sign of potential ventricular tachyarrhythmia, was also seen in the MONALEESA-2 trial, and EKG monitoring is recommended during the first 6 weeks of treatment [19]. Abemaciclib is a more potent inhibitor for CDK4 than for CDK6, and due to this selective inhibition, diarrhea is the most common adverse event (13% G3) in addition to lower neutropenia (20–30%) unlike the other CDK4/6 inhibitors (about 60% G3 neutropenia).

With regard to predictive biomarkers for efficacy, the benefit of CDK4/6 inhibitors seems to be similar in all biomarker subgroups evaluated. These include cell cycle markers evaluated for protein expression by IHC in PALOMA-2 (ER, RB, p-16, cyclin-D1) [17] or by mRNA levels in the MONALEESA-2 trial (ESR-1, CDK2, CCNE1, PI3K, MAPK, and cell cycle control genes) [19]. Thus, there is no additional biomarker at this time that would suggest a lack of benefit from these agents added to endocrine therapy. Subgroup analyses from these trials and an FDA analysis by age confirm that all subgroups in pivotal trials benefit from the addition of CDK4/6 inhibitors and it may not be appropriate to deny these agents to seemingly unworthy candidates such as the elderly with bone-only metastases.

Aberrant signaling via the PI3K/Akt/mTOR pathway is a common mechanism by which BC cells attain resistance to endocrine and HER2-targeted therapy [23]. Integrative profiling of tumors from HER2 overexpressing breast cancer patients showed that the presence of PIK3CA-activating mutations and loss of PTEN expression inversely correlated with the probability of response to trastuzumab therapy ($p = 0.093$ and 0.034, respectively) [24]. Conversely, the presence of activating PIK3CA mutations did not attenuate the PFS benefit of T-DM1 in a correlative analysis of the randomized comparison of T-DM1 versus lapatinib plus capecitabine (**EMILIA** trial). Thus, targeting these oncogenic mechanisms of resistance can perhaps provide an opportunity for improving efficacy of trastuzumab and other HER2 inhibitors. These mTOR inhibitors have been explored in combination therapies in mBC to improve response and extend benefit from endocrine and HER2-targeting agents in secondary resistance settings. The **BOLERO-2** Phase III trial evaluated the addition of the mTOR inhibitor everolimus to standard endocrine therapy to overcome resistance in the second line or greater mBC. The addition of everolimus to exemestane more than doubled the PFS time compared to exemestane alone (median PFS: 10.6 months vs. 4.1 months;

Table 2.2 Trials of CDK4/6 and PI3K/mTOR inhibitors in hormone-receptor-positive, HER2-negative mBC

Trial name	Target	Agent	Design	Population	Primary endpoint
BOLERO-2 [25]	mTOR	Exemestane ± **Everolimus**	Phase III Randomized 2:1 Double-blind Placebo-controlled	Second-line Postmenopausal ≤1 prior chemo Any lines of ET *N* = 724	PFS: 6.9 months versus 2.8 months HR: 0.43 95% CI (0.35–0.54)
PALOMA-1/ TRIO-18 [80]	CDK4/6	Letrozole ± **Palbocilcib**	Phase II Randomized 1:1 Open-label Placebo-controlled	First-line Postmenopausal *N* = 165	PFS: 20.2 months versus 10.2 months HR: 0.488 95% CI (0.32–0.75)
PALOMA-2 [17]	CDK4/6	Letrozole ± **Palbocilcib**	Phase III Randomized 2:1 Double-blind Placebo-controlled	First-line Postmenopausal *N* = 666 patients	PFS: 24.8 months versus 14.5 months HR: 0.58 95% CI (0.46–0.72)
PALOMA-3 [20]	CDK4/6	Fulvestrant ± **Palbocilcib**	Phase III Randomized 2:1 Double-blind Placebo-control	Second-line Any menopausal status** ≤1 prior chemo Any lines of ET *N* = 521	PFS: 9.5 months versus 4.6 months HR: 0.46 95% CI (0.36–0.59)
MONARCH-1 [22]	CDK4/6	**Abemaciclib**	Phase II Single-arm Open label	Heavily treated 1 or 2 prior chemo *N* = 132	ORR 19.7% 95% CI (13.3–27.5) PFS: 6 months
MONARCH-2 [21]	CDK4/6	Fulvestrant ± **Abemaciclib**	Phase III Randomized 2:1 Double-blind Placebo-controlled	Second-line Any menopausal status** No prior chemo 1 prior line of ET *N* = 669 patients	PFS: 16.4 months versus 9.3 months HR: 0.55 95% CI (0.45–0.68)
MONARCH-3 [18]	CDK4/6	NSAI ±	Phase III Randomized 2:1	First-line Postmenopausal	PFS: NR versus 14.7 months

(continued)

Table 2.2 (continued)

Trial name	Target	Agent	Design	Population	Primary endpoint
		Abemaciclib	Double-blind Placebo-controlled	$N = 493$	HR: 0.54 95% CI (0.41–0.72)
MONALEESA-2 [19]	CDK4/6	Letrozole ± **Ribociclib**	Phase III Randomized 1:1 Double-blind Placebo-controlled	First-line Postmenopausal $N = 668$	PFS: 25.3 months versus 16.0 months HR: 0.56 95% CI (0.43–0.72)
MONALEESA-7 [81]	CDK4/6	Tamoxifen or NSAI with Goserelin ± **Ribociclib**	Phase III Randomized 1:1 Double-blind Placebo-controlled	First-/Second-line Premenopausal ≤1 prior chemo $N = 672$ patients	PFS: 23.8 months versus 13 months HR: 0.55 95% CI (0.44–0.69)
BELLE-2 [29]	PI3K	Fulvestrant ± **Buparlisib**	Phase III Randomized 1:1 Double-blind Placebo-controlled	Second-line Postmenopausal ≤1 prior chemo $N = 1147$	PFS: 6.9 months versus 5.0 months HR: 0.78 95% CI (0.67–8.89)
BELLE-3 [30]	PI3K	Fulvestrant ± **Buparlisib**	Phase III Randomized 2:1 Double-blind Placebo-controlled	Second line Postmenopausal ≤ 1 ≤1 prior chemo Prior mTOR inhibitor $N = 432$	PFS: 3.9 months versus 1.8 months HR: 0.67 95% CI (0.53–0.84)
SANDPIPER	PI3K	Fulvestrant ± **Taselisib**	Phase III Randomized 2:1 Double-blind Placebo-controlled	Second-line Postmenopausal ≤ 1 ≤1 prior chemo Prior mTOR inhibitor $N = 516$	PFS: 7.4 months versus 5.4 months HR: 0.70 95% CI (0.56–0.89)

NSAI: non-steroidal aromatase inhibitor
ET: endocrine therapy
NR: not reach
**If premenopausal, they required ovarian suppression

HR: 0.36; 95% CI: 0.27–0.47; $p < 0.001$) [25]. The **BOLERO-3** trial also showed a benefit, though more modest, with the addition of everolimus to chemotherapy plus trastuzumab in previously treated trastuzumab-resistant HER2-positive mBC (median PFS: 7.0 months vs. 5.78 months; HR: 0.78; 95% CI: 0·65–0·95; $p = 0.0067$) [26]. In the first-line HER2-positive mBC setting, however (**BOLERO-1** trial), the PFS for the overall population with everolimus added to trastuzumab and weekly paclitaxel was not statistically better than the control arm without everolimus (median PFS: 14.95 months vs. 14.49 months; HR: 0.89; 95% CI: 0.73–1.08; $p = 0.1166$). There was a trend toward greater benefit with everolimus in the HR-negative, HER2-positive population, though not statistically significant (median PFS: 20.27 months vs. 13.08 months; HR = 0.66; 95% CI: 0.48–0.91; *p*: NS) [27].

The different efficacy signals seen in the first line versus later lines of treatment with mTOR inhibition added to anti-HER2 treatments may suggest that the PI3K/mTOR signaling pathway is important in an acquired resistance setting as opposed to primary resistance. In addition, the functional significance of alterations in this pathway may be different in the context of different biology of disease, i.e., hormone-receptor-negative, HER2-positive disease (HER2-enriched subtype) versus hormone-receptor-positive, HER2-positive (Luminal B) disease. A joint biomarker analysis of the BOLERO-1 and 3 trials showed that patients with tumors that had PI3K pathway activation (mutations in pathway genes detected by NGS, or loss of PTEN expression by IHC) derived greater benefit from everolimus than those without these alterations [28]. Neither of these trials was prospectively enriched for these tumors however.

In addition to mTOR inhibitors, a variety of inhibitors of the PIK3CA isoforms (pan-inhibitors or alpha isoform-specific) are also under investigation for the treatment of endocrine-resistant hormone-receptor-positive mBC. Buparlisib (a pan PIK3CA inhibitor) was evaluated in combination with fulvestrant in the **BELLE-2** trial in patients with prior progression on endocrine therapy. Serious adverse events occurred in 23% of patients on buparlisib versus 16% in the placebo group [29]. The combination was marginally better than single-agent fulvestrant (median PFS: 6.9 months vs. 5.0 months; HR: 0.78; $p < 0.001$) but at the cost of increased toxicity [Grade 3/4 toxicities (buparlisib vs. placebo): hyperglycemia (15% vs. <1%), increased liver enzymes (18% vs. none), and rash (8% vs. none)], dampening the enthusiasm for clinical use.

Patients who initially respond to mTOR inhibitors also develop resistance, likely through compensatory phosphorylation of AKT that occurs through a feedback loop which can be abrogated by PI3K inhibitors. The **BELLE-3** trial evaluated the efficacy of fulvestrant + the PI3K inhibitor buparlisib in advanced or metastatic ER + BC patients previously treated with or currently progressing on mTOR inhibitors. Despite showing modest benefit in the overall population with regard to prolonged PFS (3.9 months vs. 1.8 months; HR: 0.67; 95% CI: 0.53–0.84) in the combination arm, the trial was discontinued due to increased number of adverse events with the combination including serious adverse events and deaths [30]. In both BELLE-2 and BELLE-3 trials, patients identified to have a PIK3CA mutation either in archival tumor tissue or by circulating tumor DNA (ctDNA) showed a more meaningful difference in PFS with the combination compared to those who were PIK3CA wild type. The HR for PFS for the combination arm versus single-agent fulvestrant in the BELLE-2 trial was 0.56 ($p < 0.001$) for ctDNA PIK3CA mutation positive and 1.05 ($p = 0.642$) for the PIK3CA wild subgroup. Similarly, the HR for the combination was more favorable in the BELLE-3 trial for the PIK3CA mutation-positive subset. These data, though exploratory, do suggest that perhaps a real-time biomarker-based selection strategy with ctDNA could result in a better risk–benefit ratio for these agents allowing them to be integrated into the treatment of a subset of PIK3CA-mutant hormone-receptor-positive breast cancers.

The Phase III **SandPiper** trial was recently reported evaluating a combination of fulvestrant with or without the beta-sparing PI3K inhibitor taselisib in post-menopausal women with hormone-receptor-positive mBC who had progressed on an aromatase inhibitor and no more than 1 prior line of chemotherapy [31]. The trial enrolled two cohorts, one with PIK3CA mutation-positive tumors (archival tissue for central testing) and another without. Both cohorts were separately randomized 2:1 to taselisib or placebo in combination with fulvestrant. The primary endpoint of investigator-assessed PFS in the ITT population (PIK3CA-mutant group) was met with median PFS of 7.4 months versus 5.4 months in the taselisib versus placebo groups, respectively (HR: 0.70; 95% CI: 0.56–0.89; $p = 0.0037$). There was no clear benefit in the PIK3CA wild-type group (HR: 0.69; 95% CI: 0.44–1.08). Though this trial met its primary endpoint in a biologically defined group, there were toxicity concerns as with other PI3K inhibitors which will be a barrier to rapid adoption of this class of drugs in the clinic. Nevertheless, this trial does support in principle that a biomarker-enrichment strategy for enrollment is feasible and can be further improved upon perhaps both by better technology like ctDNA for capturing in real time the tumors that continue to be addicted to an oncogenic driver (overcoming clonal heterogeneity between primary and recurrent tumors) and drugs with a more favorable therapeutic index.

These data also provide evidence that due to the dynamic and heterogeneous nature of cancer cell genomes, transcriptomes, and proteomes, a single snapshot of the histology or multi-omic profile of a tumor is not indicative of the tumor over time and may miss populations that may emerge as a result of treatment pressure from a given targeted therapy. Isolation and interrogation of these treatment-emergent-mutant subpopulations via improved technology platforms can provide a therapeutic opportunity for application of precision medicine in the treatment of mBC.

The circulating tumor DNA (ctDNA) analysis is one such platform by which the mutational status of tumors can be tracked longitudinally for a patient in both primary and metastatic setting and is increasingly incorporated for correlative analyses as highlighted above. Chandarlapaty et al. profiled ctDNA from participants in the BOLERO-2 trial for two specific mutations in the ESR1 gene [13]. They found that 21.1 and 13.3% of patients screened positive for the ESR1 mutations D538G and Y537S, respectively. Both mutations correlated with more aggressive cancer phenotypes and poor outcomes. Wild-type and D538G ESR1 patients appeared to respond to everolimus, but no clear benefit was observed for Y537S patients.

2.4 Precision Medicine Applications of Multi-omic Profiling

The advent and availability of DNA sequencing, mRNA micro-arrays, NGS, and an array of proteomics assays have allowed profiling of large numbers of tumors based on mutational profiles and aberrant gene and protein expression. Profiling can be performed by genomic sequencing, transcriptomic profiling, or via combinatorial multi-omic platforms. Genomic profiling is primarily performed on tumor cells to uncover somatic mutations (single-nucleotide variants, indels), copy-number changes, or oncogenic fusions. Transcriptomic and proteomic profiling including phospho-protein profiling, on the other hand, provide information on the pathway activation status, providing another avenue for targeted therapies. A large amount of transcriptome data generated by large-scale research efforts has allowed for non-biased segregation of breast cancers into molecular subtypes that appear to loosely but not directly mirror histological characterization [2]. The subtypes that have emerged appear to provide some opportunities for precision medicine and targeted therapies (Table 2.1).

Further analysis of large populations of breast cancer tissues revealed additional complexity and molecular subgroups. For instance, a meta-analysis of data obtained by the METABRIC (Molecular Taxonomy of Breast Cancer International Consortium) revealed 10 different molecularly defined subgroups that correlated with different prognoses [3]. These studies highlight the great potential but also the tremendous complexity for precision medicine including difficulties in the accumulation of sufficient patient numbers to test select treatments in a specific subgroup.

While whole-genome sequencing is an excellent tool for discovery research that aims to find novel tumor-associated genes that identify a specific subgroup or offer new drug targets for precision medicine, it remains expensive and time-consuming for widespread clinical application outside of clinical trials. Because most actionable mutations can be determined from a smaller-scale sampling of the tumor, a number of commercially developed assays sequence a smaller number of the most relevant genomic alterations for diagnostic purposes. The oncogenic mutations for breast cancer can be divided into recurrent mutations (1–10% frequency) in 10–20 relevant genes and rare mutations (0–1% frequency in ≥ 100 genes) underscoring the difficulty in developing targeted therapies for such a molecularly heterogeneous disease.

By its definition, precision medicine aims to precisely match each individual's unique genomic alterations to an effective therapy. Novel precision medicine trial designs such as basket and umbrella trials can help address some of the inherent difficulties in accruing sufficiently large numbers within any molecular subgroup to evaluate a matched therapy of choice. Basket trial designs are agnostic to site of origin of the tumor and seek to cluster and treat tumors with a therapy that targets a common biologic variable such as an activating oncogenic mutation, copy-number variation or fusion. Basket trials can be designed for one therapeutic agent of choice or can test multiple simultaneous targets and therapies. The NCI-MATCH and ASCO-sponsored TAPUR trials (Molecular Analysis for Therapy Choice) are examples of basket trials. The MATCH trial is designed to screen 6000 patients to identify unique targets of interest in individual patients and assign patients, irrespective of histology, to a pre-selected therapeutic against that target. In this large-scale effort, patients' tumors are biopsied and profiled by a standardized panel including NGS, IHC, and other methods. Patients appropriate for a specific arm are identified by standardized informatics tools generated by the NCI Center for Biomedical Informatics and Information Technology (CBIIT). Treatment is initiated with the targeted therapy specified for the patient's arm. Once disease progresses after treatment the tumor is again biopsied for profiling. If another actionable mutation is detected, another iteration of treatment is initiated, this time with the new targeted therapy [32]. As many as 40 different therapeutic agents/arms with 35 patients each are being evaluated simultaneously in this trial. Promising results of this approach have been presented for a few of the arms, like the efficacy of the immune checkpoint inhibitor nivolumab in microsatellite instability high (MSI high) non-colorectal tumors, while pembrolizumab is already approved for this indication [33]. In contrast, umbrella trial designs aim to dive deeply into a single tumor type or histologic organ of origin and segregate tumors based on inter-tumor heterogeneity. By doing this, treatment is individualized for tumors based on their unique molecular thumbprint so that individual patients with breast cancer, for example, can expect to receive different treatments despite a common histology. Such a design leads to the possibility of adaptive trials, which allow for changes in randomization ratios and rearrangement of treatment arms based on data obtained in the initial phases of the trial. A few of these umbrella designs have been conducted and reported by different groups that included variable numbers of patients with metastatic breast cancer (Table 2.3) that demonstrate that this approach is feasible.

The largest effort of its kind in breast cancer is in the neoadjuvant setting, whereby the **I-SPY2** trial is a platform for testing up to five novel agents in parallel in combination with standard chemotherapy for locally advanced breast cancers that are all molecularly typed upon study entry. The trial has an adaptive randomization design, whereby agents can be quickly evaluated for efficacy with a short-term endpoint of pathologic complete remission (pCR) utilizing pretest predictors of efficacy. An agent that crosses this predetermined threshold of efficacy can then "graduate on" with a high probability of success in a given molecular subtype in a future randomized study. One of the most recent agents to graduate this initial test of feasibility is pembrolizumab in the triple-negative breast cancer (TNBC) subset. A large randomized neoadjuvant/adjuvant trial of pembrolizumab in TNBC is now underway (**KEYNOTE-522**).

Table 2.3 Reported multi-omic profiling trials with breast cancer cohorts

Trial (or location)	Disease	Technology	*N* screened	Matched therapy	Outcome
SAFIR01 [82]	Metastatic breast cancer	CGH/Sanger	423	55 (13%)	30% OR and/or SD > 4 months
MOSCATO 01 [83]	Metastatic solid tumors	CGH/NGS	843	199 (23%)	11% OR, longer PFS in 33% versus previous
MOSCATO 02 (NCT01566019)	Metastatic solid tumors	CGH/NGS	1050 (estimated)	TBA	PFS
MDACC [84]	Metastatic breast and crc	Panel of 11, 46, or 50 gene hotspots (MS or NGS)	2000	11% of genomically matched trials, 15% on other trials	Not reported
Princess Margaret [85]	Metastatic breast cancer with good performance status	Panel of 48 genes	440 genotyped	15% matched 9% non-matched	Time on treatment 3.6 versus 3.8 months RR = 16% versus 10%
T-Gen [86]	Refractory metastatic cancer	IHC, FISH, micorarray	86	66 (76%)	27% PFS ratio* $\geq$ 1.3
SHIVA [87]	Refractory metastatic cancer	NGS	741	195 (26%)	Targeted therapy did not improve PFS (2.3 months vs. 2 months)
Sideout 1 [88]	Refractory metastatic breast cancer	Multi-omic molecular profiling	28	25 (89%)	Met objective 44% had GMI** $\geq$ 1.3

*PFS ratio: PFS on molecular profiling-based therapy/PFS on most recent therapy
** GMI: same definition as the PFS ratio

The molecular profiling utilized in various studies ranges from immunohistochemistry to high-throughput multigene sequencing. Regardless of the platform utilized or cancer type investigated, there are some common limitations that emerge from the results of these trials as discussed above. The first and perhaps most important one is that less than 1 in 5 patients whose tumors are profiled are actually matched to a therapeutic agent despite a quarter to one-third of them having an identifiable genomic alteration. Roughly half of that number (approximately 10%) of patients is able to be treated with a targeted drug currently on the market or on a clinical trial seeking a particular genomic alteration. Factors influencing this low "match" rate include lack of specific drugs to target the alteration, barriers to clinical trial eligibility, payers who are often unwilling to pay for off-label uses of expensive cancers therapies, etc. Well-designed trials with strong academic/pharmaceutical partnerships are necessary to overcome some of these barriers. An example of a "just-in-time" approach to improve access to clinical trial agents for patients across different clinical settings is illustrated by the Signature trial. Patients are enrolled at any research-experienced site based only on the presence of an actionable mutation, and the protocol is activated at that site once a suitable patient is pre-screened as potentially eligible to receive the trial treatment, with a central IRB and a non-negotiable contract resulting in a 15 d timeline.

Big data initiatives like CancerLinq (https://cancerlinq.org) and TAPUR (Targeted Agent and Profiling Utilization Registry) are additional approaches to collect and analyze real-world data in the practice settings that can expand the reach of precision medicine for patients with tumor types and genetic changes that would not otherwise be feasible to be tested in a clinical trial design.

With these large-scale molecular profiling efforts, tumor heterogeneity, both inter-tumor and intra-tumor, has emerged as another cause for lack of matched therapies or only modest benefit from a given matched therapy for the entire treatment group at an individual trial level. Furthermore, clonal evolution and change of putative drivers between the primary and metastatic sites of disease can lead to lack of response or emergence of treatment resistance. Besides the exceptional responders (defined by the NCI as patients who have a unique response to treatments that are not effective for most other patients) for the 10–25% of overall patients who are initially shown to have a response to personally matched therapies, emergence of resistance in the short term remains a formidable challenge.

A recent meta-analysis of reported Phase II clinical trials across multiple tumor types (570 studies; 32,149 patients), however, did show that a personalized therapy approach compared with a non-personalized approach demonstrated an overall higher response rate (31% vs. 10.5%, $p < 0.001$), prolonged median progression-free survival (5.9 months vs. 2.7 months, $p < 0.001$), and prolonged overall survival (13.7 months vs. 8.9 months, $p < 0.001$). Further inspection of the data revealed that personalized therapy arms based on genomic markers outperformed those based on protein biomarkers [34].

2.5 Targeting DNA Repair Deficiencies in Breast Cancer

The promise of precision medicine lies in the rapid translation of scientific discoveries into better treatment options for patients and tailoring therapy to those most likely to benefit from them. In breast cancer, this promise has been realized for patients with germline mutations in the BRCA1/2 genes (hereditary breast cancer) with the recent approval of the PARP inhibitor olaparib for the treatment of mBC in these patients. Olaparib and two other PARP inhibitors (rucaparib and niraparib) are also approved for the treatment of recurrent ovarian cancer in patients with BRCA mutations. The biological basis of this investigation and the trials leading to the approvals are briefly discussed in this section.

2.5.1 PARP Inhibitors

Like all dividing cells, cancer cells experience numerous "nicks" or single-strand breaks in the course of DNA replication. PARP (Poly(ADP-ribose) polymerase) 1 and 2 are zinc finger-binding proteins that are activated in response to DNA damage and bind and repair single-strand breaks through the base excision repair program. If left unrepaired, these single-strand breaks become double-strand breaks and threaten to induce apoptosis. PARP-inhibiting drugs make cancer cells, particularly breast cancer cells with defects in the double-strand break repair protein BRCA, more susceptible to the cytotoxic effects of DNA-damaging drugs or radiation (Fig. 2.2).

There are two major forms of DNA damage: single-strand breaks (SSBs) and double-strand breaks (DSBs). For the SSBs, the major forms of DNA repair are mismatch repair, nucleotide excision repair, base excision repair, and translesional

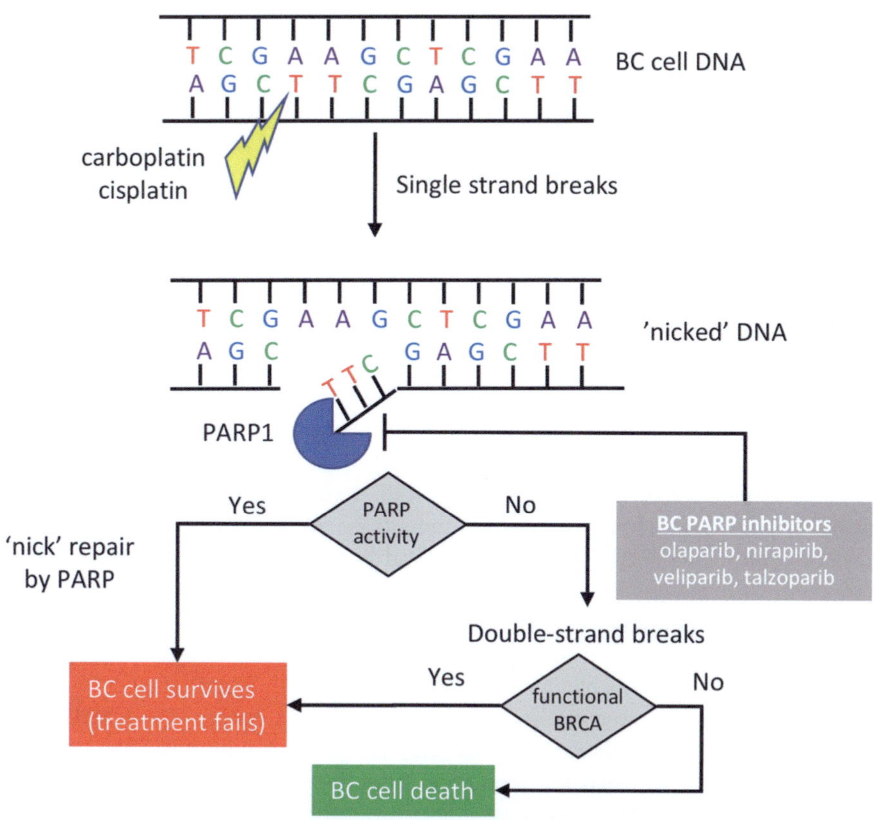

Fig. 2.2 Platinum agents act by introducing single-strand breaks into the DNA. PARP enzymes repair breaks that may accumulate. In the absence of BRCA double-strand break repair. PARP inhibitors can lead to cancer cell death

synthesis. For the DSBs, the two major forms of repair are nonhomologous end-joining repair and homologous recombination repair [35].

BRCA1 and BRCA2 are tumor suppressor genes that are involved in homologous recombination repair. Germline mutations in these genes lead to an increased risk of breast cancer. Poly(ADP-ribose) polymerases (PARPs) are nuclear enzymes that are involved in DNA repair, specifically base excision repair. When there is damage to the DNA causing a SSB, the PARP enzyme is activated and repairs the site of the SSB. In the presence of a PARP inhibitor, this repair mechanism is jeopardized. This leads to an increased amount of SSB and stalling of the replication fork leading to DSB. If the cell also has a homologous recombination defect like BRCA-mutant cancers do, the DSBs will accumulate and lead to cell death. This is the concept of synthetic lethality [36]. This susceptibility to DNA-damaging agents has led to clinical trials to explore PARP inhibitors in patients with BRCA mutations.

Olaparib

Olaparib is a PARP inhibitor that is approved for the treatment of ovarian and breast cancer with germline mutations in the BRCA gene. The **Olympiad** trial was the registration Phase III trial that leads to its recent approval for the treatment of mBC in patients with BRCA mutations. This was a randomized trial for patients with mBC and germline BRCA mutations who had received less than two previous chemotherapy regimens for their metastatic disease. A total of 302 patients were randomized (2:1) to either monotherapy with olaparib at a dose of 300 mg twice a day or standard therapy with single-agent chemotherapy of physician's choice. The primary endpoint was PFS. About a quarter of the patients in both arms had received prior platinum therapy. The median PFS was 7 months for olaparib and 4.2 months for standard therapy (HR: 0.58; 95% CI: 0.43–0.80; $p < 0.001$). The benefit of olaparib was noted across all subgroups including BRCA1 and BRCA2 mutation, hormone-receptor status, or prior platinum exposure. There was no difference in overall survival, but it is to too early to assess. The response rate was more than double in the olaparib arm compared to the chemotherapy arm (60% vs. 29%). The side-effect profile and the overall toxicity rate favored the olaparib group. There was more nausea, anemia, and fatigue in the olaparib group, but lower rates of neutropenia and overall grade $\geq$ 3 adverse events (AEs) [37]. This trial is noteworthy for having led to the approval of the first oral targeted therapy for a subset of TNBC patients, i.e., those with BRCA mutations.

Talazoparib

Talazoparib is a dual-mechanism PARP inhibitor and PARP trapper that also reported positive data recently in the treatment of breast cancer. The **EMBRACA** trial is a Phase III trial that randomized (2:1) 431 patients with mBC and germline BRCA mutations who had received $\leq$ 3 prior lines of chemotherapy to either talazoparib (1 mg daily) or standard single-agent chemotherapy. The median PFS favored the talazoparib group (8.6 months vs. 5.6 months) with a HR of 0.54 (95% CI: 0.41–0.71; $p < 0.0001$). Response rates were nearly double of the chemotherapy group as well. Interestingly, a subset analysis showed that patients with central

Table 2.4 Select Phase II/III trials of PARP inhibitors in breast cancer

NCT	Phase	Design	Patient population
NCT01905592	III	Physician choice versus niraparib (BRAVO)	BRCA mutation, HER2−
NCT02163694	III	Carboplatin/Paclitaxel ± veliparib (BROCADE-3)	BRCA mutation, HER2−
NCT02595905	II	Cisplatin ± veliparib (SWOG 1416)	Triple-negative breast cancer and/or BRCA-mutated
NCT02032823	III	Adjuvant: olympia: olaparib versus placebo for 12 months	BRCA-mutated Post-adjuvant: high-risk Post-neoadjuvant: with residual disease

nervous metastasis had a more profound benefit (HR: 0.32; 95% CI: 0.15–0.88), but this finding is considered exploratory and needs further investigation. Compared to the control arm, anemia, requiring transfusion support, was more prominent with talazoparib, but the rate of neutropenia and grade 3 neutropenia was lower. Global QOL scores were significantly better in patients randomized to talazoparib compared to chemotherapy [38]. An NDA for talazoparib for the treatment of BRCA mutation-positive mBC has been submitted. Other PARP inhibitors like veliparib are also being evaluated in this setting. A few of the noteworthy Phase II and III ongoing trials are listed in Table 2.4.

2.5.2 Targeting BRCA-like Tumors

Besides breast cancers with germline BRCA mutations, other breast cancers have been noted to have BRCA-like functional abnormalities. This can be due to somatic BRCA mutations, BRCA gene promoter methylation or mutations in other genes that are important in the homologous recombination pathway. BRCAness is a term used to describe tumors that behave similar to BRCA-mutated tumors, such that they have high responses to platinum and other DNA-damaging drugs like topoisomerase inhibitors and/or have a specific gene expression profile [15, 39]. Patients with homologous recombination deficiency (HRD) theoretically have good response to platinum agents in particular [40]. A HRD score has been put forth that involves measuring loss of heterozygosity, large-scale state transitions, and telomeric allelic imbalance in several genes involved in the homologous recombination pathway. New therapeutic options targeting the vulnerability of the tumors with ineffective DSB repair are under evaluation with many ongoing studies including a broad set of tumors defined by their “BRCAness”.

The HRD score has been evaluated retrospectively in triple-negative breast cancer patients as a predictive marker for response to DNA-damaging drugs like platinum chemotherapy. Nearly half of TNBC tumors can have the "BRCAness" genotype. The **TNT** trial is a Phase III trial that randomized 376 patients with locally advanced or metastatic triple-negative breast cancer to either six cycles of docetaxel or six cycles of carboplatin. There was no difference in progression-free survival between treatment arms except for patients with BRCA 1 or BRCA 2 mutations where carboplatin was superior to docetaxel. The authors also studied other biomarkers of platinum sensitivity including BRCA1 promoter methylation, and high HRD score, none of which were shown to be predictive of response to carboplatin. In fact, patients without germline BRCA1/2 mutations faired better with docetaxel compared to carboplatin [41]. This result contrasts the findings of Telli et al. that showed that a high HRD predicts response to platinum drugs in the neoadjuvant setting [40]. Though these data are intriguing, HRD score requires further validation as a precision medicine tool before it can be routinely employed in clinical practice.

2.6 Precision in Chemotherapy Delivery: Antibody-Drug Conjugates (ADCs)

ADCs are an excellent tool for precision medicine. Taking advantage of known cell surface proteins overexpressed in a particular cancer of interest, ADCs consist of a monoclonal antibody (Mab) directed against that antigen, a linker region, and the payload, typically a cytotoxic drug (Fig. 2.3). After binding to the cell surface antigen, the ADC is endocytosed. At that time, some linkers are cleaved due to the intracellular conditions of the cell of interest, typically the tumor cell, and the active

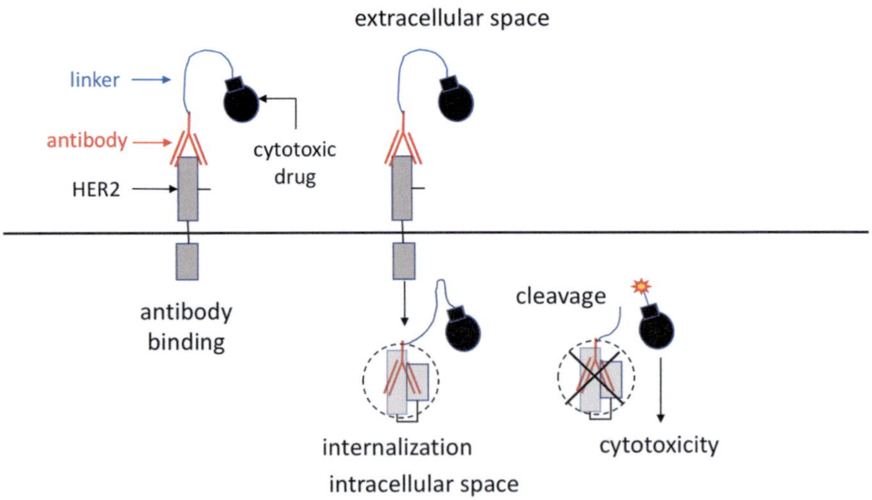

Fig. 2.3 Mechanism of action of ADCs (example T-DM1). (1) Targeting antibody binds cell surface target (HER2). (2) Complex is internalized. (3) Linker is cleaved, releasing payload to exert anti-tumor effect

drug is released others such as T-DM1 employ a non-cleavable linker region and are only released after the Mab is degraded in the lysosome. ADCs allow a large dose of cytotoxic drug to be delivered specifically to the tumor cell, increasing tumor cell death and reducing the negative effects on other cells caused by systemic administration (though some nonspecific uptake in other tissues can be seen). It should be noted that, while the original cell surface antigen selected for targeting should be enriched on the target cell, the antibody chosen to bind it need not have clinical efficacy on its own.

The earliest ADCs developed for breast cancer focused on HER2+ tumors, using the well-established HER2+ antagonistic antibody trastuzumab. In 2014, trastuzumab–emtansine (abbreviated T-DM1) became the first FDA-approved ADC for the treatment of metastatic HER2+ breast cancer; the ADC consists of trastuzumab conjugated to emtansine, an anti-microtubule drug too toxic for any systemic administration. Encouragingly, adverse events to T-DM1 (primarily thrombocytopenia and mild hepatotoxicity) were better tolerated than control treatment. The Phase III EMILIA trial showed that T-DM1 increased PFS in previously treated metastatic HER2 + breast cancer by 50% (median PFS: 9.6 months vs. 6.4 months; HR = 0.65; 95% CI: 0.55–0.77; $p < 0.001$) over the standard control treatment arm (capecitabine + lapatinib) [42] and led to FDA approval. In the first-line metastatic setting, however, the Phase III **MARIANNE** trial did not demonstrate superiority of T-DM1 alone or T-DM1 plus pertuzumab over standard trastuzumab plus taxane, though the safety profile was more favorable with T-DM1 and the PFS in both T-DM1 arms was non-inferior to the control arm. Thus, T-DM1 could be a reasonable alternative first-line regimen in select patients with HER2-positive mBC [43].

Since that time trials have been conducted for a number of other ADCs in breast cancer, including a number that target TNBC (Table 2.5). Some, such as sacituzumab govitecan and glembatumumab vedotin, have entered late phase clinical trials. In a Phase III trial (NCT01631552) of heavily treated metastatic TNBC (mTNBC) patients, an objective response rate of 34% was seen [44]. This drug is now being evaluated in the Phase III **ASCENT** trial in which patients with mTNBC with ≥ 2 lines of treatment will be randomized 2:1 to sacituzumab govitecan or chemotherapy of physicians' choice. (NCT02574455). Glembatumumab vedotin was evaluated in the randomized Phase II **METRIC** trial in GPNMB-expressing TNBC patients with capecitabine as the control arm. This trial unfortunately did not meet its primary endpoint of PFS or ORR compared to capecitabine, and further development has been halted by the manufacturer.

Additional HER2-targeted ADCs seek to deliver either a different, more effective payload including DNA-damaging agents; others have modified targeting strategies including a separate epitope on HER2; and some seek to improve both aspects for improved therapeutic efficacy [45]. DS-8201 {trastuzumab-deruxtecan (a topoisomerase-1 inhibitor)} and SYD985 {trastuzumab-duocarmycin (an alkylating agent)} are novel HER2-binding ADCs that have completed Phase 1 testing and demonstrated encouraging activity in HER2-pretreated and HER2 low mBC.

Table 2.5 Antibody-drug conjugates in development for breast cancer

Name [45]	Ab target	Cytotoxic agent (active payload)	Indication	Phase (clinicaltrials.gov ID)
T-DM1	HER2	Maytansinoid	HER2+ metastatic	Approved
MEDI-4276	HER2	Tubulysin	HER2+ advanced	Phase 1/2: (NCT02576548)
XMT-1522	HER2	Auristatin	HER2+	Phase 1 (NCT02952729)
ARX788	HER2	Auristatin	Solid tumors with HER2 expression	Phase 1 (NCT03255070)
DS-8201a	HER2	Exatecan	HER2+ unresectable/metastatic	Phase 2 (NCT03248492)
SYD985	HER2	Duocarmycin	HER2+ mBC	Phase 3 (NCT03262935)
ADCT-502	HER2	PBD dimer	HER2+	Phase 1 (NCT03125200)
Sacituzumab govitecan IMMU-132	TROP2	Irontecan	TNBC	Phase 3 (NCT02574455)
Glembatumumab vedotin	GPNMB	Auristatin	TNBC	Phase 2—completed (NCT01156753)
SAR566658 anti-CA6-DM4	Tumor-associated sialoglycotope CA6	Maytansinoid	CA6+ TNBC	Phase 2 (NCT02984683)
SGN-LIV1A	LIV1 SLC39A6	Auristatin	LIV-1 expressing	Phase 1 (NCT01969643)
PF-06647020	PTK7	Auristatin	PTK7+ TNBC	Phase 1 in combination w/gedatolisib (NCT03243331)
SAR428926	LAMP-1	Maytansinoid	HER2−	Phase 1 (NCT02575781)
PCA062	P-Cadherin/cadherin3	Maytansinoid	pCAD+ TNBC	Phase 1 (NCT02375958)

2.7 Tumor Micro-Environment Targeting Approaches: Harnessing the Immune System

That the immune responses of the host to cancer cells can augment the anticancer effect of cancer therapeutics has been known in HER2-positive breast cancer since the development of trastuzumab that employs ADCC (antibody-dependent cellular cytotoxicity) as one of its mechanism of action. In recent years, novel immunotherapeutic agents called immune checkpoint inhibitors have been developed and been very successful in the treatment of solid tumors like melanoma, RCC, and NSCLC. Herein, we will discuss the emerging data and ongoing evaluation of checkpoint inhibitors in breast cancer (see Fig. 2.4).

2.7.1 Immune Checkpoint Inhibitors

2.7.1.1 PDL-1/PD-1 Inhibitors

The programmed death ligand 1 (PDL-1) and its corresponding receptor on T cells (PD-1) allow tumors to escape immune surveillance. By inhibiting this checkpoint pathway, T-cell-mediated immunity is enhanced [46]. Checkpoint inhibitors have made tremendous strides in the treatment of metastatic melanoma, NSCLC, bladder cancer, RCC and MSI high tumors. Several of these are also being investigated as single agents or on various combinations for the treatment of breast cancer.

Pembrolizumab

Pembrolizumab is a humanized antibody that inhibits PD-1 and has some early data of activity in breast cancer:

Keynote-012: This was a multicenter phase 1b study of single-agent pembrolizumab in patients with advanced TNBC, head and neck cancer, urothelial cancer, and gastric cancer. Patients had to have PD-L1 expression (expression in stroma or $\geq 1\%$ tumor cell expression by immunohistochemistry). Thirty-two patients with TNBC were enrolled. The dose was 10 mg/kg of pembrolizumab administered intravenously every 2 weeks. Patients received a median of 5 doses (range 1–36 doses). The reported response rate was 18.5%. The toxicity profile was similar to that observed with pembrolizumab in other tumors. The authors concluded that pembrolizumab had an acceptable safety profile and clinical activity in patients with TNBC warranting additional investigation [47].

Keynote-086: This is a multicohort single-arm Phase II study of pembrolizumab monotherapy in mTNBC. Part one: Cohort A included patients with at least one systemic treatment for mBC. PD-L1 expression was not required; Cohort B included patients with no prior systemic therapy for mBC and with positive PD-L1 expression (tumor PDL-1 combined positive score [CPS] $\geq$ 1). Part two was an expansion of cohort A with the exception that enrolled patients had to have strong

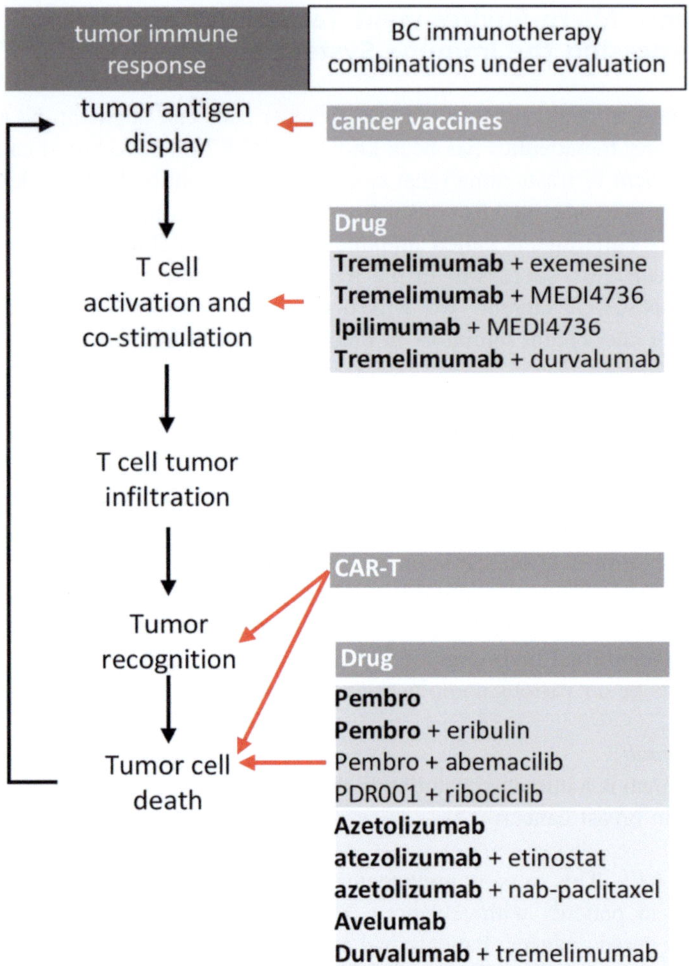

Fig. 2.4 List of the major steps of the tumor immune response and the immunotherapy treatments (and treatment combinations) that act on each step

PD-L1 expression. Pembrolizumab was given at a dose of 200 mg IV every 3 weeks for up to 24 months. Results of cohorts A and B were presented in 2017:

Cohort A: A total of 170 patients were enrolled. Sixty percent of the screened PD-L1 patients had PD-L1-positive tumors. The overall response rate was 5% regardless of PD-L1 expression. The median duration of response was 6.3 months. Sixty-three percent of the responders had long responses with no progression at data cutoff. The safety profile was manageable [48].

Cohort B: A higher response rate was seen in patients with untreated mTNBC in cohort B. Of the 128 patients that had tumor PDL-1 $\geq$ 1, 84 patients met eligibility criteria and were enrolled. The overall response rate was 23% (3 CRs and 16 PRs;

95% CI: 15–33). The median duration of response was 8.4 months with several durable responses, and a 6-month PFS and OS of 26 and 83%, respectively [49].

Keynote-028: This is a multicohort, Phase Ib study that evaluates the efficacy and safety of pembrolizumab in patients with advanced biomarker-positive tumors of different histologies (CPS $\geq$ 1). The cohort of estrogen receptor-positive, HER2-negative breast cancer included 261 patients who were screened for PDL-1 expression. The results from 25 patients who were PDL-1 positive and met all eligibility criteria to be finally enrolled in this cohort were recently published [50]. This was a very heavily treated group with a median of nine prior lines of therapy. The ORR was 12% (three patients had a partial response) with a clinical benefit rate of 20%. As in other trials, the patients who responded had a durable response with a median duration of response of 12 months.

Pembrolizumab/Eribulin

Enhance1/Keynote-150. A Phase Ib/II trial that enrolled patients with TNBC who had been previously treated with two or less lines of chemotherapy established the recommended Phase II dose as 1.4 mg/m^2 of eribulin on days 1, 8 plus 200 mg of pembrolizumab on Day 1 of a 21 d cycle (Tolaney, SABC 2016 Abstract P5-15-02) [51]. A total of 104 patients were enrolled in the Phase II portion, and the data from 82 evaluable patients were reported in 2017 [49]. The ORR was 25.5%. The combination had manageable toxicities consistent with the individual agent's safety profile; the most common were fatigue, nausea, and neuropathy [49].

Atezolizumab

Atezolizumab is a humanized antibody that inhibits PD-L1 and has shown encouraging activity in patients with triple-negative breast cancer.

A Phase I trial evaluated the activity of single-agent atezolizumab in 115 patients with metastatic triple-negative breast cancer who were heavily pretreated. They received 15 or 20 mg/kg or 1200 mg of atezolizumab intravenously every 3 weeks for up to 16 cycles. The overall response rate was 10%. Here again, the patients who responded had a prolonged disease-free survival (21.1 months). Higher response rate seemed to be associated with higher levels of tumor-infiltrating lymphocytes, PD-L1 expression, and CD8 T cells [52].

Atezolizumab was evaluated in combination with nab-paclitaxel in a Phase Ib trial of TNBC patients who had received $\leq$ 2 lines of therapy for metastatic disease. The ORR for this combination among the 24 patients evaluable for efficacy was 42%, and 67% among patients that received this regimen as first line, with 8% of patients having a complete response [48]. This was the first trial in TNBC patients to report the efficacy of combination chemotherapy + checkpoint inhibitor therapy and led to the development of Phase III trials of the combination in the first-line metastatic (Impassion130) and neoadjuvant settings (Impassion031). Results from these trials are highly anticipated to see if a chemotherapy–checkpoint combination therapy is the ideal way to incorporate checkpoint inhibitor therapy in the treatment paradigm for TNBC.

Avelumab
Avelumab is another PD-L1 antibody that has entered clinical investigation in mBC.

JAVELIN Solid Tumor Study: This is a Phase I trial in patients with advanced solid malignancies. A total of 168 heavily pretreated patients with mBC including 58 patients with TNBC have been enrolled. The ORR was 3% in the whole group, and 5.5% in the TNBC subset. Exploratory analysis showed a trend toward higher response in patients with PD-L1-positive tumors (16.7% vs. 1.6%) and patients with triple-negative breast cancer (22% vs. 2.6%) [53].

2.7.1.2 Other Molecules

Taking the lead from other tumor types like NSCLC and melanoma, other molecules that stimulate T-cell immunity are currently being studied in breast cancer as well, such as antibodies that target the T-cell immunoglobulin and immunoreceptor tyrosine-based inhibitory motif (TIGIT), antibodies that target the T-cell costimulatory protein (ICOS), antibodies that target tumor necrosis factor superfamily member 4 (OX40), antibodies against the lymphocyte activation gene-3 (LAG3), etc. [54].

2.7.2 Improving Immune Checkpoint Inhibitor Activity

As highlighted by the data from various trials and in different breast cancer histologic types, monotherapy in breast cancer is only effective in a small subset of patients, especially in pretreated patients. For this reason, several strategies are being developed to improve the activity of checkpoint inhibitors. In general, breast cancer immune phenotypes range from poorly immunogenic to an inflamed immunogenic type. Approximately one-third of basal-like and HER2-enriched tumors in the TCGA database were noted to express a favorable immune tumor phenotype based on gene expression data, whereas only 5 and 10% of Luminal A and B tumors, respectively, were represented in the favorable group [55]. Consistent with other studies that have shown that a higher proportion of tumor-infiltrating lymphocytes are associated with better prognosis in breast cancer [16], this study also showed improved survival for patients with favorable immune profiles. Thus, there is ongoing enthusiasm for identifying those breast cancers that are inherently more likely to respond to immunotherapy as well as approaches to make less immunogenic tumors more immunogenic to increase their likelihood of response (convert “cold” tumors to “hot” ones).

One of the strategies is to combine checkpoint inhibitors with agents that can generate and deliver tumor-associated antigens (neoantigens) to antigen-presenting cells.

The use of CDK4/6 inhibitors in combination with PD-1 inhibitors is based on this principle. CDK4/6 inhibitors augment antigen presentation. The combination of pembrolizumab with abemaciclib (**JPCE** trial) is currently being studied in a Phase

Ib parallel assignment study. Preclinical data showed that abemaciclib increases T-cell infiltration in tumors and could enhance the activity of pembrolizumab. In this trial, patients with non-small cell lung cancer and hormone-receptor-positive breast cancer were enrolled. Twenty-eight patients had ER+ mBC. The ORR was 14.3% (at a 16-week analysis). The combination had an acceptable safety profile [56]. Another trial is testing the combination of ribociclib with PDR001 (an anti-PD-1 agent) in patients with hormone-receptor-positive breast cancer or ovarian cancer (NCT03294694).

Another trial that recently reported encouraging data in TNBC patients is looking at a PARP inhibitor (niraparib) in combination with pembrolizumab (**TOPACIO/Keynote 162** trial). Among 54 enrolled patients with TNBC who had received a median of 1 prior treatment, an ORR of 29% (3 CRs and 10 PRs) and a disease control rate (DCR) of 49% were reported. The ORR and DCR in BRCA mutation-positive patients were higher at 67 and 75%, respectively. Prior platinum exposure or PDL-1 status did not impact efficacy to the combination. This trial offers a possible strategy to not only improve checkpoint inhibitor therapy efficacy but also potentially overcome platinum and PARP resistance in TNBC patients [57].

Combining different immune checkpoint inhibitors together like CTLA-4 inhibitors with a PD-1 inhibitor can augment tumor T-cell trafficking and improve efficacy. Tremelimumab in combination with durvalumab in patients with triple-negative or hormone-receptor +/HER2− breast cancer was studied in a single-arm pilot study [58]. A total of 18 patients were accrued with a 17% response rate, limited to the TNBC patients. A higher tumor mutational load was associated with response to therapy.

Other ways to augment immunogeneity that are underway are to combine checkpoint inhibitors with other drugs such as histone deacetylase (HDAC) inhibitors, radiotherapy, or cryotherapy to enhance the release of tumor neoantigens [54].

2.8 Adjuvant or Early Breast Cancer Setting

Precision medicine has also impacted treatment in patients with early-stage breast cancer. In the past, most patients with invasive breast cancer were advised adjuvant chemotherapy regardless of hormone receptor, nodal or menopausal status [59]. In 2005, the Early Breast Cancer Trialists Collaborative Group (EBCTCG) meta-analysis demonstrated that the proportional and absolute benefit from poly-chemotherapy was higher in ER-negative disease and in pre-menopausal women as compared to postmenopausal ER-positive disease [7]. There were still no good risk stratification tools beyond clinic-pathologic factors like age, tumor size, nodal status, and grade that could identify ER/PR-positive patients who were less likely to benefit from adjuvant chemotherapy in addition to adjuvant endocrine therapy. Over the past 10–15 years, multiple genomic predictors, mostly prognostic but some predictive, have been developed to guide the use of chemotherapy in early-stage ER/PR-positive, HER2-negative breast cancer.

2.8.1 Molecular Profiling

The use of multigene molecular signatures has allowed us to predict the risk of distant recurrence in patients with ER-positive breast cancer and predict to some extent which patients are unlikely to benefit from adjuvant chemotherapy.

The use of a 21-gene expression assay (Oncotype DX) uses reverse transcriptase–polymerase chain reaction (RT-PCR) to quantify gene expression in paraffin-embedded tumor tissue. Based on the expression of the genes (16 cancer-related and 5-reference genes), a recurrence score (RS) is calculated. The patients are then categorized into three groups: low risk (RS < 18), intermediate (RS: 18–30), and high risk (RS: >30) [60]. The signature was validated for its prognostic and predictive role by applying the signature retrospectively to prospectively collected outcomes data from the NSABPB-20 trial. Patients who had a high RS had the greatest absolute benefit from chemotherapy (increase in 10-year distant recurrence-free survival of 27.6% ± 8%) while those with a low RS derived minimal benefit from addition of chemotherapy (CMF) to tamoxifen (10-year DRFS increase −1.1% ± 2.2%) [60]. This led to the rapid adoption of the 21-gene RS into adjuvant therapy decision making for node-negative hormone-receptor-positive, HER2-negative breast cancer ahead of the availability of level-1 prospective randomized trial data.

TAILORx was the prospective randomized Phase III trial that evaluated the need of chemotherapy in patients with hormone-receptor-positive, HER2-negative breast cancer. Patients with tumors of 1.1–5 cm (of 0.6–1 cm if intermediate or high tumor grade) and no lymph node metastasis are eligible [61]. It is important to note that this trial shifted the cutoffs for low-, intermediate-, and high-risk groups. Patients with a score <10 were not randomized and were treated with endocrine therapy alone. Excellent 5-year invasive disease-free survival {93.8% (95% CI: 92.4–94.9)} and overall survival {98% (95% CI: 97.1–98.6)} for this low-risk group were recently reported [61]. The results of the randomized population in the study, those with an intermediate RS (11–25), were recently published and showed that endocrine therapy alone was non-inferior to the addition of chemotherapy in patients with an intermediated score with a HR for invasive disease-free survival of 1.08 (95% CI: 0.94–1.24). Exploratory analysis by age suggested that there was some potential benefit of chemotherapy in younger women (50 years or younger) with scores of 16–25 [61] with decreased distant recurrence risk especially in women with scores between 21 and 25. Whether those benefits would still hold true if optimal endocrine therapy, i.e., ovarian ablation plus an aromatase inhibitor as opposed to tamoxifen alone were employed in this high-risk premenopausal group of women (as supported by the joint analysis of the SOFT and TEXT trials) remains an open question.

Some evidence exists that the 21-gene expression assay may be useful in patient with positive lymph nodes and that patients with a low score might not require chemotherapy [62–64]. Available tumor blocks from the SWOG 8814 study of node-positive hormone-receptor-positive patients were profiled for risk of recurrence and correlated with prospectively collected outcome data [65]. Patients in the low RS category did not benefit from addition of anthracycline-based chemotherapy (CAF) to tamoxifen (HR: 1.02; logrank $p = 0.97$). Those in the high RS group, however, derived significant benefit from CAF (HR: 0.59; $p = 0.03$). The prospective trial investigating this question is ongoing at this time (SWOG 0017, RxPONDER trial).

The 70-gene signature test (MammaPrint) is another tool being used to determine which patients will benefit from adjuvant chemotherapy. This test uses DNA microarray analysis of 70 genes to categorize patients as poor or good prognosis [66, 67]. A randomized Phase III study (**MINDACT** trial) evaluated the clinical utility of this test in patients with early node-negative or node-positive (1–3 positive nodes) breast cancer. The genomic risk and the clinical risk were determined using the 70-gene signature and a modified version of adjuvant online. Patients with low clinical and low genomic risk did not receive chemotherapy and patients with high clinical and high genomic risk received chemotherapy. Patients with discordant scores in either the genomic or the clinical risks were used to determine the need for or not for chemotherapy. The primary aim of this study was to determine whether patients with high clinical risk and low genomic risk could avoid chemotherapy (if a 5-year distant disease-free survival of 92% or greater without chemotherapy could be demonstrated in this group). This study reached its endpoint demonstrating that the absolute benefit of chemotherapy in this genomically low-risk group despite traditional high-risk clinic-pathologic factors was minimal and these patients do just as well when treated with endocrine therapy alone [68].

Other commercially available genomic signature tools include the PAM-50-based Prosigna risk of recurrence, EndoPredict, and the breast cancer index. These tests differ in the number of genes tested, and the specific genes that constitute the gene signature, but overall are able to select out a group of tumors with favorable biology that have a low risk of recurrence. A retrospective study compared the different genomic signatures for predicting distant and late recurrences along with two clinicopathological algorithms: the clinical treatment score (nodal status, tumor size, age, grade, and endocrine treatment) and a 4-marker immunohistochemical score. A total of 774 postmenopausal women who were enrolled in the ATAC study (Anastrozole vs. Tamoxifen) trial had tumor blocks available for this analysis. Patients who received chemotherapy or who had 4 or more positive lymph nodes were excluded. The study found that each of the gene signatures provided additional independent prognostic information in node-negative patients compared to the clinical treatment score and IHC-4 score. However, the performance of the genomic signatures tested was limited in node-positive patients. This analysis did not assess the benefit from chemotherapy or extended endocrine therapy though some assays like the breast cancer index have been evaluated in that setting to predict which patients may have significant residual risk of late distant recurrences to warrant extended endocrine therapy [69, 70].

The use of precision medicine tools has also changed the current staging system in breast cancer. In 2018, the AJCC published the new staging system introducing for the first time a prognostic stage group based on different biomarkers such as receptor status, tumor grade, and multigene molecular profiling. This change was made due to the fact that biology impacts survival in BC. Patients with tumors of the same size and same number of lymph node involvement have different outcomes depending on their tumor markers. Using this new staging system, many hormone-receptor-positive, HER2-negative breast cancers with a low recurrence score will be down-staged to reflect their excellent prognosis. This also highlights that, now more than ever, there is a tremendous need for selective decision making regarding adjuvant therapy in hormone-receptor-positive early-stage breast cancer.

2.8.2 HER2-Positive Breast Cancer

HER2-directed therapy has dramatically changed the outcome of patients with HER2 positive BC. After the approval of trastuzumab in metastatic HER2-positive BC, it was evaluated in the adjuvant setting. There were four large Phase III randomized trials that studied trastuzumab in the adjuvant setting and all of them showed improvements in disease-free survival (relative reduction in hazard of 30–35% for trastuzumab-containing arms) and overall survival (relative reduction in hazard of 25–30% for the trastuzumab-containing arms) which led to the approval of trastuzumab for the adjuvant treatment of HER2-positive BC [71–73].

Pertuzumab is another monoclonal antibody that showed impressive improvements in progression-free survival and overall survival in the metastatic setting and was then studied in the neoadjuvant and adjuvant settings. The **NeoSphere** clinical trial was a multicenter open-label Phase II randomized trial that randomized patients to four arms: A: trastuzumab plus docetaxel; B: pertuzumab and trastuzumab plus docetaxel; C: pertuzumab and trastuzumab; D: pertuzumab and docetaxel. This was followed by surgery and three cycles of FEC (5-fluorouracil, epirubicin, and cyclophosphamide) and trastuzumab to complete one year. The primary endpoint was pathological complete response. The trial showed a statistically significant improvement in pathologic complete response in arm B compared with arm A (39.3% vs. 21.5%) [74]. This leads to its approval in the neoadjuvant setting. Even though there was improvement in the pathologic complete response, there was no difference in progression-free survival. In 2017, results from the **APHINITY** trial were published. It was a randomized Phase III trial of standard adjuvant chemotherapy for 18 weeks plus one year of trastuzumab with either placebo or pertuzumab. The 3-year disease-free survival (DFS) was 94.1% versus 93.2% favoring the pertuzumab arm which leads to its approval in the adjuvant setting. High-risk patients like those with hormone-receptor-negative and node-positive patients derived greater benefit from dual HER2 blockade compared to the hormone-receptor-positive subset [75].

There are no clinically useful biomarkers that have emerged which can help predict benefit or lack thereof from single or dual HER2-targeted therapy in the early-stage setting. Some interesting observations, however, are worth mentioning. In the neoadjuvant setting, tumors with a high HER2 mRNA expression [76] and those with a HER2-enriched genotype on the PAM50 assay [77] have been shown to have higher pCR rates when treated with HER2-directed therapy. Conversely, tumors with a Luminal B genotype characterized by a high expression of ESR1 and intermediate expression of ERBB2 genes derive the least benefit from adjuvant trastuzumab [78]. These observations would need validation in additional data sets to help define their utility for therapy selection in HER2-positive breast cancer.

2.9 Conclusions

The emergence of novel technology, data sharing tools, and creative clinical trial designs has pushed precision medicine into the forefront of drug development and care for oncology patients and established new drug approval paradigms. In 2017, 16 new small molecule and biologic applications were approved by the FDA, 5 of those with breast cancer indications, highlighting the rapid pace at which novel therapies are becoming available to our patients. This progress and expansion of knowledge have also brought forth several new challenges. To name a few: identifying functionally significant targets from the gigabytes of genomic/proteomic data, selecting patients most likely to benefit from targeted therapies, securing access to therapy for individual patients, overcoming treatment-emergent resistance and toxicities associated with new therapies like the checkpoint inhibitors that are just now finding their way into breast cancer treatment protocols, and showing limited application. Ongoing collaborative research, cross-discipline resource and knowledge sharing, and setting a higher bar for clinically meaningful clinical trial endpoints will ensure that precision medicine will ultimately deliver on its promise of better treatments and outcomes for breast cancer patients.

References

1. Ellsworth RE et al (2017) Molecular heterogeneity in breast cancer: state of the science and implications for patient care. Semin Cell Dev Biol 64:65–72
2. Perou CM et al (2000) Molecular portraits of human breast tumours. Nature 406(6797): 747–752
3. Curtis C et al (2012) The genomic and transcriptomic architecture of 2000 breast tumours reveals novel subgroups. Nature 486(7403):346–352
4. Lerner HJ et al (1976) Phase II study of tamoxifen: report of 74 patients with stage IV breast cancer. Cancer Treat Rep 60(10):1431–1435
5. Wiggans RG et al (1979) Phase-II trial of tamoxifen in advanced breast cancer. Cancer Chemother Pharmacol 3(1):45–48
6. Gradishar WJ et al (2015) NCCN guidelines insights breast cancer, version 1.2016. J Natl Compr Canc Netw 13(12):1475–1485

7. Early Breast Cancer Trialists' Collaborative Group (2005) Effects of chemotherapy and hormonal therapy for early breast cancer on recurrence and 15-year survival: an overview of the randomised trials. Lancet 365(9472):1687–717
8. Slamon DJ et al (2001) Use of chemotherapy plus a monoclonal antibody against HER2 for metastatic breast cancer that overexpresses HER2. N Engl J Med 344(11):783–792
9. Baselga J et al (2012) Pertuzumab plus trastuzumab plus docetaxel for metastatic breast cancer. N Engl J Med 366(2):109–119
10. Cardoso F et al (2014) ESO-ESMO 2nd international consensus guidelines for advanced breast cancer (ABC2). Breast 23(5):489–502
11. Wilken JA, Maihle NJ (2010) Primary trastuzumab resistance: new tricks for an old drug. Ann NY Acad Sci 1210:53–65
12. Robinson DR et al (2013) Activating ESR1 mutations in hormone-resistant metastatic breast cancer. Nat Genet 45(12):1446–1451
13. Chandarlapaty S et al (2016) Prevalence of ESR1 mutations in cell-free DNA and outcomes in metastatic breast cancer: a secondary analysis of the BOLERO-2 clinical trial. JAMA Oncol 2 (10):1310–1315
14. Fribbens C et al (2016) Plasma ESR1 mutations and the treatment of estrogen receptor-positive advanced breast cancer. J Clin Oncol 34(25):2961–2968
15. Turner N, Tutt A, Ashworth A (2004) Hallmarks of 'BRCAness' in sporadic cancers. Nat Rev Cancer 4(10):814–819
16. Thangavel C et al (2011) Therapeutically activating RB: reestablishing cell cycle control in endocrine therapy-resistant breast cancer. Endocr Relat Cancer 18(3):333–345
17. Finn RS et al (2016) Palbociclib and letrozole in advanced breast cancer. N Engl J Med 375 (20):1925–1936
18. Goetz MP et al (2017) MONARCH 3: abemaciclib as initial therapy for advanced breast cancer. J Clin Oncol 35(32):3638–3646
19. Hortobagyi GN et al (2016) Ribociclib as first-line therapy for HR-positive, advanced breast cancer. N Engl J Med 375(18):1738–1748
20. Cristofanilli M et al (2016) Fulvestrant plus palbociclib versus fulvestrant plus placebo for treatment of hormone-receptor-positive, HER2-negative metastatic breast cancer that progressed on previous endocrine therapy (PALOMA-3): final analysis of the multicentre, double-blind, phase 3 randomised controlled trial. Lancet Oncol 17(4):425–439
21. George W, Sledge J et al (2017) MONARCH 2: abemaciclib in combination with fulvestrant in women with HR+/HER2− advanced breast cancer who had progressed while receiving endocrine therapy. J Clin Oncol 35(25):2875–2884
22. Dickler MN et al (2017) MONARCH 1, a phase 2 study of abemaciclib, a CDK4 and CDK6 inhibitor, as a single agent, in patients with refractory HR+/HER2− metastatic breast cancer. Clin Cancer Res
23. Beeram M et al (2007) Akt-induced endocrine therapy resistance is reversed by inhibition of mTOR signaling. Ann Oncol 18(8):1323–1328
24. Sueta A et al (2014) An integrative analysis of PIK3CA mutation, PTEN, and INPP4B expression in terms of trastuzumab efficacy in HER2-positive breast cancer. PLoS ONE 9(12): e116054
25. Baselga J et al (2012) Everolimus in postmenopausal hormone-receptor-positive advanced breast cancer. N Engl J Med 366(6):520–529
26. Andre F et al (2014) Everolimus for women with trastuzumab-resistant, HER2-positive, advanced breast cancer (BOLERO-3): a randomised, double-blind, placebo-controlled phase 3 trial. Lancet Oncol 15(6):580–591
27. Hurvitz SA et al (2015) Combination of everolimus with trastuzumab plus paclitaxel as first-line treatment for patients with HER2-positive advanced breast cancer (BOLERO-1): a phase 3, randomised, double-blind, multicentre trial. Lancet Oncol 16(7):816–829

28. Andre F et al (2016) Molecular alterations and everolimus efficacy in human epidermal growth factor receptor 2-overexpressing metastatic breast cancers: combined exploratory biomarker analysis from BOLERO-1 and BOLERO-3. J Clin Oncol 34(18):2115–2124
29. Baselga J et al (2017) Buparlisib plus fulvestrant versus placebo plus fulvestrant in postmenopausal, hormone receptor-positive, HER2-negative, advanced breast cancer (BELLE-2): a randomised, double-blind, placebo-controlled, phase 3 trial. Lancet Oncol 18 (7):904–916
30. Di Leo A et al (2018) Buparlisib plus fulvestrant in postmenopausal women with hormone-receptor-positive, HER2-negative, advanced breast cancer progressing on or after mTOR inhibition (BELLE-3): a randomised, double-blind, placebo-controlled, phase 3 trial. Lancet Oncol 19(1):87–100
31. Baselga J, Dent SF, Cortés J, Im Y-H, Diéras V, Harbeck N, Krop IE, Verma S, Wilson TR, Jin H, Wang L, Schimmoller F, Hsu JY, He J, DeLaurentiis M, Drullinsky P, Jacot W (2018) Phase III study of taselisib (GDC-0032) + fulvestrant (FULV) versus FULV in patients (pts) with estrogen receptor (ER)-positive, PIK3CA-mutant (MUT), locally advanced or metastatic breast cancer (MBC): primary analysis from SANDPIPER. In: 2018 ASCO annual meeting
32. Conley BA, Chen AP, O'Dwyer PJ, Arteaga CL, Hamilton SR, Williams PM, Little RF, Takebe N, Patton D, Sazali K, Zhang J, Zwiebel JA, Mitchell EP, Gray RJ, McShane L, Li S, Rubinstein L, Flaherty K (2016) NCI-MATCH (Molecular analysis for therapy choice)—a national signal finding trial. In: 2016 ASCO annual meeting
33. Azad N, Overman M, Gray R, Schoenfeld J, Arteaga C, Coffey B, Patton D, Li S, McShane L, Rubenstein L, Harris L, Comis R, Abrams J, Williams PM, Mitchell E, Zweibel J, Sharon E, Streicher H, Dwyer PJ, Hamilton S, Conley B, Chen AP, Flaherty K (2017) Nivolumab in mismatch-repair deficient (MMR-d) cancers: NCI-MATCH Trial (Molecular analysis for therapy choice) arm Z1D preliminary results. In: SITC 2017
34. Schwaederle M et al (2015) Impact of precision medicine in diverse cancers: a meta-analysis of phase II clinical trials. J Clin Oncol 33(32):3817–3825
35. del Rivero J, Kohn EC (2017) PARP inhibitors: the cornerstone of DNA repair-targeted therapies. Oncology (Williston Park) 31(4):265–273
36. Livraghi L, Garber JE (2015) PARP inhibitors in the management of breast cancer: current data and future prospects. BMC Med 13:188
37. Robson M et al (2017) Olaparib for metastatic breast cancer in patients with a germline BRCA mutation. N Engl J Med 377(6):523–533
38. Litton JK et al (2017) A feasibility study of neoadjuvant talazoparib for operable breast cancer patients with a germline BRCA mutation demonstrates marked activity. NPJ Breast Cancer 3:49
39. Konstantinopoulos PA et al (2010) Gene expression profile of BRCAness that correlates with responsiveness to chemotherapy and with outcome in patients with epithelial ovarian cancer. J Clin Oncol 28(22):3555–3561
40. Telli ML et al (2016) Homologous recombination deficiency (HRD) score predicts response to platinum-containing neoadjuvant chemotherapy in patients with triple-negative breast cancer. Clin Cancer Res 22(15):3764–3773
41. Tutt A, Ellis P, Kilbum L (2014) TNT: a randomized phase III trial of carboplatin compared with docetaxel for patients with metastatic or recurrent locally advanced triple negative or BRCA 1/2 breast cancer. In: 2014 San Antonio breast cancer symposium
42. Verma S et al (2012) Trastuzumab emtansine for HER2-positive advanced breast cancer. N Engl J Med 367(19):1783–1791
43. Perez EA et al (2017) Trastuzumab emtansine with or without pertuzumab versus trastuzumab plus taxane for human epidermal growth factor receptor 2-positive, advanced breast cancer: primary results from the phase III MARIANNE study. J Clin Oncol 35(2):141–148

44. Bardia A, Vahdat LT, Diamond J, Kalinsky K, O'Shaughnessy J, Moroose RL, Isakoff SJ, Tolaney SM, Santin AD, Abramson V, Shah NC, Govindan SV, Maliakal P, Sharkey RM, Wegener WA, Goldenberg DM, Mayer IA (2017) Sacituzumab govitecan (IMMU-132), an anti-Trop-2-SN-38 antibody-drug conjugate, as $\geq$ 3rd-line therapeutic option for patients with relapsed/refractory metastatic triple-negative breast cancer (mTNBC): efficacy results. In: 2017 San Antonio breast cancer symposium
45. Trail PA, Dubowchik GM, Lowinger TB (2018) Antibody drug conjugates for treatment of breast cancer: novel targets and diverse approaches in ADC design. Pharmacol Ther 181: 126–142
46. Alsaab HO et al (2017) PD-1 and PD-L1 checkpoint signaling inhibition for cancer immunotherapy: mechanism, combinations, and clinical outcome. Front Pharmacol 8:561
47. Nanda R et al (2016) Pembrolizumab in patients with advanced triple-negative breast cancer: phase Ib KEYNOTE-012 study. J Clin Oncol 34(21):2460–2467
48. Adams S et al (2016) Phase Ib trial of atezolizumab in combination with nab-paclitaxel in patients with metastatic triple-negative breast cancer (mTNBC). J Clin Oncol 34 (15_suppl):1009
49. Tolaney S et al (2018) Abstract PD6-13: Phase 1b/2 study to evaluate eribulin mesylate in combination with pembrolizumab in patients with metastatic triple-negative breast cancer. Cancer Res 78(4 Supplement):PD6-13
50. Rugo HS et al (2018) Safety and antitumor activity of pembrolizumab in patients with estrogen receptor-positive/human epidermal growth factor receptor 2-negative advanced breast cancer. Clin Cancer Res 24(12):2804–2811
51. Tolaney S et al (2017) Abstract P5-15-02: Phase 1b/2 study to evaluate eribulin mesylate in combination with pembrolizumab in patients with metastatic triple-negative breast cancer. Cancer Res 77(4 Supplement):P5-15-02
52. Schmid P, Cruz C, Braiteh FS, Eder JP, Tolaney S, Kuter I, Nanda R, Chung C, Cassier P, Delord J-P, Gordon M, Li Y, Liu B, O'Hear C, Fasso M, Molinero L, Emens LA (2017) Atezolizumab in metastatic TNBC (mTNBC): long-term clinical outcomes and biomarker analyses. In: 2017 AACR annual meeting
53. Dirix LY et al (2018) Avelumab, an anti-PD-L1 antibody, in patients with locally advanced or metastatic breast cancer: a phase 1b JAVELIN solid tumor study. Breast Cancer Res Treat 167(3):671–686
54. Kwa MJ, Adams S (2018) Checkpoint inhibitors in triple-negative breast cancer (TNBC): Where to go from here. Cancer 124(10):2086–2103
55. Hendrickx W et al (2017) Identification of genetic determinants of breast cancer immune phenotypes by integrative genome-scale analysis. Oncoimmunology 6(2):e1253654
56. Rugo H et al (2018) Abstract P1-09-01: A phase 1b study of abemaciclib plus pembrolizumab for patients with hormone receptor-positive (HR+), human epidermal growth factor receptor 2-negative (HER2-) metastatic breast cancer (MBC). Cancer Res 78(4 Supplement):P1-09-01
57. Vinayak S et al (2018) TOPACIO/Keynote-162: niraparib plus pembrolizumab in patients (pts) with metastatic triple-negative breast cancer (TNBC), a phase 2 trial. J Clin Oncol 36 (15):abstr 1011
58. Santa-Maria CA et al (2018) A pilot study of durvalumab and tremelimumab and immunogenomic dynamics in metastatic breast cancer. Oncotarget 9(27):18985–18996
59. Adjuvant therapy for breast cancer (2000) NIH Consens Statement 17(4):1–35
60. Paik S et al (2004) A multigene assay to predict recurrence of tamoxifen-treated, node-negative breast cancer. N Engl J Med 351(27):2817–2826
61. Sparano JA et al (2015) Prospective validation of a 21-gene expression assay in breast cancer. N Engl J Med 373(21):2005–2014
62. Albain KS et al (2010) Prognostic and predictive value of the 21-gene recurrence score assay in postmenopausal women with node-positive, oestrogen-receptor-positive breast cancer on chemotherapy: a retrospective analysis of a randomised trial. Lancet Oncol 11(1):55–65

63. Nitz U et al (2017) Reducing chemotherapy use in clinically high-risk, genomically low-risk pN0 and pN1 early breast cancer patients: five-year data from the prospective, randomised phase 3 West German Study Group (WSG) PlanB trial. Breast Cancer Res Treat 165(3):573–583
64. Roberts MC et al (2017) Breast cancer-specific survival in patients with lymph node-positive hormone receptor-positive invasive breast cancer and oncotype DX recurrence score results in the SEER database. Breast Cancer Res Treat 163(2):303–310
65. Albain KS et al (2010) Prognostic and predictive value of the 21-gene recurrence score assay in a randomized trial of chemotherapy for post-menopausal, node-positive, estrogen receptor-positive breast cancer. Lancet Oncol 11(1):55–65
66. Van 't Veer LJ et al (2002) Gene expression profiling predicts clinical outcome of breast cancer. Nature 415(6871):530–536
67. van de Vijver MJ et al (2002) A gene-expression signature as a predictor of survival in breast cancer. N Engl J Med 347(25):1999–2009
68. Cardoso F et al (2016) 70-Gene signature as an aid to treatment decisions in early-stage breast cancer. N Engl J Med 375(8):717–729
69. Sestak I et al (2018) Comparison of the performance of 6 prognostic signatures for estrogen receptor-positive breast cancer: a secondary analysis of a randomized clinical trial. JAMA Oncol
70. Sgroi DC et al (2013) Prediction of late distant recurrence in patients with oestrogen-receptor-positive breast cancer: a prospective comparison of the breast-cancer index (BCI) assay, 21-gene recurrence score, and IHC4 in the TransATAC study population. Lancet Oncol 14 (11):1067–1076
71. Cameron D et al (2017) 11 years' follow-up of trastuzumab after adjuvant chemotherapy in HER2-positive early breast cancer: final analysis of the HERceptin Adjuvant (HERA) trial. Lancet 389(10075):1195–1205
72. Perez EA et al (2014) Trastuzumab plus adjuvant chemotherapy for human epidermal growth factor receptor 2-positive breast cancer: planned joint analysis of overall survival from NSABP B-31 and NCCTG N9831. J Clin Oncol 32(33):3744–3752
73. Slamon, D et al (2016) Abstract S5-04: Ten year follow-up of BCIRG-006 comparing doxorubicin plus cyclophosphamide followed by docetaxel (AC → T) with doxorubicin plus cyclophosphamide followed by docetaxel and trastuzumab (AC → TH) with docetaxel, carboplatin and trastuzumab (TCH) in HER2+ early breast cancer. Cancer Res 76(4 Supplement):S5-04
74. Gianni L et al (2016) 5-year analysis of neoadjuvant pertuzumab and trastuzumab in patients with locally advanced, inflammatory, or early-stage HER2-positive breast cancer (Neo-Sphere): a multicentre, open-label, phase 2 randomised trial. Lancet Oncol 17(6):791–800
75. von Minckwitz G et al (2017) Adjuvant pertuzumab and trastuzumab in early HER2-positive breast cancer. N Engl J Med 377(2):122–131
76. Schneeweiss A et al (2014) Evaluating the predictive value of biomarkers for efficacy outcomes in response to pertuzumab- and trastuzumab-based therapy: an exploratory analysis of the TRYPHAENA study. Breast Cancer Res 16(4):R73
77. Prat A et al (2014) Research-based PAM50 subtype predictor identifies higher responses and improved survival outcomes in HER2-positive breast cancer in the NOAH study. Clin Cancer Res 20(2):511–521
78. Pogue-Geile KL et al (2013) Predicting degree of benefit from adjuvant trastuzumab in NSABP trial B-31. J Natl Cancer Inst 105(23):1782–1788
79. Cancer Genome Atlas Network (2012) Comprehensive molecular portraits of human breast tumours. Nature 490(7418):61–70
80. Finn RS et al (2015) The cyclin-dependent kinase 4/6 inhibitor palbociclib in combination with letrozole versus letrozole alone as first-line treatment of oestrogen receptor-positive, HER2-negative, advanced breast cancer (PALOMA-1/TRIO-18): a randomised phase 2 study. Lancet Oncol 16(1):25–35

81. Tripathy D et al, Ribociclib plus endocrine therapy for premenopausal women with hormone-receptor-positive, advanced breast cancer (MONALEESA-7): a randomised phase 3 trial. Lancet Oncol
82. Andre F et al (2014) Comparative genomic hybridisation array and DNA sequencing to direct treatment of metastatic breast cancer: a multicentre, prospective trial (SAFIR01/UNICANCER). Lancet Oncol 15(3):267–274
83. Massard C et al (2017) High-throughput genomics and clinical outcome in hard-to-treat advanced cancers: results of the MOSCATO 01 trial. Cancer Discov 7(6):586–595
84. Meric-Bernstam F et al (2015) Feasibility of large-scale genomic testing to facilitate enrollment onto genomically matched clinical trials. J Clin Oncol 33(25):2753–2762
85. Pezo RC et al (2018) Impact of multi-gene mutational profiling on clinical trial outcomes in metastatic breast cancer. Breast Cancer Res Treat 168(1):159–168
86. Von Hoff DD et al (2010) Pilot study using molecular profiling of patients' tumors to find potential targets and select treatments for their refractory cancers. J Clin Oncol 28(33):4877–4883
87. Le Tourneau C et al (2015) Molecularly targeted therapy based on tumour molecular profiling versus conventional therapy for advanced cancer (SHIVA): a multicentre, open-label, proof-of-concept, randomised, controlled phase 2 trial. Lancet Oncol 16(13):1324–1334
88. Jameson GS et al (2014) A pilot study utilizing multi-omic molecular profiling to find potential targets and select individualized treatments for patients with previously treated metastatic breast cancer. Breast Cancer Res Treat 147(3):579–588

The Role of Precision Medicine in the Diagnosis and Treatment of Patients with Rare Cancers

3

Michael J. Demeure

Contents

M. J. Demeure (✉)
Hoag Family Cancer Institute, Newport Beach, CA, USA
e-mail: Michael.Demeure@hoag.org

M. J. Demeure
Translational Genomics Research Institute, Phoenix, AZ, USA

D. D. Von Hoff and H. Han (eds.), *Precision Medicine in Cancer Therapy*,
Cancer Treatment and Research 178, https://doi.org/10.1007/978-3-030-16391-4_3

3.1 Introduction

Rare cancers pose a unique opportunity to harness the potential of precision medicine. Precision medicine offers a new paradigm for the development of new cancer treatments. It promises more effective treatments with less toxicity for patients with cancer. Fulfillment of these promises would be particularly welcome to patients with a rare cancer. Patients with a rare cancers face the challenges that patients with more common cancers do but also must contend with a relative lack of information available to them and their physicians to guide treatment. Patients may have difficulty finding an expert or have to travel to get care from physicians with experience treating their type of cancer. With refractory or recurrent rare cancers when there is an absence of large prospective clinical trial data to guide chemotherapy choices, genomic analysis of tumors or precision medicine offers the opportunity to expose therapeutic options. Genomic sequencing to guide treatment has become tractable in recent times due to the rapidly decreasing cost, increasing evidence of clinical utility, and the increasing willingness of payers to provide for tumor profiling. This chapter delves into the problems posed by rare cancers and explores how precision medicine may improve patient care and outcomes.

3.2 Unique Problems for Patients with Rare Cancers

There is no generally accepted definition of rare cancers [1]. It is clear, however, that in the aggregate, rare cancers are not really rare. Rare cancers are defined as cancers with an incidence of less than 15 cases per 100,000 per year. There are less than 40,000 new cases per year in the USA [2]. Using another perspective, if one tabulates sixty of the least common of the 71 cancer types listed in the Cancer in North America (CINA) database [3], these cancers account for 25% of all adult cancers. Rare cancers tend to occur in patients who are younger, nonwhite, and more often of Hispanic origin, when compared to patients with more common cancers. Patients with rare cancers often face unique challenges in addition to those encountered by patients with more common cancers [4]. These include delay or difficulty in establishing a correct diagnosis, a possibility of previous errors in diagnosis, encountering physicians who are unfamiliar with their cancer or offer conflicting treatment recommendations, in addition to the need to research, find and travel to seek care from expert providers. The internet is a valuable and powerful resource for patients to find information regarding their cancers, establish contact with other patients and advocacy groups, and to identify expert physicians. On the other hand, it can also harm patients by exposing vulnerable patients to contradictory or inaccurate information and dubious claims of miraculous results from expensive treatments. Many rare cancers are aggressive and often fatal. Survival rates for adult patients with rare cancers are generally poorer than for those with common cancers [5, 6]. Patients and caregivers have limited evidence upon which to base decisions for treatment, and the literature offering guidance for care is frequently based on case reports or small single-institution series. For more common cancers, knowledge is gained from a traditional and progressive series of clinical trials to establish the optimum care regimens. Prospective randomized phase III studies to identify a standard treatment are uncommon when a disease is rare because accrual of sufficient numbers of patients for such studies may not be possible or may take years. The First International Randomized Trial in Locally Advanced and Metastatic Adrenocortical Carcinoma Treatment (FIRM-ACT) study to establish a multi-drug regimen as first-line therapy for advanced adrenocortical cancer took over 5 years to accrue 304 patients from 12 countries treated at 40 centers [7]. Financial support for such studies is lacking as pharmaceutical firms seek larger markets for agents in their pipelines and governmental agencies prioritize funding for more common cancers. Funding may be left to nonprofit disease-focused advocacy groups. In general, fewer investigators study rare cancers than more common cancers due to reasons such as access to grant funding or availability of biospecimens. Genomics and related studies can be employed to overcome these hurdles. It is hoped that insight from genomic interrogation of an individual patient's tumor will lead to improved outcomes. Indeed, notable examples of remarkable advances based on the study of small numbers of patients have resulted in paradigm shifts in the care of certain cancers.

3.3 Genomics for Diagnosis and Treatment

Cancer has traditionally been diagnosed based on tissue of origin and histologic features, as in adenocarcinoma of the lung. Molecular genetic and genomic aberrations have been elucidated and implicated in the oncogenic process (Table 3.1). Molecular analysis has changed the process of determining a diagnosis for many cancers because molecular characteristics may alter the clinical behavior and outcome as well as the response to proffered treatments (Table 3.2). This section is meant to illustrate examples of the use of molecular techniques to improve the diagnosis and the development of molecularly targeted agents against rare cancers. The paradigm is repeated increasingly often in medical oncology to the benefit of patients.

Nowhere is the role of molecular analysis, including cytogenetics and the study of molecular alterations, more relevant than in the classification of sarcomas [8]. Genomic classification is now fundamental and has expanded the repertoire of subtypes of sarcomas to many more than was previously appreciated by histopathology [9]. There are now over 50 distinct histologic subtypes of sarcomas as described by the World Health Organization [10]. Advances in immunohistochemistry and molecular genetic analysis to identify characteristic markers, mutations, and gene fusions have resulted in refined diagnostic criteria in a more recent iteration of the WHO report [11]. Furthermore, molecular testing, in one study, altered the diagnosis in 14% of cases initially reviewed by experienced pathologists at sarcoma referral centers [12]. The molecular diagnosis then becomes determinative in the treatment of patients, as in when a KIT mutation is discovered in a

Table 3.1 Definition of terms related to genomics

Term	Definition	Reference
Genetics	The study of heredity including limited number of genes and their functions	63
Genomics	The study of genome, the complete genetic information of an organism	77 (p. 496)
Mutation	A permanent change in genomic DNA sequence	77 (p. 500)
Indel	An insertion or deletion of one or more bases in the genome	77 (p. 498)
Copy number variant (CNV)	Presence or absence of a section of DNA	77 (p. 492)
Amplification	Increased number of copies of a gene or DNA fragments	3
Deletion	Loss of DNA sequence from a chromosome that may vary by length, ranging from a single base pair to a large segment of chromosome	77 (p. 493)
Loss of heterozygosity (LOH)	Loss of one normal allele (wild-type) of a gene, while the second allele is inactive	77 (p. 499)
Fusion genes	Combination of genes or parts of two genes resulting from structural rearrangements such as translocations known as drivers of cancer	53 (p. 324), 64
Driver genes	Genes that frequently carry somatic mutations in different cancer types, while passenger gene mutations appear to be non-recurrent in specific cancer types and are not directly causing cancer development and progression. Driver genes are classified in two different categories: tumor suppressor genes and activated oncogenes	77 (p. 314, p. 494, and p. 502)
Tumor suppressor genes	Genes that are known to be involved in the regulation of cell proliferation, where loss of function mutations in these genes result in tumor development or progression	77 (p. 314)
Oncogenes	Genes that are responsible for tumor development or progression when activated	77 (p. 501)

gastrointestinal stromal tumor (GIST). An exon 9 or 11 KIT mutation suggests sensitivity to imatinib, a tyrosine kinase inhibitor [13]. Conversely, secondary KIT mutations in exons 13, 14, 17, or 18 that may be seen commonly seen after treatment and confer resistance to treatment [14, 15]. An understanding of the functional consequences of identified genomic aberrations associated with particular sarcomas can identify potential new treatments. Recently, an exploration of the EWS-FL11 translocation characteristic of Ewing sarcoma showed it blocks the function of BRCA1-mediated DNA repair and offers an explanation for the sensitivity of this cancer to chemotherapy including etoposide and PARP inhibitors [16]. Additionally, patients with sarcomas may harbor germline mutations such as TP53 in Li-Fraumeni syndrome. These patients are at increased risk of other

Table 3.2 Classification of sequence variants (adapted from Reference 93)

	Classification	Definition
A	Pathogenic mutation	A variant with sufficient evidence to cause a disease
B	Likely pathogenic variant (VLP)	A variant has strong evidence toward pathogenicity
C	Variant of uncertain significance (VUS)	A variant with conflicting or limited evidence to be disease causing
D	Benign or likely benign variants	Variants with very strong or strong evidence against pathogenicity
E	Pathogenic mutation	A variant with sufficient evidence to cause a disease
F	Likely pathogenic variant (VLP)	A variant has strong evidence toward pathogenicity
G	Variant of uncertain significance (VUS)	A variant with conflicting or limited evidence to be disease causing
H	Benign or likely benign variants	Variants with very strong or strong evidence against pathogenicity

Table 3.3 Levels of evidence for reporting of somatic variants (adapted from Reference 67)

	Biomarkers	Reference
A	Biomarkers that predict response or resistance to an FDA-approved treatment for a specific tumor type, on that have included in guidelines from professional organizations. An example is detection of an EGFR mutation in lung cancer	70
B	Biomarkers that predict response or resistance to treatments based on well-powered clinical studies with expert consensus. An example would be BRAF mutation in Hairy Cell Leukemia	114
C	Biomarkers that predict response or resistance to treatments approved by the FDA or recommended by professional organizations for a different tumor type, an off-label indication. An example is the identification of an ALK fusion in thyroid cancer	22
D	Biomarkers that show a logical significance based on pathway, preclinical studies or limited experience consisting of small series or case reports, with no consensus. An example is the identification of an FGFR2 gene fusions in cholangiocarcinomas	94

cancers as well, so screening for other tumors should be done. Family members of affected patients then should also receive genetic counseling and testing.

Gene mutations in rare cancers such as brain tumors can inform prognosis and be important for guiding treatment (Table 3.3). Malignant brain tumors occur with annual incidence of 8.62 per 100,000 adults in the USA [17]. Of these, the most common are gliomas which account for approximately 15%. Glioblastoma is the most deadly and common type of glioma in adults. Grade I gliomas are curable with complete resection, but those that transform into higher grade tumors have a poor prognosis. Although the distinction has prognostic import, it is difficult to determine by histopathology a secondary glioblastoma arising from a low-grade glioma from a primary glioblastoma [18]. Mutations in the isodehydrogenase 1 gene (IDH1) occur in approximately 12% of gliomas and are thought to drive the progression of these tumors to high-grade glioblastoma multiforme [19]. Gliomas, as well as anaplastic astrocytomas, that harbor a mutant IDH1 or IHD2 gene have a significantly better outcome than is associated with tumors with wild-type IDH genes [20]. Wild-type IDH genes were a feature of primary high-grade tumors, leading the investigators to suggest that determination of IDH mutation status could be a diagnostic aid.

In hematologic cancers, molecular characterization contributes routinely in clinical practice to the diagnosis, assessment of prognosis, and in the determination of treatment plans. For example, a mutation in the Janus Kinase 2 gene (JAK2 V617F) has been reported in 97% of cases of polycythemia vera and 50% of cases of primary myelofibrosis [21]. Polycythemia vera is a myeloproliferative neoplasia that may on occasion, undergo leukemic transformation which is then associated with a bleak median survival of approximately 5 months [22]. Functional studies showed the JAK2 V617F mutation results in constitutive activation. The later finding of patients undergoing leukemic transformation often had JAK2 V617F negative blast cells suggests that this mutation is not the initiating single-hit event for this neoplasia [23]. First-line therapy in polycythemia vera has been phlebotomy and hydroxyurea. Ruxolitinib, a JAK2 inhibitor, was studied in a cohort of 222 patients with polycythemia vera who had either unacceptable toxicity or inadequate response to hydroxyurea and was found to be effective in 60% of patients and overall was superior to continued standard treatment [24]. In this series, complete hematologic remission was seen in 24% of patients.

An unusual subgroup of lymphoid and myeloid neoplasms is characterized by eosinophilia and translocations in PDGFRA, PDGFRB, or FGFR1 resulting in activation of these tyrosine kinase pathways [25]. Patients who harbor translocations in PDGFRA or PDGFRB respond very well to imatinib, whereas patients with FGFR1 translocations do not [26, 27]. Early treatment of myeloid and lymphoid neoplasms associated with eosinophilia if they have PDGFRA or PDGFRB rearrangements is warranted because progression to a more aggressive disease is likely. Treatment with imatinib typically results in complete remission and prevents progression to leukemic transformation [28]. Conversely, FGFR1-rearranged disease is associated with a high incidence of T cell lymphoblastic lymphoma with progression to acute myeloid leukemia and requires early aggressive combination chemotherapy followed by allogeneic hematopoietic cell transplant [29].

Anaplastic large-cell lymphoma (ALCL) accounts for 10–15% of all childhood lymphoma [30]. The great majority of these tumors harbor a gene rearrangement in the anaplastic lymphoma kinase (ALK) gene. Initial reports showed that translocations involving ALK were also present in nearly half of the cases of inflammatory myofibroblastic tumors, a rare mesenchymal tumor of children and adolescents. Subsequently, next-generation sequencing showed that additional ALK fusions could be detected as well as actionable kinase fusions involving ROS1 and PDGFRB in the majority of cases initially classified as ALK fusion negative [31]. ALK and ROS1 fusions are sensitive to treatment with crizotinib, a drug that was developed for ALK fusion-positive lung cancer [32]. These findings led to a clinical trial using crizotinib involving 26 patients with relapsed or refractory ALK position anaplastic large-cell lymphoma and 14 patients with inoperable or metastatic inflammatory myofibroblastic tumors. The overall response rates were 83–90% for ALCL depending on the dose used and 86% for IMT [33].

In chronic lymphocytic leukemia (CLL), treatment with chemotherapy and immunotherapy has been associated with remissions but recurrences have high-risk disease features and chemotherapy has increased toxicity in elderly patients. The orally administered agent ibrutinib inhibits Bruton tyrosine kinase that mediates signaling through the B cell receptor and thus induces apoptosis [34]. Ibrutinib is proving to be a major advance in the treatment of CLL. Particularly encouraging are the responses to ibrutinib seen in the subgroup of patients with deletion of chromosome 17p13.1 that have a poor response to standard first-line chemoimmunotherapy. For patients with relapsed or refractory CLL, treatment with ibrutinib treatment led to durable responses with a 26-month estimated rate of progression-free survival and an overall survival rate of 83% [35]. In this study, the response rate in patients with a 17p13.1 deletion was 68%, including one complete response. Most recently, an inhibitor of BCL-2, venetoclax, in combination with rituximab, was demonstrated to be more effective than standard therapy with bendamustine plus rituximab in patients with prior treatment [36]. Currently, a phase II trial is ongoing to look at the combination of venetoclax and ibrutinib in refractory or relapsed CLL or in untreated patients with high-risk genetic features (NCT02756897).

Another illustrative example of a remarkably effective precision medication targeted against a rare cancer with a specific gene mutation is vismodegib. This drug is an inhibitor of the smoothened homologue (SMO) gene. Cyclopamine blocks hedgehog pathway signaling by binding to SMO and blocking activation of GLI and other downstream genes [37]. Cyclopamine has poor oral solubility, and its lack of specificity of action results in off-target toxicity [38]. High-throughput screening of a chemical library and subsequent development by medicinal chemistry led to the discovery of vismodegib, a more potent inhibitor with more desirable pharmaceutical properties [39]. Basal cell carcinomas (BCCs) of the skin are typically cured by surgical excision but may on occasion progress into invasive or metastatic cancers. Almost all BCCs harbor genetic aberrations in the sonic hedgehog (SHH) pathway, most commonly a loss of function mutation in the patched homologue 1 (PTCH1) gene which normally acts to suppress activation of SMO. The loss of function mutation releases inhibition of SMO with resultant downstream gene activation. Vismodegib was remarkably effective from the onset [40]. In the initial study of 33 patients, objective responses were seen in 18 patients including 2 with complete responses. Of the other patients, 11 had stable disease, and 4 had progressive disease. A later larger study showed a median overall survival for patients with advanced basal cell carcinoma treated with vismodegib was 33.4 months [41] which compares very favorably to the 8-month median survival time previously reported with systemic chemotherapy [42]. Mutations in PTCH1 are also a common feature of medulloblastomas, a rare malignant tumor of the cerebellum occurring in children or young adults [43]. Relapse or progression after primary therapy is associated with a median survival of less than 6 months and a

2-year survival rate of only 9% [44]. Efficacy of vismodegib in SHH aberrant medulloblastoma was demonstrated in phase II trials but its beneficial effect was negated by the coexistence of mutations in the TP53 tumor suppressor gene. There was also no benefit if SHH mutations were absent [45]. The side effects of this agent are generally well-tolerated but show on target effects of SHH inhibition such as the loss of taste and smell [46].

3.4 Genomics in the Development of Novel Treatment for Rare Cancers

In precision medicine, one can learn from exceptional responders. A patient with bladder cancer enrolled in a phase II clinical trial achieved a durable complete response to treatment with everolimus, a drug that targets mTOR overactivation. Although the study was unsuccessful overall in that it failed to meet its projected endpoint, the investigators did whole genome sequencing (WGS) to discern why that particular patient did so well [47]. Loss of function mutations was identified in TSC1 and in NF2 which in preclinical models have been associated with mTORC1 dependence [48]. Testing of other patients' tumors showed that indeed, mutations in TSC1 were associated with improved response to treatment with everolimus. Other rare mutations are identified in cancers that may expose effective therapeutic opportunities. In non-small-cell lung cancer (NSCLC), an ALK fusion is a fortuitous finding. In ALK-positive NSCLC, first-line targeted treatment with crizotinib is associated with better progression-free survival, greater response rates and less toxicity than is associated with standard chemotherapy [49]. Crizotinib is also more effective than chemotherapy in ALK-positive NSCLC in patients who have previously been treated with a platinum-based regimen [50]. ALK fusions have also been described as low-frequency oncogenic events in other cancers including those of the thyroid, kidney, bladder, and rectum [51–53]. Another uncommon somatic event is the occurrence of fusions of the NTRK gene in approximately 1% of all cancers, but they are targetable driver events [53]. Several NTRK inhibitors are under development and showing encouraging results in multiple tumor types [54].

Precision medicine using genomic analysis of patients' tumor DNA may expose options for off-label use of FDA-approved drugs or clinical trials with novel agents. The routine use of next-generation sequencing in a coordinated fashion in rare cancers is beginning. Initial institutional experiences suggest that actionable variants are commonly found leading to beneficial results with targeted therapy. The University of California San Diego published their results of tumor and plasma circulating tumor DNA sequence analysis and immunohistochemistry for drug targets with 40 patients presenting to their rare tumors clinic [55]. In all 37 (92%) of their patients had a least one target identified that corresponded to FDA-approved drug or an investigational agent. Several commercial and academic laboratories were used so molecular analysis varied. In this series, twelve of their patients did have data available to assess progression in matched treatment compared to time to progression on their most recent prior treatment. These patients had significant improvement on matched therapy. This endpoint was previously reported in the Bisgrove Trial as significantly improved or greater than 1.3-fold longer progression-free survival in 27% of patients receiving drug treatment matched to the identified molecular target in their tumors [56]. The tumor analysis in this study uses immunohistochemistry to predictive markers and gene expression array. While most of these patients had breast or colorectal cancer the study did show benefit, however, in patients with cholangiocarcinoma, mesothelioma, eccrine sweat gland cancer, and a gastrointestinal stromal tumor. Another widely cited report is the retrospective analysis by the Intermountain Healthcare team, showing that for a matched cohort group of 72 patients with a variety of advanced cancers, the average progression-free survival for the group treated with a precision medicine approach was 22.9 weeks compared to 12 weeks for the control group [57]. In a subset analysis where the information was available because patients received their care within their system, the precision medicine group's charges were $4665 per week compared to $5000 per week for the control group of patients. In this study, the testing was done by the in house laboratory using a 96 cancer-related hotspot gene panel. The systematic study of the potential benefits of a more comprehensive molecular analysis using full exon comprehensive gene panels or even whole exome sequencing needs to be done to broadly to assess outcomes and the impact on value, quality, and cost of care.

Given the potential for benefit, consideration is needed for how one uses genomic data to identify a potential drug for treatment. A consensus statement from the Association for Molecular Pathology, the American Society of Clinical Oncology and the College of American Pathologists set standards for the reporting and interpretation of gene sequence variants in cancer [58]. Reporting of somatic variants should be categorized based on their clinical impact with Tier I variants having strong clinical significance. An example is the PML-RARα fusion between promyelocytic leukemia gene and retinoic acid receptor α which is pathognomonic for promyelocytic leukemia [59] and is associated with a good prognosis and response to all-trans retinoic acid or arsenic [60]. Tier II variants are of potential clinical significance. Tier III variants are of unknown clinical significance, and Tier IV variants are benign or likely benign. When the variants are tied to drug response or resistance, these genes would fall stratified based on levels of evidence. The highest level of evidence associates either response or resistance to an FDA-approved drug for an approved indication based on the gene variant. Lower levels of evidence are assigned based on predicted response or resistance based on well-powered studies with consensus from expert in the field, then for therapies based on a biomarker but for different type of tumor than for which the drug is approved. The lowest levels of evidence are assigned to results of small series or case reports and plausible therapeutic import based on preclinical studies [58].

3.5 Basket and Umbrella Trials

Basket and umbrella trials are seeking to clarify the clinical utility of the application of molecular analysis into routine care. As previously explained, patients with rare cancers for which there are no approved drug treatments often lack available clinical trials. Drugs developed to target a mutation in one type of cancer may be found to be effective in the treatment of other cancers that harbor the same mutation. For these reasons, increasingly trials are open to multiple tumor types harboring a particular gene mutation to which the study agent is designed to target. Ideally, patients with rare tumors will be entered into basket trials that are designed to test the efficacy of a drug on tumor harboring a particular mutation. The trials are open to a variety of tumors and test therapeutic agents based on the presence of a relevant mutation or predicted molecular target, irrespective of the tumor histology [61]. Examples of basket trials include the National Cancer Institute Molecular Analysis for Therapy Choice trial (NCI-MATCH) and the American Society of Clinical Oncology Targeted Agent and Profiling Utilization Registry (TAPUR) study. Drugs are assigned based on levels of evidence, and for example, priority for gene to drug matching has been articulated for the NCI-MATCH trial [62, 63]. Pharmaceutical companies including Genentech (My Pathway) and Novartis (Signature) also are sponsoring basket trials. In this way, a series of baskets are included in the trial design each evaluating a particular mutation and corresponding drug that targets that mutation. One may learn whether the drug has any efficacy and whether the effect is context specific [64].

One advantage is that if a treatment is approved in another disease, efficacy in another tumor type may be quickly seen. This was the case for vemurafenib, a BRAF inhibitor, which targets the V600E mutation in BRAF common in melanoma. A basket trial included patients with Erdheim–Chester disease (ECD), a rare slow-growing blood cancer that originates in the bone marrow [65, 66]. ECD is estimated to affect 600–700 patients worldwide. BRAF V600 mutation has been reported in 54% of patients with ECD [67] and treatment with vemurafenib was associated with response rates of 43% in patients with Erdheim–Chester disease or Langerhans cell histiocytosis [66]. This led the US Food and Drug Administration to approve vemurafenib for the treatment of BRAF V600 mutant ECD in 2017. Responses were also seen in other tumors with BRAF mutations including anaplastic thyroid cancer, cholangiocarcinoma, salivary duct carcinoma, anaplastic pleomorphic xanthoastrocytoma, serous ovarian cancer, and a thoracic clear cell sarcoma [66].

The umbrella trial design differs from a basket trial in that umbrella trials focus on patients with a particular tumor type or histology. Patients are assigned to a treatment based on the genomic analysis of their tumor. Multiple treatment arms are available for the tumor histology. This trial design recognizes that all cancers of similar histology are not genomically identical, but rather they may differ in their mutational profile. A successful umbrella trial was the Biomarker-Integrated Approaches of Targeted Therapy for Lung Cancer Elimination or BATTLE trial

[68]. Patients were assigned to one of four different treatment arms based on a required biopsy at the start of the trial. A limitation of the umbrella design, however, is that even for common cancers such as non-small-cell lung cancer, an umbrella trial may fail to accrue sufficient patients with rare mutations in their corresponding arms [69].

With the expanding armamentarium of targeted agents available and underdevelopment, there are more options and greater opportunities to assign patients to clinical trials based on their tumor genomics. A meta-analysis of phase II clinical trials supported this approach by concluding that a precision medicine approach toward selecting trials for patients based on the mutations present in their tumors results in higher median response rates and improved progression-free and overall survival when compared to a non-selective assignment to clinical trials [70]. Moreover, a targeted approach was associated with fewer toxic deaths. Given the difficulty in conducting traditional disease-focused clinical trials for rare cancers, the alternative basket trial approach offers a path forward.

3.6 Genetics to Identify Patients at High Risk for Cancer

Investigators are beginning to demonstrate frequent germline mutations in cancer predisposition genes in patients presenting with apparently sporadic cancers. In a large screening program of 1120 patients with cancer younger than age 20, using either whole genome or whole exome sequence analysis, pathogenic or likely pathogenic mutations were identified in 8.5 of the patients [71]. The most commonly mutated genes were TP53, APC, BRCA, NF1, RB1, and RUNX1. In patients with germline mutations, only 40% had a family history of cancer. Of these, only half had a family history that was consistent with the observed cancer predisposition syndrome. Our team observed that similar findings have been observed in adults with cancer [72].

Datasets from tumor profiling using matched tumor–normal samples to filter for true somatic events and improve variant calls allow researchers to query the burden of unsuspected germline mutations in patients with advanced cancer. In one series from Memorial Sloan Kettering Cancer Center, 12.6% of patients had germline mutations in cancer susceptibility genes [73]. As was seen in the pediatric population, the germline finding was concordant with the patients' known cancer type in less than half of the cases. Additionally in this study, almost all patients had at least one variant of uncertain significance among the 187 curated genes in their panel. Even if one restricts the calls to the cancer gene set endorsed by the American College of Medical Genetics and Genomics (ACMG), 5% of patients had germline mutations. Others have similarly found unsuspected germline mutations when testing patients with advanced cancer [74]. These findings may alert the physician to the need to screen the patient for other cancers or refer family members for genetic testing. It may also inform one regarding potential treatment modalities. Nearly 12% of men with metastatic prostate cancer harbor germline mutations in

DNA repair genes including BRCA1 and BRCA2, ATM, CHEK2 [75]. Men with metastatic prostate cancer and DNA-repair gene mutations may have a favorable response to treatment with poly (ADP-ribose) polymerase (PARP) inhibitors [76] and platinum-based chemotherapy [77].

Knowledge of germline mutations can be used to improve patient care by appropriate screening for tumors, early intervention, and in some cases, preventative treatments. Rare cancers are a feature of the Li-Fraumeni syndrome (LFS). It is a relatively uncommon inherited disorder in which affected individuals have a germline TP53 mutation. These affected individuals are at increased risk for a variety of cancers including soft tissue and bone sarcomas, breast cancer, adrenocortical cancers, and central nervous system cancers including gliomas, neuroblastomas, and choroid plexus carcinomas. Less commonly, these patients may develop lung cancers, leukemias, kidney cancers bladder cancer, esophageal cancer, stomach cancer, thyroid cancers, melanomas, pancreatic or colon cancer [78]. A registry at the National Cancer Institute shows that women with LFS have an approximately 50% chance of developing cancer by age 31 years, and men have a 50% risk by age 46 [79]. Nearly all affected individuals develop cancer by age 70. Many individuals with LFS develop two or more primary cancers over their lifetimes. Several centers, including our own, have instituted periodic rapid whole-body magnetic resonance imaging in order to screen affected LFS individuals harboring germline TP53 mutations for early cancers. At initial screening, the prevalence of detected new primary cancers has been 7–13% [80, 81]. In one series, 34% of patients had abnormalities on initial screen that required further evaluation, and 7% of patients had new primary cancers [82].

Medullary thyroid cancer (MTC) is a tumor of the C cells [83] and accounts for less than 5% of all thyroid cancers and is a familial cancer in approximately 25% of the cases [84]. MTC is a feature of the familial medullary thyroid cancer (FMTC) and the multiple endocrine neoplasia type 2 (MEN2) syndromes. The etiology is an inherited autosomal dominant mutation of the RET proto-oncogene. There is a certainty that patients who inherit the RET mutation will develop MTC [85]. Prophylactic thyroidectomy in childhood prevents the development of this cancer, and the patients can be well-managed by oral thyroid hormone replacement [86]. Prophylactic thyroidectomy based on genetic testing has proven to be a safe and effective method of management of condition. Prior to the discovery of the causative germline mutation in RET, all patients with a family history of medullary thyroid cancer or MEN2 had to undergo biochemical screening tests to measure pentagastrin-stimulated calcitonin levels annually as they had a 50% of harboring the disease. Now, as a result of having genetic testing, unaffected patients need not be screened and those affected can undergo prophylactic surgery [87]. Furthermore, the clinical behavior and aggressiveness of tumors associated with particular mutation are being elucidated. Patients with a germline RET M918T mutation have particularly early-onset tumors, so total thyroidectomy is recommended in the first year of life [87].

Another less certain but notable example of germline mutations predisposing a rare cancer occurs in the hereditary diffuse gastric cancer syndrome (HDGC). This syndrome features diffuse gastric cancer and lobular cancer of the breast. Mutations in the CDH1 gene, encoding epithelial cadherin or E-cadherin (CDH1), are identified in affected members of these kindreds. In a series of 183 index cases who met clinical criteria for HDGC, 31 distinct pathogenic germline mutations in CHD1 were identified in 34 subjects (19%) [88]. The cumulative risk of gastric cancer occurring in CDH1 carriers by the age of 80 was 70% for men and 56% for women. In CDH1 negative patients, an additional 11% of the probands had pathogenic mutations in other known candidate cancer genes including CTNNA1, BRCA2, STK11, SDHB, PRSS1, ATM, MSR1, and PALB2. Members of affected HDGC kindreds who test positive for a pathogenic mutation in CDH1 should strongly consider a prophylactic gastrectomy [89]. This decision, however, is not as straightforward as the case put forth for prophylactic thyroidectomy in MEN2-affected individuals. As noted above, the penetrance of CDH1 for HDGC, although high, is not 100%. The risk of the surgical gastrectomy procedure and the long-term consequences of living without one's stomach are more impactful than living without a thyroid gland. The optimal timing for gastrectomy in unknown but some suggest it should be done by age 20 [90]. Those that choose to delay or forego surgery should undergo frequent endoscopic surveillance with multiple biopsies ideally in experienced centers with established protocols [91]. Affected patients should also be screened for the development of lobular breast cancer with breast MRI. Prophylactic mastectomy is not generally recommended but may be a consideration for some women [89]. An unresolved question centers around the patient who does not have a family history of gastric cancer or lobular breast cancer who undergoes germline panel testing for another reason and is found to have a germline CDH1 coding variant, particularly if the variant does not result in a premature stop codon and a truncated E-cadherin protein [89].

An increasing appreciation for the clinical utility of the identification of cancer-related germline variants for screening and treatment has led to interest in the potential for reporting these variants based on tumor profiling. The most straightforward approach is to assess the germline sequences from assays that due to tumor normal sequencing such as is done by with the groups at Memorial Sloan Kettering with their MSK-IMPACT™ assay or by Ashion®, the Translational Genomics Research Institute's® clinical laboratory. This approach garnered significant interest when the group at Johns Hopkins showed a false positive rate of 31% in reporting of somatic mutations that proved to be in fact germline mutations (after filtering for common germline variants e.g., BRCA1) using a targeted panel and 65% for exome sequencing [74]. Of particular concern is that in many cases, the germline would have been falsely reported as an actionable somatic mutation if a tumor-only approach was used. In this series notably, analysis of the matched normal DNA identified germline alterations in genes associated with cancer predisposition in 3% of patients thought to have sporadic tumors. Leading commercial laboratories including Foundation Medicine and Caris Life Sciences offer solid tumor analysis featuring tumor-only sequencing. The advantage of reporting tumor-only sequencing results is decreased cost as only one reaction is done. Additionally, one does not need to obtain patient's informed consent as one must for germline sequence reporting, and one does not need to ask the patient to undergo genetic counseling. One may suspect a reported variant observed on tumor only sequencing is a germline mutation if it is represented in a high number of sequencing reads-that is having a high variant allele frequency (VAF). Putatively, if VAF is in excess of 50%, one might suspect a heterozygous germline mutation and if 100%, then a homozygous germline variant is likely. When tested, however, this approach was not reliable [92]. Results were affected by tumor content in the sample and loss of heterozygosity. Recently, Foundation Medicine investigators reported a computational algorithm that seeks to identify potential germline variants from tumor-only sequencing [93]. The method depends on at least 10% normal non-tumor cells in the specimen sequenced. The authors reported call rates of 85% and accuracy rates of 95–99% in distinguishing somatic from germline variants in their validation set. This approach, however, has not been verified by other investigators and remains at best an indirect surrogate for direct germline sequence analysis. Tumor-only approaches carry some risk of misclassifying somatic and germline variants, and treating physicians must be aware of this limitation in commonly used commercial tests.

The American College of Medical Genetics and Genomics (ACMG) has published guidelines for reporting of incidental findings in clinical sequencing [94]. Constitutional mutations in a published list of well-curated variants in a list of 56 genes associated with cancer and other diseases should be reported by the testing laboratory to the ordering physician who, in turn, has the responsibility to provide comprehensive counseling to the patient, or in case of children, their parents, or guardian. The ACMG later amended their recommendations to state patients should have the option to opt out of being informed [95]. Updated recommendations referred to secondary findings rather than incidental findings because these genes where intentionally being analyzed [96]. The number of genes that should be reported increased to 59 as a result of additional curation efforts, adding 4 while eliminating one gene from the list. At this point in time, patients with suspected germline mutations in cancer-related genes identified by tumor profiling should be referred to a genetic counselor and offered verification of the germline variant by additional testing.

3.7 Database Efforts

As stated previously for rare cancers, finding an expert with experience treating the disease may be difficult for patients. Large central databases detailing epidemiology, clinical practices, treatment modalities, and outcomes offer the opportunity for collective learning and experience that translate into benefits for patients. Furthermore, annotation of genomic changes observed with treatment outcomes can provide real-time improvement in the curation of genomic aberrations. Many patients receive treatment with targeted drugs that may have been approved for another cancer, based on detection of a genomic mutation seen on next-generation sequence analysis. If this occurs outside of a clinical trial, in the absence of a database designed to collect outcome data, this experience with a particular patient with a tumor harboring a particular patient receiving a drug is lost and does not benefit other patients. Data-sharing efforts for rare cancers are beginning. The National Cancer Institute recently funded the Kids First Pediatric Data Resource Center designed to discover causes of pediatric cancers and birth defects through the use of WGS and big data. There are many disease-focused databases and registries, as well as those devoted to a group of rare cancers, including the Rare Cancer Genetics Registry. Advocacy groups have participated to develop registries to include genomic profiles of particular cancers. For example, the Multiple Myeloma Research Foundation launched their effort called the CoMMpass (Relating Clinical Outcomes in MM to Personal Assessment of Genetic Profile). The CoMMpass study includes over 1000 patients with newly diagnosed treatment naïve multiple myeloma from more than 100 sites in the USA, Canada, and the European Union. Researchers are following the clinical course of patients and collecting sequential tissue biopsies in order to learn how a patient's molecular profile may affect his or her clinical progression and individual response to treatment. Commercial sequencing companies who do tumor cancer-related gene panel testing have registries to collect clinical data and outcomes related to patients whose tumors they have tested. Examples include Foundation Medicine's Foundation CORE™ and Caris Life Sciences' Precision Oncology Alliance™. A promising result of these efforts could be that an oncologist could query the database to learn from collective experience treating a rare cancer harboring a targetable gene mutation.

3.8 Future Advances in Genomics

The next advances in the understanding of the genomics of rare cancers will come from more extensive molecular analysis, decreasing costs, improved analytics, and access to a greater repertoire of targeted agents. The current most commonly used genomic profiling test employs large gene panels consisting of approximately 400–600 cancer-relevant genes. Testing may or may not employ germline analysis for determination of true somatic variants or increased accuracy of the calling of copy number alterations. Because cancer development may be influenced by oncogenic genomic events in noncoding regions of the genome or due to epigenetic alterations, important information would be learned by WGS and RNA sequencing as well determination of the methylome (our unpublished data). These sequencing technologies are available, but these tests are generally not yet CLIA certified and thus not available for the care of patients. As a result of large-scale sequencing research projects such as The Cancer Genome Atlas and the International Cancer Genome Consortium, researchers are turning toward the investigation of rare mutated driver genes and the study of rare variants of driver genes [97, 98]. While there exists now an extensive accumulation of available exome sequencing data, there is a limited amount of information regarding somatic oncogenic mutations in noncoding regions of the human genome. WGS would elucidate the role of aberrations in introns, promoters, regulatory elements, noncoding functional RNA, and mitochondrial genes [99]. WGS may also elucidate the etiology of some cancers by demonstrating, for example, viral DNA in the sequence of a patient's tumor. WGS analysis of liver cancer has detected integration of the hepatitis B virus into the regions of the TERT and MLL4 genes [100, 101]. Similarly, investigators have shown human papillomavirus genomic sequences integrated into the genome of cervical cancer cells [102]. Mutations in noncoding DNA have been linked to disease [103]. Mutations in expression quantity trait loci (eQTLs) altering expression of known cancer genes have been shown in melanoma, lung, colon, and many other cancers by studying the WGS of paired normal and tumor tissues in 930 patients across 22 types of cancer from TCGA [104]. These findings may allow one to identify therapeutic targets in patients for whom standard limited gene panel testing does not [105].

Improved analytics of multiple datasets such as whole genome sequencing, methylome, RNA sequencing, and proteomics, in other words, a multi-omic analysis of tumors will also lead to a greater understanding of the pathogenesis of various rare cancers and one to prioritize among potential therapeutic targets. An assessment of RNA can show that mutations may not be expressed or conversely a mutation may be dominantly expressed and therefore may present a better therapeutic target. Methylation or other epigenomic changes may affect gene expression. Mutations in noncoding regions of genes have been shown to alter gene expression [104]. A greater understanding of the functional consequence of a set of mutations requires one to move beyond a linear pathway model to a network model. Combinations of mutations may interact to cause cancer or expose therapeutic vulnerabilities. Different combinations of genomic events may be associated with a cancer etiology forming a mutational signature [106]. In the case of a rare cancer, one might be able to map a genome to one of the identified signatures seen in tumors harboring inactivation mutations in BRCA even in the absence of a BRCA mutation, or BRCAness. One might surmise then that treatments including PARP inhibitors that show efficacy in tumors harboring a BRCAness signature might then also work in such a rare cancer having the same signature [107, 108]. Enhanced resources to better define druggable genes and define drug–gene interactions to support drug development and patient care are being developed [109]. These need to include better paradigms for matching drugs to multiple pathways, and mutational signatures will move beyond the current simplistic single-gene mutation to corresponding drug model. These approaches may include metronomic dosing [110] or synthetic lethal considerations as well [111, 112].

Molecular profiles from WGS and RNA sequencing may better predict response to immunotherapy as well. Current predictive biomarkers including total mutational burden on gene panels and PDL1 immunostaining are suboptimal. Somatic mutations have been identified that would appear to confer resistance to immunotherapy, including in APLNR and the Janus Kinases [113]. Mapping mutated sequences derived from transcriptomes to known HLA-specific MHC binding motifs might also predict the immunogenicity of a particular tumor [114]. Identification of the burden and character of such neoantigens in individual tumors will one day allow for more effective tumor vaccines and immunotherapy [115, 116].

3.9 Hurdles to Be Overcome

Barriers to widespread adoption of genomic analysis remain. One must demonstrate clinical utility of the precision medicine approach to treating patients with cancer. In other words, do the findings of genomic analysis alter treatment plans devised by physicians and do the patients derive a benefit as a result? While costs are declining for sequencing, payers have not agreed on criteria for testing [117]. The evidence for clinical utility is accumulating which will prompt payers to reimburse genomic testing and just as importantly, pay for the targeted treatments prescribed and the perception that costs will increase may not be true. An early report notably showed no increase in cost associated with treatment based on molecular profiling as well as a significantly prolonged progression-free survival [57]. The rapid development of complex testing and its interpretation vexes many physicians who might have a fairly rudimentary knowledge of genomics and little understanding of sequencing technologies. Testing platforms vary with different coverage of genes, such as entire exon coverage or hotspot testing, as well as differences in sensitivity or false positive rates. Hence, the selection of appropriate genomic tests based on advantages and limitations of the particular testing method may result in failures to identify or correctly interpret genomic aberrations. Similarly, payers may not be sufficiently informed to understand differences in tests. Multi-disciplinary molecular tumor boards established by institutions are one way to assist in patient management (see sidebar). Such molecular tumor boards would include the traditional medical specialties but would also include molecular pathologists, clinical genomics scientists, and research pharmacists. Case presentations would highlight the results of genomic testing and the therapeutic implications to assist doctors in developing treatment plans. Additionally, hospitals and professional societies must develop continuing education programs for physicians and other healthcare providers. Lastly, there are potential legal liabilities associated with either the failure to order genetic testing when appropriate or with the incorrect interpretation of test results [118, 119].

3.10 Summary

Application of precision medicine to the treatment of rare cancers in clinical practice at present requires a dedicated effort. A team approach of physicians is needed to include not only medical oncologists, surgeons, radiation oncologists, radiologists, and pathologists but also experts in molecular genetics, variant scientists, genetic counselors, pharmacologists as well as billing and insurance specialists. There is little doubt that genomics is the future and for many rare cancers, the future is now. The pace of discovery and progress driven by more in-depth sequencing and integrative analysis of multi-omic tumor profiling will accelerate. Even common cancers may have rare variants that should be identified as in non-small-cell lung cancers that harbor an EML4-ALK gene rearrangement which impacts greatly on treatment decisions and outcome. Rare cancers may share genetic aberrations with more common and better-studied cancers so that treatments developed for more common cases, as was the case for BRAF mutant melanoma, may be repurposed to the treatment patients with the rare cancer. There remains a need for more therapeutic agents to exploit the identified targets. Genomics presents a path forward to overcome many of the impairments to the development of more effective and less toxic treatments for patients with rare cancers.

Acknowledgements The author wishes to express his gratitude to Sourat Darabi, Ph.D. for her editorial review and assistance with creation of tables.

A Case Report from a Rare Cancer Precision Medicine Tumor Board

Sourat Darabi
Hoag Family Cancer CenterNewport Beach, CA 92603, USA

A 41-year-old woman with no family history of cancer was diagnosed with moderately differentiated serous adenocarcinoma of ovary. She underwent a radical hysterectomy with tumor debulking, followed by chemotherapy with carboplatin and paclitaxel (paclitaxel/carboplatin). The patient later developed recurrence of her cancer and was treated with carboplatin heated intraperitoneal chemotherapy.

A comprehensive somatic 592-gene sequencing panel tumor profiling (Caris Life Sciences, Phoenix AZ) was performed on the patient's tumor. The results showed no microsatellite instability (MSI), proficient mismatch repair by immunohistochemistry, estrogen receptor positive immunostaining, and a pathogenic variant in *BRCA1* gene, p.K1254fs (Table 3.4). The gene encodes BRCA1 protein that is involved in DNA damage repair. Pathogenic variants in this gene have been associated with increased risk of several types of cancer, including hereditary breast and ovarian cancer. Somatic *BRCA1* mutations are illustrated in Fig. 3.1 with 63 truncating mutations from The Cancer Genome Atlas (TCGA) [120]. The specific loss of function *BRCA1* mutation identified in this patient's tumor could be a potential germline variant, so referral to a genetic counselor and germline testing is recommended. Individuals who harbor germline mutations in *BRCA1* are at increased risk for cancers of the breast, ovary, prostate, pancreas, and possibly colon and other cancers.

Table 3.4 Highlights of patient's tumor profiling results

Biomarker	Method	Results
Total mutational load	NGS	Low → 6 mutations/Mb
MSI	NGS	Stable
Mismatch repair status	Presence or absence of MLH1, MSH2, MSH6, and PMS2 proteins by IHC	Proficient
ER	IHC	Positive
ERCC1	IHC	Negative
TUBB3	IHC	Negative
BRCA1	**NGS**	**Pathogenic mutation → p.K1254fs**
BRCA2	NGS	No pathogenic mutation identified
ATM	NGS	No pathogenic mutation identified

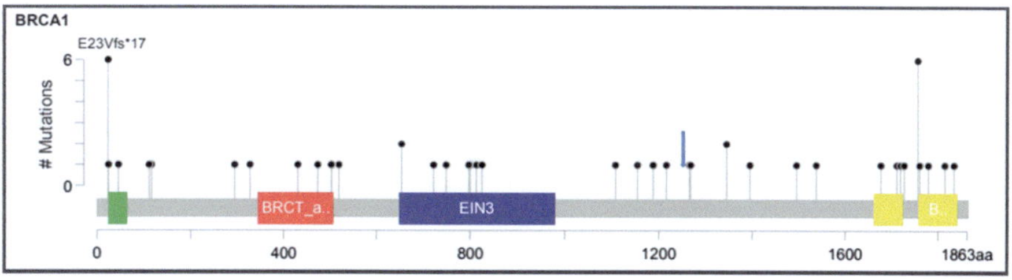

Fig. 3.1 Spectrum of reported *BRCA1* truncating mutations in cBIo portal [120]. The blue arrow indicates the approximate region where the p.K1254fs variant identified in this patient occurred. The horizontal axis displays the identified truncating mutations in 1754 samples (from three different TCGA datasets), and the boxes are BRCA1 domains. The vertical axis indicates the frequency of the identified variants

Ovarian cancer is estimated to be responsible for approximately 2.3% of all cancer deaths in the USA in 2018 [121]. Approximately half of tumors in patients with high-grade serous ovarian cancer have homologous recombination repair deficiencies, which are most often caused by pathogenic mutations in the *BRCA1* or *BRCA2* genes [122]. Germline mutations in *BRCA1* and *BRCA2* are also frequently seen in patients with high-grade serous ovarian cancer [123]. Homologous recombination repair deficiencies lead to insufficient double-stranded DNA breaks repair [124]. Poly (ADP-ribose) polymerase (PARP) enzymes repair single-stranded DNA breaks with a mechanism called base excision repair (BER). Inhibition of PARP in tumors with homologous recombination repair deficiencies causes inaccurate DNA repair leading to cell cycle arrest and apoptosis, as it is illustrated in Fig. 3.2 [124, 125].

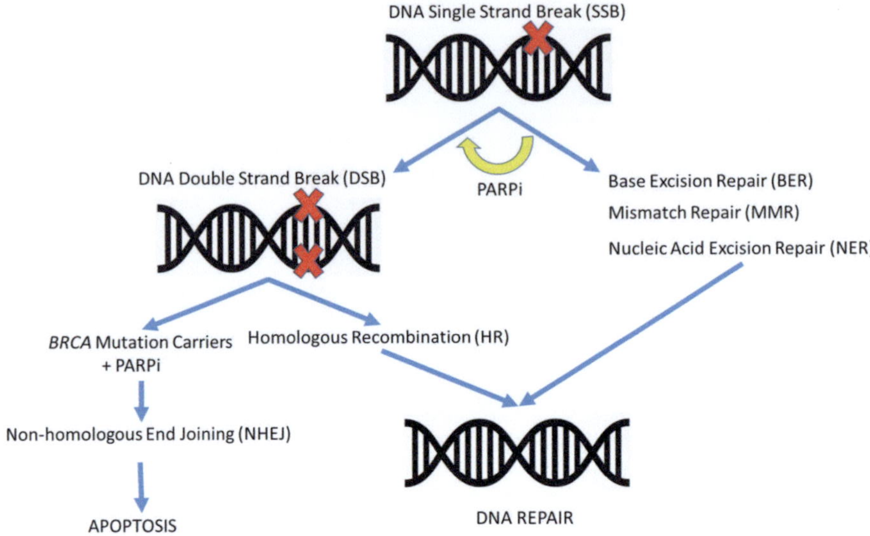

Fig. 3.2 Molecular mechanism of PARP inhibition (PARPi). Single-strand break (SSB) DNA repair is carried by mismatch repair (MMR), nucleic acid excision repair (NER), and base excision repair (BER) mechanisms. PARPi impairs BER, so an SSB becomes a double-strand break (DSB). Non-homologous end joining (NHEJ) and homologous recombination (HR) mechanisms are involved in DSB repair. When PARP inhibition occurs in a patient who has a homologous recombination repair (HR) deficiency, due to a *BRCA* mutation, then a DSB cannot be repaired and cell death or apoptosis results [125, 131]

Olaparib is a PARP inhibitor and is approved to treat patients with ovarian cancer that harbor *BRCA1* or *BRCA2* mutations. Patients with platinum-sensitive high-grade serous ovarian cancer and somatic or germline *BRCA1/2* mutations benefit similarly from olaparib treatment; progression-free survival (PFS) is illustrated in Fig. 3.3 [123]. A combination of olaparib with chemotherapy (carboplatin and paclitaxel) in patients with an advanced breast and ovarian cancer showed significant results [126–128]. There are other PARP inhibitors on the market such as niraparib and rucaparib. In a randomized, placebo control phase III clinical trial, niraparib increased PFS in patients with recurrent ovarian cancer [129]. The AREL3 study, a randomized, placebo control double-blinded phase III study, showed rucaparib in patients with platinum-sensitive ovarian cancer improved PFS [130].

Thus, the results from tumor profiling, along with the outcomes from several clinical trials, provide valuable information to help clinicians offer a personalized precision care for this patient. If the BRCA1 mutation proves to be a germline mutation, then family members should be referred for genetic counseling as well.

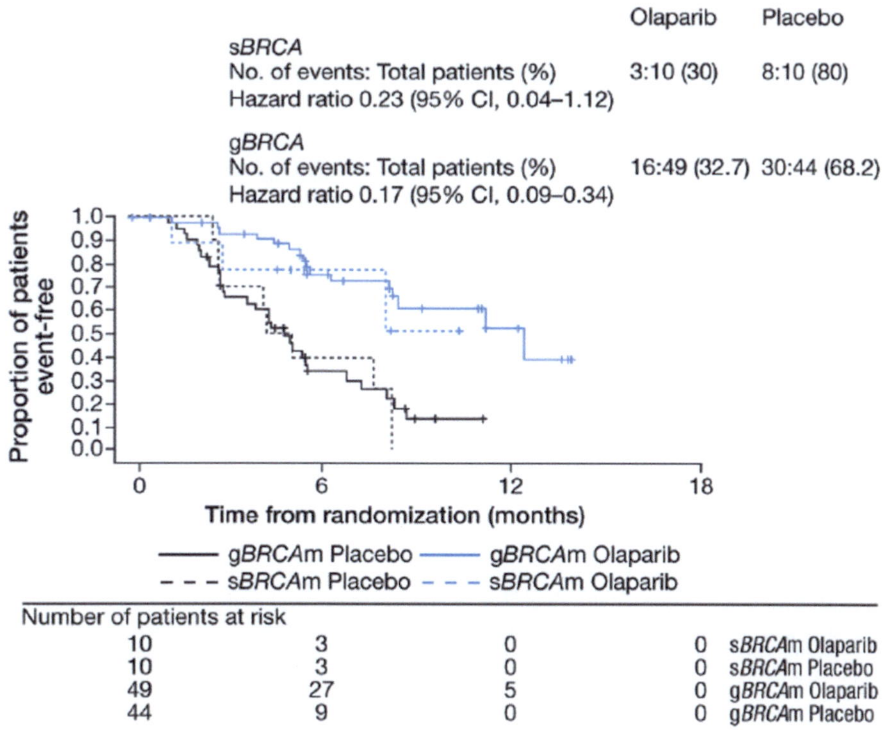

Fig. 3.3 Progression-free survival of patients with *BRCA1/2* somatic mutations compared with the ones with germline mutations treated with olaparib or placebo. The blue line is the group treated with olaparib, and the black line is for the placebo group (from Dougherty [123])

Take Home Points

(1) Referral to genetic counseling for germline testing is recommended based on the tumor profiling results;

(2) Consider PARPi to treat the patient according to the data, showing the efficacy of PARPi in patients with BRCA mutations.

References

1. Pillai RK, Jayasree K (2017) Rare cancers: challenges & issues. Indian J Med Res 145:17–27
2. Greenlee RT, Goodman MT, Lynch CF et al (2010) The occurrence of rare cancers in U.S. adults, 1995–2004. Public Health Rep 125:28–43
3. Tucker TC, Howe HL (2001) Measuring the quality of population-based cancer registries: the NAACR perspective. J Reg Manag 28:41–44

4. Trice Loggers E, Prigerson HG (2014) The end-of-life experience of patients with rare cancers and their caregivers. Rare Tumors 6:24–27
5. DeSantis CE, Kramer JL, Jemal A (2017) The burden of rare cancers in the United States. CA Cancer J Clin 67:261–272
6. Gatta C, Ciccolallo L, Kunkler I et al (2006) Survival from rare cancer in adults: a population-based study. Lancet Oncol 7:132–140
7. Fassnacht M, Terzolo M, Allolio B et al (2012) Combination chemotherapy in advanced adrenocortical carcinoma. N Engl J Med 366:2189–2197
8. Smith SM, Coleman J, Bridge JA, Iwenofu OH (2015) Molecular diagnostics in soft tissue sarcoma and gastrointestinal stromal tumors. J Surg Oncol 111:520–531
9. Schaefer IM, Cote GM, Hornick JL (2017) Contemporary sarcoma diagnosis, genetics, and genomics. J Clin Oncol 36:101–110
10. Fletcher CDM, Unni KK, Mertens F (2002) WHO classification of tumours of soft tissue and bone, 3rd edn. IARC Press, Lyon, France
11. Fletcher CD, Hogendoorn P, Mertens F, Bridge J (2013) WHO classification of tumours of soft tissue and bone, 4th edn. IARC Press, Lyon, France
12. Italiano A, Di Mauro I, Rapp J et al (2016) Clinical effect of molecular methods in sarcoma diagnosis (GENSARC): a prospective, multicenter, observational study. Lancet Oncol 17:532–538
13. Joensuu H, Wardelmann E, Sihto H et al (2017) Effect of KIT and PDGFRA mutations on survival in patients with gastrointestinal stromal tumors treated with adjuvant imatinib: an exploratory analysis of a randomized clinical trial. JAMA Oncol 3:602–609
14. Gunawan B, Bergmann F, Höer J et al (2002) Biological and clinical significance of cytogenetic abnormalities in low-risk and high-risk gastrointestinal stromal tumors. Hum Pathol 33:316–321
15. Raut CP et al (2006) Surgical management of advanced gastrointestinal stromal tumors after treatment with targeted systemic therapy using kinase inhibitors. J Clin Oncol 24:2325–2331
16. Gorthi A, Romero JC, Loranc E et al (2018) EWS-FL11 increases transcription to cause R-loops and block BRCA repair in Ewing sarcoma. Nature, 87–391
17. Ostrom QT, Gittleman H, Liao P et al (2017) CBTRUS statistical report: primary brain and other central nervous system tumors diagnosed in the United States in 2010–2014. Neuro-Oncology 19(supp 5): v1–v88
18. Ohgaki H, Kleihues P (2007) Genetic pathways to primary and secondary glioblastoma. Am J Pathol 170:1445–1453
19. Parsons DW, Jones S, Zhang X et al (2008) An integrated genomic analysis of human glioblastoma multiforme. Science 321:1807–1812
20. Yan H, Parsons W, Jim G et al (2009) IHD1 and IDH2 mutations in gliomas. N Engl J Med 360:765–773
21. Baxter EJ, Scott LM, Campbell PJ et al (2005) Cancer genome project: acquired mutation of the tyrosine kinase JAK2 in human myeloproliferative disorders. Lancet 365:1054–1061
22. Tam CS, Nussenzveig RM, Popat U et al (2008) The natural history and treatment outcome of blast phase BCR-ABL- myeloproliferative neoplasms. Blood 112:1628–1637
23. Theocharides A, Boissinot M, Girodon F et al (2007) Leukemic blasts in transformed JAK2-V617F-positive myeloproliferative disorders are frequently negative for the JAK2-V617F mutation. Blood 110:375–379
24. Vannucchi A, Kiladjian JJ, Griesshammer M et al (2015) Ruxolitinib versus standard therapy for the treatment of polycythemia vera. N Engl J Med 372:426–435
25. Vega F, Medeiros LJ, Bueso-Ramos CE et al (2015) Hematolymphoid neoplasms associated with rearrangements of PDGFRA, PDGFRB, and FGFR1. Am J Clin Path 144:377–392
26. Apperley JF, Gardembs M, Melo JC et al (2002) Response to imatinib mesylate in patients with chronic myeloproliferative diseases with rearrangements of the platelet-derived growth factor receptor beta. N Engl J Med 347:481–487

27. Baccarani M, Cilloni D, Rondoni M et al (2007) The efficacy of imatinib mesylate in patients with FIP1L1-PDGFRalpha-positive hypereosinophilic syndrome. Results of a multicenter prospective study. Haematologica 92:1173–1179
28. Klion AD, Robyn J, Akin C et al (2004) Molecular remission and reversal of myelofibrosis in response to imatinib mesylate treatment in patients with the myeloproliferative variant of hypereosinophilic syndrome. Blood 15:473–478
29. Tefferi A, Gotlib J, Pardanani A (2010) Hypereosinophilic syndrome and clonal eosinophilia: point-of-care diagnostic algorithm and treatment update. Mayo Clin Proc 85:158–164
30. Wright D, McKeever P, Carter R (1997) Childhood non-Hodgkin lymphomas in the United Kingdom: findings from the UK Children's Cancer Study Group. J Clin Pathol 50:128–134
31. Lovly CM, Gupta A, Lipson D et al (2014) Inflammatory myofibroblastic tumors harbor multiple potentially actionable kinase fusions. Cancer Discov 4:889–895
32. Kwak EL, Bang YJ, Camidge Dr et al (2010) Anaplastic lymphoma kinase inhibition in non-small-cell lung cancer. N Engl J Med 363:1693–1703
33. Mossé YP, Voss SD, Lim MS et al (2017) Targeting ALK with crizotinib in pediatric anaplastic large cell lymphoma and inflammatory myofibroblastic tumor: A Children's Oncology Group Study. J Clin Oncol 35:3215–3221
34. Maddocks K, Jones JA (2016) Bruton tyrosine kinase inhibition in chronic lymphocytic leukemia. Semin Oncol 43:251–259
35. Byrd MC, Furman RR, Coutre SE et al (2013) Targeting BTK with ibrutinib in relapsed chronic lymphocytic leukemia. N Engl J Med 369:32–42
36. Seymour JF, Kipps TJ, Eichhorst B et al (2018) Venetoclax–rituximab in relapsed or refractory chronic lymphocytic leukemia. N Engl J Med 378:1107–1120
37. Chen JK, Taipale J, Cooper MK et al (2002) Inhibition of hedgehog signaling by direct binding of cyclopamine to smoothened. Genes Dev 16:2743–2748
38. Tremblay MR, Nevalainen M, Nair SJ et al (2008) Semisynthetic cyclopamine analogues as potent and orally bioavailable hedgehog pathway antagonists. J Med Chem 51:6646–6649
39. Gould SE, Low JA, Marsters JC Jr et al (2014) Discovery and preclinical development of vismodegib. Expert Opin Drug Discov 9:969–984
40. Von Hoff DD, LoRusso PM, Rudin CM et al (2009) Inhibition of the hedgehog pathway in advanced basal-cell carcinoma. N Engl J Med 361:1164–1172
41. Sekulic A, Migden MR, Basset-Sequin N et al (2017) Long-term safety and efficacy of vismodegib in patients with advanced basal cell carcinoma: final update of the pivotal ERIVANCE BCC study. BMC Cancer 17:332–341
42. Pfeiffer P, Hansen RO, Rose C (1990) Systemic cytotoxic therapy of basal cell carcinoma: a review of the literature. Eur J Cancer 26:73–77
43. Raffel C, Jenkins RB, Frederick L et al (1997) Sporadic medulloblastomas contain PTCH mutations. Cancer Res 57:842–845
44. Zeltzer PM, Boyett JM, Finlay JL et al (1999) Metastasis stage, adjuvant treatment, and residual tumor are prognostic factors for medulloblastoma in children: conclusions From the Children's Cancer Group 921 randomized phase III study 17:832–845
45. Robinson GW, Orr BA, Wu G et al (2015) Vismodegib exerts targeted efficacy against recurrent sonic hedgehog-subgroup medulloblastoma: Results from phase II pediatric brain tumor consortium studies PBTC-025B and PBTC-032. J Clin Oncol 33:2646–2654
46. Henkin RI, Hosein S, Stateman WA, Knoppel AB (2016) Sonic Hedgehog in nasal mucous is a biomarker for smell loss in patients with hyposmia. Cell Mol Med 2:1–5
47. Iyer G, Hanrahan AJ, Milowsky MI et al (2012) Genome sequencing identifies a basis for everolimus sensitivity. Science 338:221–223
48. López-Lago MA, Okada T, Murillo MM et al (2009) Loss of the tumor suppressor gene NF2, encoding merlin, constitutively activates integrin-dependent mTORC1 signaling. Mol Cell Biol 29(15):4235–49

49. Solomon BJ, Mok T, Kim D-W et al (2014) First-Line crizotinib versus chemotherapy in ALK-positive lung cancer. N Engl J Med 371:2167–2177
50. Shaw AT, Kim DW, Nakagawa K et al (2013) Crizotinib versus chemotherapy in advanced ALK-positive lung cancer. N Engl J Med 368:2385–2394
51. Demeure MJ, Aziz M, Rosenberg R, Gurley SD, Bussey KJ, Carpten JD (2014) Whole-genome sequencing of an aggressive BRAF wild-type papillary thyroid cancer identified EML4-ALK translocation as a therapeutic target. World J Surg 38:1296–1305
52. Kelly LM, Barila G, Liu P et al (2014) Identification of the transforming STRN-ALK fusion as a potential therapeutic target in the aggressive forms of thyroid cancer. Proc Natl Acad Sci 111:4233–4238
53. Stransky N, Cerami E, Schalm S, Kim JL, Lengauer C (2014) The landscape of kinase fusions in cancer. Nature Commun 5:4846. https://doi.org/10.1038/ncomms5846
54. Amatu A, Sartore-Bianchi A, Siena S (2016) NTRK gene fusions as novel targets of cancer therapy across multiple tumour types. ESMO Open.1:e000023. eCollection 2016
55. Kato S, Kurasaki K, Ikeda S, Kurzrock R (2017) Rare Tumor Clinic: The University of California San Diego Moores Cancer Center experience with precision medicine approach. Oncologist 22:1–8
56. Von Hoff DD, Stephenson JJ Jr, Rosen P et al (2010) Pilot study using molecular profiling of patients' tumors to find potential targets and select treatments for their refractory cancers. J Clin Oncol 28:4877–4883
57. Haslem DS, Van Norman SB, Fulde G et al (2017) A retrospective analysis of precision medicine outcomes in patients with advanced cancer reveals improved progression-free survival without increased health care costs. J Oncol Pract 13:108–119
58. Li MM, Datto M, Duncavage EJ et al (2017) standards and guidelines for the interpretation and reporting of sequence variants in cancer: a joint consensus recommendation of the Association for Molecular Pathology, American Society of Clinical Oncology, and College of American Pathologists. J Mol Diagn. 19:4–23
59. Rowley JD, Golomb HM, Dougherty C (1977) 15/17 translocation, a consistent chromosomal change in acute promyelocytic leukaemia. Lancet 309:549–550
60. Wang YZ, Chen Z (2008) Acute promyelocytic leukemia: from highly fatal to highly curable. Blood 111:2505–2515
61. Redig AJ, Jänne PA (2015) Basket trials and the evolution of clinical trial design in an era of genomic medicine. J Clin Oncol 33:975–977
62. Dangi-Garimella S (2017) Innovative approach to precision medicine trial: NCI-MATCH and Beat AML. Am J Manag Care 23:sp32–sp33
63. Conley BA, Chen AP, O'Dwyer PJ et al (2016) NCI-MATCH (Molecular Analysis for Therapy Choice): a national signal finding trial. J Clin Oncol 34:15_suppl, TPS2606
64. Cunanan KM, Gonen M, Shen R et al (2017) Basket trials in oncology: a trade-off between complexity and efficiency. J Clin Oncol 35:271–275
65. Diamond EL, Subbiah B, Lockhart AC et al (2018) Vemurafenib for BRAF V600–mutant Erdheim-Chester disease and Langerhans cell histiocytosis: Analysis of data from the histology-independent, phase 2, open-label VE-BASKET study. JAMA Oncol 4:384–388
66. Hyman DM, Puzanov I, Subbiah C et al (2015) Vemurafenib in multiple nonmelanoma cancers with BRAF V600 mutations. N Engl J Med 373:726–736
67. Haroche J, Charlotte F, Arnaud L et al (2012) High prevalence of BRAF V600E mutations in Erdheim-Chester disease but not in other non-Langerhans cell histiocytoses. Blood 120:2700–2703
68. Kim ES, Herbst RS, Wistuba II et al (2011) The BATTLE trial: personalizing therapy for lung cancer. Cancer Discov 1:44–53
69. Lopez-Chavez A, Thomas A, Rajan A et al (2015) Molecular profiling and targeted therapy for advanced thoracic malignancies: a biomarker-derived, multiarm, multihistology phase II basket trial. J Clin Oncol 33(9):1000–1007

70. Schwaederle M, Zhao M, Lee JJ et al (2015) Impact of precision medicine in diverse cancers: a meta-analysis of phase II clinical trials. J Clin Oncol 33:3817–3825
71. Zhang J, Walsh MF, Wu G et al (2015) Germline mutations in predisposition genes in pediatric cancer. N Engl J Med 373:2336–2346
72. Krishnan S, Basu G, Gonzalez-Malerva L et al (2016) Germline findings in targeted tumor sequencing using matched normal DNA. Cancer Res 76(14 Suppl), Abstract nr 4493
73. Schrader KA, Cheng DT, Joseph V et al (2016) Germline variants in targeted tumor sequencing using matched normal DNA. JAMA Oncol 2:104–111
74. Jones S, Anagnostou V, Lytle K et al (2015) Personalized genomic analyses for cancer mutation discovery and interpretation. Sci Transl Med 7(283):283ra53. https://doi.org/10.1126/scitranslmed.aaa7161
75. Pritchard CC, Mateo J, Walsh MF et al (2016) Inherited DNA-repair gene mutations in men with metastatic prostate cancer. N Engl J Med 375:443–453
76. Mateo J, Carreira S, Sandhu S et al (2015) DNA-repair defects and olaparib in metastatic prostate cancer. N Engl J Med 373:1697–1708
77. Cheng HH, Pritchard CC, Boyd T, Nelson PS, Montgomery B (2016) Biallelic inactivation of BRCA2 in platinum-sensitive metastatic castration-resistant prostate cancer. Eur Urol 69:992–995
78. Hisada M, Garber JE, Fung CY, Fraumeni JF Jr, Li FP (1998) Multiple primary cancers in families with Li-Fraumeni syndrome. J Natl Cancer Inst 90:606–611
79. Mai PL, Best AF, Peters JA et al (2016) Risks of first and subsequent cancers among TP53 mutation carriers in the national cancer institute Li-Fraumeni syndrome cohort. Cancer 122:3673–3681
80. Ballinger ML, Best A, Pai ML et al (2017) Baseline surveillance in Li-Faumeni syndrome using whole-body magnetic resonance imaging: a meta-analysis. JAMA Oncol 3:1634
81. Bojadzieva J, Amini B, Day SF et al (2018) Whole body magnetic resonance imaging (WB-MRI) and brain MRI baseline surveillance in TP53 germline mutation carriers: experience from the Li-Fraumeni syndrome education and early detection (LEAD) clinic. Fam Cancer. 17:287–294
82. Pai ML, Kincha PP, Toud JT et al (2017) Prevalence of cancer at baseline screening in the national cancer institute Li-Fraumeni syndrome cohort. JAMA Oncol 3:1640
83. Williams ED (1966) Histogenesis of medullary carcinoma of the thyroid. J Clin Pathol 19:114–118
84. Al-Rawi M, Wheeler MH (2006) Medullary thyroid cancer: update and present management controversies. Ann R Coll Surg Engl 88:433–438
85. Wells SA Jr, Chi DD, Toshima K et al (1994) Predictive DNA testing and prophylactic thyroidectomy in patients at risk for Multiple Endocrine Neoplasia Type 2A. Ann Surg 220:237–250
86. Wells SA Jr, Skinner MA (1998) Prophylactic thyroidectomy, based on direct genetic testing, in patients at risk for the multiple endocrine neoplasia type 2 syndromes. Exp Clin Endocrinol Diabetes 106:29–34
87. Wells SA Jr, Asa SL, Dralle H et al (2015) Revised American Thyroid Association guidelines for the management of medullary thyroid carcinoma. Thyroid 25:567–610
88. Hansford S, Kaurah P, Li-Chang H et al (2015) Hereditary diffuse gastric cancer syndrome: CDH1 mutations and beyond. JAMA Oncol 1:23–32
89. van der Post RS, Vogelaar IP, Carneiro F et al (2015) Hereditary diffuse gastric cancer: updated clinical guidelines with an emphasis on germline CDH1 mutation carriers. J Med Genet 52:361–74
90. Blair V, Martin I, Shaw D et al (2006) Hereditary diffuse gastric cancer: diagnosis and management. Clin Gastroenterol Hepatol 4(3):262–75
91. Fitzgerald RC, Hardwick R, Huntsman D et al (2010) Hereditary diffuse gastric cancer: updated consensus guidelines for clinical management and directions for future research. J Med Genet 47:436–444

92. Montgomery ND, Selitsky SR, Patel NM et al (2018) Identification of germline variants in tumor Genomic sequencing analysis. J Mol Diagn 20:123–125
93. Sun JX, He Y, Sanford E et al (2018 Feb 7) A computational approach to distinguish somatic vs. germline origin of genomic alterations from deep sequencing of cancer specimens without a matched normal. PLOS Comput Biol. https://doi.org/10.1371/journal.pcbi.1005965
94. Green RC, Berg JS, Grody WW et al (2013) ACMG recommendations for reporting of incidental findings in clinical exome and genome sequencing. Genet Med 15:565–574
95. ACMG Board of Directors (2015) ACMG policy statement: updated recommendations regarding analysis and reporting of secondary findings in clinical genome-scale sequencing. Genet Med 17:68–69
96. Kalia SS, Adelman K, Bale SJ et al (2017) Recommendations for reporting of secondary findings in clinical exome and genome sequencing, 2016 update (ACMG SF v2.0): a policy statement of the American College of Medical Genetics and Genomics. Genet Med 19:249–255
97. Garraway LA, Lander ES (2013) Lessons from the cancer genome. Cell 153:17–37
98. Leiserson MD, Vandin F, Wu H et al (2015) Pan-cancer network analysis identifies combinations of rare somatic mutations across pathways and protein complexes. Nat Genet 47:106–114
99. Nakagawa H, Fujita M (2018) Whole genome sequencing analysis for cancer genomics and precision medicine. Cancer Sci 109:513–522
100. Fujimoto A, Furuta M, Totoki Y et al (2016) Whole genome mutational landscape and characterization of non-coding and structural mutations in liver cancer. Nat Genet 48:500–509
101. Sung WK, Zheng H, Li S et al (2012) Genome-wide survery of recurrent HBV integration in hepatocellular carcinoma. Nat Genet 44:765–769
102. Ojesina AI, Lichtenstein L, Freeman SS et al (2014) Landscape of genomic alterations in cervical carcinomas. Nature 506:371–375
103. Tewhey R, Kotliar D, Park DS et al (2016) Direct identification of hundreds of expression-modifying variants using a multiplexed reporter assay. Cell 165:1519–1529
104. Zhang W, Bojorquez-Gomez A, Velez DO et al (2018) A global transcriptional network connecting noncoding mutations to changes in tumor gene expression. Nat Genet 50:613–620
105. Johannessen CM, Boehm JS (2017) Progress toward precision functional genomics in cancer. Curr Opinion in Sys Biol 2:74–83
106. Alexandrov LB, Nik-Zainal S, Wedge DC et al (2013) Signatures of mutational processes in human cancer. Nature 500:415–421
107. Engert F, Kovac M, Baumhoer D, Nathrath M, Fuida S (2017) Osteosarcoma cells with genetic signatures of BRCAness are susceptible to the PARP inhibitor talazoparib alone or in combination with chemotherapeutics. Oncotarget 8:48794–48806
108. Fong PC, Boss DS, Yap TA et al (2009) Inhibition of poly(ADP-ribose) polymerase in tumors from BRCA mutation carriers. N Engl J Med 361:123–134
109. Wagner AH, Coffman AC, Ainscough BJ et al (2016) DGIdb 2.0: mining clinically relevant drug-gene interactions. Nucleic Acids Res 44:D1036–D1044
110. Scharovsky OG, Mainetti LE, Rozados VR (2009) Metronomic chemotherapy: changing the paradigm that more is better. Curr Oncol 16:7–15
111. Hartwell LH, Szankasi P, Robets CJ, Murray AW, Friend SH (1997) Integrating genetic approaches into the discovery of anticancer drugs. Science 278:1064–1068
112. Ye H, Zhang X, Chen Y, Liu Q, Wei J (2016) Ranking novel cancer driving synthetic lethal gene pairs using TCGA data. Oncotarget 7:55352–55367
113. Patel SJ, Sanjana NE, Kishton RJ et al (2017) Identification of essential genes for cancer immunotherapy. Nature, 537–545

114. Fortier MH, Caron E, Hardy MP et al (2008) The MHC class I peptide repertoire is molded by the transcriptome. J Exp Med 205:595–610
115. Karasaki T, Nagayama K, Kuwano K et al (2017) Prediction and prioritization of neoantigens: intergration of RNA sequencing data with whole-exome sequencing. Cancer Sci 108:170–177
116. Wirth TC, Kühnel (2017) Neoantigen targeting—dawn of a new era in cancer immunotherapy. Front Immunol 8:1–16
117. Phillips KA, Deverka PA, Trosman JR et al (2017) Payer coverage policies for multigene tests. Nat Biotechnol 35:614–617
118. Kurian AW, Li Y, Hamilton AS et al (2017) Gaps in incorporating germline genetic testing into treatment decision-making for early-stage breast cancer. J Clin Oncol 35:2232–2239
119. Merchant GE, Lindor RA (2013) Personalized medicine and genetic malpractice. Genet Med 15:921–922. https://doi.org/10.1038/gim.2013.142
120. Cerami et al (2012 May) The cBio cancer genomics portal: an open platform for exploring multidimensional cancer genomics data. Cancer Discov 2:401
121. Surveillance, Epidemiology, and End Results (SEER) Program populations (1969–2016) (www.seer.cancer.gov/popdata). National Cancer Institute, DCCPS, Surveillance Research Program, released December 2017
122. Cancer Genome Atlas Research Network (2011) Integrated genomic analyses of ovarian carcinoma. Nature 474(7353):609
123. Dougherty BA, Lai Z, Hodgson DR, Orr MC, Hawryluk M, Sun J … Fielding A (2017) Biological and clinical evidence for somatic mutations in BRCA1 and BRCA2 as predictive markers for olaparib response in high-grade serous ovarian cancers in the maintenance setting. Oncotarget 8(27):43653–43661
124. Oza AM, Cibula D, Benzaquen AO, Poole C, Mathijssen RH, Sonke GS, … Mahner S (2015) Olaparib combined with chemotherapy for recurrent platinum-sensitive ovarian cancer: a randomised phase 2 trial. Lancet Oncol 16(1):87–97
125. Cortesi L, Toss A, Cucinotto I (2018) Parp inhibitors for the treatment of ovarian cancer. Current cancer drug targets. (Epub ahead of print)
126. Balmana J, Tung NM, Isakoff SJ, Grana B, Ryan PD, Saura C, … Garber JE (2014) Phase I trial of olaparib in combination with cisplatin for the treatment of patients with advanced breast, ovarian and other solid tumors. Ann Oncol 25(8):1656–1663
127. Del Conte G, Sessa C, Von Moos R, Vigano L, Digena T, Locatelli A … Gianni L (2014) Phase I study of olaparib in combination with liposomal doxorubicin in patients with advanced solid tumours. Br J Cancer 111(4):651
128. Lee JM, Hays JL, Annunziata CM, Noonan AM, Minasian L, Zujewski J A … Figg WD (2014) Phase I/Ib study of olaparib and carboplatin in BRCA1 or BRCA2 mutation-associated breast or ovarian cancer with biomarker analyses. J Natl Cancer Inst 106(6), dju089
129. Mirza MR, Monk BJ, Herrstedt J, Oza AM, Mahner S, Redondo A, Fabbro M et al (2016) Niraparib maintenance therapy in platinum-sensitive, recurrent ovarian cancer. N Engl J Med 375(22):2154–2164
130. Coleman RL, Oza AM, Lorusso D, Aghajanian C, Oaknin A, Dean A, … Leary A (2017) Rucaparib maintenance treatment for recurrent ovarian carcinoma after response to platinum therapy (ARIEL3): a randomised, double-blind, placebo-controlled, phase 3 trial. The Lancet 390(10106):1949–1961
131. Toss A, Cortesi L (2013) Molecular mechanisms of PARP inhibitors in BRCA-related ovarian cancer. J Cancer Sci Therapy 5(11):409–416
132. Albertson DG (2006) Gene amplification in cancer. Trends Genet 22:447–455
133. Jorde, LB, Carey, JC, Bamshad MJ (2015) Medical genetics e-Book. Elsevier Health Sciences (Page 324)
134. Laskar BZ, Majumder S (2017) Gene expression programming. In: Bio-inspired computing for information retrieval applications. IGI Global, pp 269–292 (Page 270)

135. Latysheva NS, Babu MM (2016) Discovering and understanding oncogenic gene fusions through data intensive computational approaches. Nucleic Acids Res 44:4487–4503
136. Lynch TJ, Bell DW, Sordella R et al (2004) Activating mutations in the epidermal growth factor receptor underlying responsiveness of non-small-cell lung cancer to gefitinib. N Engl J Med 350:2129–2139
137. Nussbaum RL, McInnes RR, Willard HF (2016) Thompson & Thompson genetics in medicine, 8th edn. Elsevier Health Sciences, Philadephia, pp 314–502
138. Richards S, Aziz N, Bale S et al (2015) Standards and guidelines for the interpretation of sequence variants: a joint consensus recommendation of the American College of Medical Genetics and Genomics and the Association for Molecular Pathology. Genet Med. 17:405–424
139. Rizvi S, Borad MJ (2016) The rise of the FGFR inhibitor in advanced biliary cancer: the next cover of time magazine? J Gastrointest Oncol. 7(5):789–796
140. Tiacci E, Trifonov V, Schiavoni G et al (2011) BRAF mutations in hairy-cell leukemia. N Engl J Med 364:2305–2315

Part II
Currently Available Techniques

Immunohistochemistry-Enabled Precision Medicine

4

Zoran Gatalica, Rebecca Feldman, Semir Vranić and David Spetzler

Contents

Z. Gatalica (✉) · R. Feldman · D. Spetzler
Caris Life Sciences, Phoenix, AZ, USA
e-mail: zgatalica@carisls.com

S. Vranić
College of Medicine, Qatar University, Doha, Qatar

D. D. Von Hoff and H. Han (eds.), *Precision Medicine in Cancer Therapy*,
Cancer Treatment and Research 178, https://doi.org/10.1007/978-3-030-16391-4_4

4.1 Methodology

Immunohistochemistry (IHC) uses specific antibodies for detection of antigens (epitopes) in tissues (cells and extracellular components) at a light microscopic level. Antigen (epitope) bound antibodies must be visualized, most commonly using a secondary detection and a chromogenic method. Localization of the color to the appropriate tissue component or subcellular compartment under microscopic examination is then subjected to various interpretation algorithms leading to diagnosis, prognosis, and/or prediction of response to therapy.

Simple qualitative interpretation (i.e., confirmation of expressed protein in its cellular/subcellular localization) forms the basis for diagnostic application of the IHC. Quantitative interpretation (usually in the form of percent of positive cancer cells, but also a proportion of specific positive non-cancerous cells in the tumor) forms the basis for prognostic and predictive (theranostic) applications of IHC [1].

Although IHC is a simple, frequently fully automated and reliable technique that is affordable to most of the pathology laboratories, it is still mostly a subjective method for which strict validation processes must be applied. Optimization, validation, and verification of clinical IHC tests must be performed by every laboratory performing these tests in the era of precision medicine [2]. The vast majority of IHC tests are developed in the individual laboratory and are designated as "laboratory-developed tests" (LDTs). Several IHC tests are now designated as "companion diagnostic" or "complimentary diagnostic" to indicate their status in regard to the FDA approval/clearance status [3].

4.2 IHC as a Diagnostic Tool in Oncology

When morphologic features observed by a pathologist using light microscopic examination are not sufficiently characteristic to assign the diagnosis, IHC is one of the most commonly used "ancillary" diagnostic techniques. Antibodies used for such purpose are traditionally divided in the "first-tier" antibodies capable of detection of antigens expressed in general tumor lineages (epithelial tumors, mesenchymal tumors, melanomas, germ cell tumors, neuroendocrine tumors and lymphomas) and "second-tier" antibodies reacting with antigens characteristically expressed in specific histologic types within the specific lineage [4, 5].

4.3 IHC in the Evaluation of a Cancer of Unknown Primary Site (CUP)

Immunohistochemistry should be applied meticulously in order to identify the tissue of origin and to exclude chemosensitive and potentially curable tumors (i.e., lymphomas and germ cell tumors) [6, 7]. However, the majority of cases (about 80%) do not belong to specific subsets, and it may be reasonable to investigate theranostic biomarkers in true CUP (those who remain without identified primary cancer after a reasonable IHC evaluation). Recent investigation in theranostic biomarkers (particularly those approved in lineage-agnostic manner [e.g., mismatch repair proteins expression for detection of MSI-H cancers, see Fig. 4.1)] may identify a subset of CUP susceptible to treatment with immune checkpoint inhibitors (also known as immuno-oncology [IO] agents) [8].

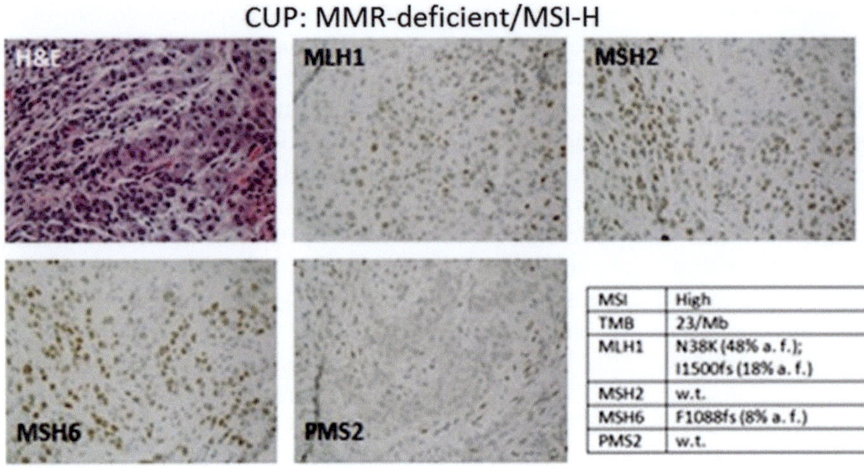

Fig. 4.1 MSI in cancer of unknown primary. This tumor showed isolated loss of PMS2 protein by immunohistochemistry (IHC) and microsatellite instability (MSI) by next generation sequencing. A pathogenic mutation, p.N38K, was detected in the MLH1 gene at a level consistent with a germline mutation. In addition, a second pathogenic MLH1 mutation (c.1499delT) was detected at a lower frequency and likely represents somatic loss of the normal allele. MLH1 missense mutations, such as p.N38K, can sometimes be associated with isolated loss of PMS2 staining by IHC

4.4 IHC in Cancer Subtyping—Breast Carcinoma

Seminal studies of Perou et al. and Sørlie et al. revealed at least four distinct molecular subtypes including basal-like, HER2-positive, luminal A, and luminal B [9–11]. This classification was validated by other researchers followed by discovery of additional molecular subtypes. Currently (at least) seven molecular subgroups have been recognized (Reviewed in: Reis-Filho and Pusztai [12]). Table 4.1 adapted from Reis-Filho and Pusztai [12] summarizes most recent classification of breast carcinomas based on molecular expression profiles.

Immunohistochemistry can effectively and practically replace gene expression array analysis to identify major subtypes using four tests. Assays for estrogen receptor (ER), progesterone receptor (PR), Ki-67 proliferation marker, and Her2 (ERBB2) (modified Table 4.2 according to Goldhirsch et al. [13]) are utilized to define the following: (1) luminal A (ER+/PR+/Her2-/Ki-67 low), (2) luminal B (two subgroups: "HER2 negative": ER+/PR+/Her2-/Ki-67 high and "HER2 positive": ER+/PR+/Her2+/any Ki-67), (3) Erb-B2 overexpression (ER-/PR-/Her2+), and (4) basal-like/triple negative (ER-/PR-/Her2-).

Table 4.1 Molecular classification of breast cancer based on the microarray data (adapted from Reis-Filho and Pusztai [12])

Molecular subtype	ER/PR/HER2 status	Histologic grade	Proliferation rate	Basal markers	Response to chemotherapy	Prognosis
Luminal A	ER+PR+ HER2-	G1/G2	Low	Negative	Poor	Good
Luminal B	ER+PR± HER2∓	G2/3	High	Negative	Intermediate	Intermediate to poor
HER2-enriched	ER-PR- HER2+	G3	High	∓	Intermediate	Poor
Basal-like	ER-PR- HER2-	G3	High	Positive	Good	Poor
Claudin-low	ER∓PR∓ HER2∓	G2/3	Intermediate	Positive	Intermediate	Intermediate
Molecular apocrine	ER-PR- HER2+ AR+	G3	High	Negative	Unknown[a]	Poor

ER: estrogen receptor; *PR:* progesterone receptor; *AR:* androgen receptor
G1–3 tumor grading: *G1:* well differentiated; *G2:* moderately differentiated; *G3:* poorly differentiated
[a]In authors' experience, apocrine carcinomas (HER2+) may have a good response to chemotherapy (including neoadjuvant) when combined with anti-HER2 treatment modalities
Note This molecular classification did not include the "normal breast-like" subtype; this subtype is poorly characterized, and most authors agree that this subtype rather represents a technical artifact caused by the high contamination with normal breast tissue during the initial microarray studies conducted in the period 2000–2003

Table 4.2 Clinical definitions of breast cancer subtypes (according to Goldhirsch et al. [13])

Molecular subtype of breast cancer	Definition
Luminal A subtype	ER positive PR positive HER2 negative Low Ki-67 expression (<14%)
Luminal B subtype	Luminal B (HER2 negative) ER and/or PR positive HER2 negative High Ki-67 (>14%) Luminal B (HER2 positive) ER and/or PR positive HER2 positive (3+ or amplified)
HER2-positive subtype	ER negative PR negative HER2 positive (3+ or amplified)
Triple-negative subtype[a]	ER negative PR negative HER2 negative

[a]80% triple-negative breast carcinomas are of basal-like subtype by microarray or immunohistochemistry (basal cytokeratins, p63, calponin, SMA, or SMM-HC positive)

From the clinical perspective, one of the most important breast cancer groups is "triple-negative breast carcinoma (TNBC)," a heterogeneous group with various molecular subtypes, of which "basal-like" being the most prominent, see Table 4.1 adapted from Metzger-Filho et al. [14]. Additional IHC biomarkers (basal cytokeratins, [e.g., CK5/6, CK14, CK17], p63, calponin, SMM-HC, SMA) may help identifying a subtype of TNBC with basal phenotype (Table 4.2).

More recently, a theranostic value of the expression of AR in TNBC was recognized and a new term "quadruple negative breast carcinoma (QNBC)" was introduced to distinguish TNBC lacking AR expression from TNBC expressing AR at the treatment relevant levels (>10%) [15, 16]. Testing for androgen receptor (AR) status has only recently become a routine for the triple-negative breast cancers, but rare breast malignancy (e.g., apocrine breast carcinomas) and some salivary gland cancers consistently over-express AR and small case series have examined the role of androgen deprivation in these patients, demonstrating clinical benefit [17, 18]. Notably, a recent, phase II study conducted by Traina et al. showed that anti-AR drug enzalutamide had a remarkable clinical activity and was well tolerated in patients with advanced AR-positive TNBC (defined as AR expression $\geq 10\%$ by IHC) [16].

Similarly, substitution of mRNA prognostic scores provided by OncotypeDX® test by a combination of morphologic cancer characteristics and select IHC tests (ER, PR, Her2, Ki-67) has been successfully achieved (e.g., Magee Equations [19, 20]).

4.5 Loss of Protein Expression as a Diagnostic Tool for Mutation Status in Breast Cancer—Loss of E-cadherin (*CDH1*) Expression in Lobular Carcinoma

Invasive lobular carcinoma (ILC) of the breast is the second most common morphological subtype of breast cancer (after invasive ductal carcinoma, NOS), comprising up to 15% of all cases. Apart from its pleomorphic variant, classical ILC is generally of a good prognostic phenotype, with a positive response to endocrine therapy (due to consistent ER+/PR+ hormone receptor status). Thus, it is important to reliably recognize this type of breast carcinoma. E-cadherin expression (encoded in *CDH1* gene and normally expressed in the cytoplasmic membrane of normal breast epithelia) has become an important diagnostic feature of ILC because approximately 90% of ILCs completely lack E-cadherin protein expression (in contrast to invasive ductal carcinomas, which retain E-cadherin expression). Somatic mutations are found in ILC and are dispersed throughout the *CDH1* coding region and are frequently truncating [21].

4.6 IHC in Cancer Classification—Gastroenteropancreatic Neuroendocrine Tumors (GEP-NETs)

Neuroendocrine tumors (NETs) can arise throughout gastrointestinal and respiratory tracts. Gastroenteropancreatic NETs are diagnosed by a characteristic cancer morphology and expression of neuroendocrine markers (e.g., synaptophysin, chromogranin A, CD56). A 2010 WHO classification of NETs incorporated Ki-67 proliferation marker IHC as a part of the classification and grading algorithm: NET Grade 1 tumors exhibit Ki-67 < 3%; Grade 2 (3–20%) while grade 3 NETs (neuroendocrine carcinomas) show >20% Ki-67 labeling [22].

In case of pulmonary neuroendocrine tumors, Ki-67 labeling is mainly used to separate the high-grade variants such as small cell (SCLC) and large cell neuroendocrine carcinomas (LCNEC) from the carcinoid tumors, especially in limited samples, e.g., a needle biopsy with extensive crush effects and necrosis [23].

4.7 Historical Examples and Some Pitfalls of Diagnostic Antigens Turned Biomarkers of Targeted Therapy

Certain biological properties related to cell of origin have successfully resulted in the development of diagnostic IHC to cell characteristic antigens. The most well-known example is the consistent expression pattern of a cell surface signaling receptor, CD117, a product of the *c-KIT* proto-oncogene, which is a defining feature of a biologically distinct group of stromal tumors of the gastrointestinal tract [24].

Prior to this knowledge, intra-abdominal mesenchymal tumors of the GI tract mostly were known to be of smooth muscle, lipomatous, neural, and vascular origin [25]. The discovery of CD117 positivity as a diagnostic criteria for gastrointestinal stromal tumors or GIST (and their origin from interstitial cells of Cajal) was a major breakthrough as CD117 staining by IHC became the new gold standard to "molecularly" subtype a broad class of tumors. Remarkably, the discovery of CD117 to define a molecular subtype of abdominal smooth muscle tumors led to translation of these findings into a clinically actionable molecular target.

Simultaneous to the identification of CD117 as diagnostic criteria for GIST, researchers also identified in these tumors activating gain-of-function mutations in the *c-KIT* gene resulting in constitutive tyrosine kinase activity [26]. It was later established that about 85% of GIST exhibit activating mutations in *c-KIT*, 10–15% exhibit mutations in platelet-derived growth factor receptor A (*PDGFRA),* and the remaining exhibit alternate mechanisms of oncogenic activation. During this time, tyrosine kinase inhibitors which block the Bcr-Abl fusion protein of chronic myeloid leukemia were also found to have activity against c-KIT and PDGFRA of the same family of receptors, providing scientific rationale to assess the clinical role of the targeted kinase inhibitor imatinib (Gleevec). After the first initial report of activity of imatinib in a metastatic GIST patient [27] and a small case series demonstrating 80% of GIST patients derive clinical response or stabilization of disease [28], imatinib was quickly approved for patients with c-KIT (CD117) positive unresectable and/or metastatic GIST in 2001, and shortly after a companion diagnostic, c-Kit pharmDx™ was also FDA-approved. To this day, the prescribing label remains unchanged despite evidence that there are exon-specific differences in survival outcome [29], whereby clinical practice guidelines now recommend a dosage increase based on data demonstrating high-dose imatinib leads to longer progression-free survival time in certain GIST subsets.

Similarly, during the early development of the anti-EGFR (epidermal growth factor receptor) monoclonal antibody cetuximab, expression levels and phosphorylation status of the target, EGFR, was hypothesized to be a predictive marker for clinical benefit. Grounded on the clinical development program assuming a strong correlation between target expression and clinical activity, in 2004, the drug was the second of its kind (followed the co-approval of HercepTest™/trastuzumab for breast cancer) to be co-approved with diagnostic test for EGFR-expressing (EGFR PharmDx™ kit) metastatic colorectal cancers (mCRC) [30]. However, this correlation was never confirmed in controlled studies and in fact, several small studies demonstrating clinical responses in EGFR-negative metastatic CRC patients challenged the use of EGFR expression to base treatment selection [31]. Subsequent studies later found mutation events in *RAS* (*KRAS/NRAS*), signal transducer downstream of EGFR, which occur in 40% of mCRC to be a negative predictive marker for clinical benefit from cetuximab [32, 33]. To this day, the prescribing information continues to include the initial approval summary regarding "EGFR-expressing" mCRC although now updated for RAS genotype.

In summary, these bench-to-bedside stories of immunohistochemically defined antigens, together with evolving scientific discoveries (e.g., activating mutation event in tumor cells), have led to a paradigm shift in the development of targeted therapies for cancer. These examples and others highlight important considerations in the identification of molecular predictors and the development of targeted therapies: (1) presence or absence of a drug target may not be the sole or best indicator for selection of patients that may benefit from targeted treatment [34], (2) pathway activation through mutations downstream of the drug target may have greater impact on treatment response than target expression, and (3) a regulatory path to update and revise prescribing labels is needed to provide the most complete source of information at the regulatory level. In total, these events promote utilization of broader molecular characterization to both define the specific disease and find optimal treatment strategy for cancers.

4.8 IHC as a Prognostic and Predictive Tool in Oncology

Immunohistochemistry-based assays to demonstrate utility in differentiating prognostic groups (e.g., early recurrence after primary treatment, aggressive phenotype, etc.) have been investigated extensively across all solid tumors. The vast majority of these studies do not meet the quality standards of large, prospective randomized trials to translate into the clinic, rather, most have been done in small cohorts with inconsistent results [35]. Some biomarkers that have been explored across cancer types are those that enable proliferative potential of cells, how cells respond to DNA damage, or are surrogates for molecular classifications that are more aggressive, such as Ki-67, p53, p16, BAP1, SDHX, and members of the HER family, including EGFR and HER2. Despite the growing pool of prognostic marker-based studies, none are routinely utilized in clinical practice [35] and those with the strongest bodies of evidence, such as Ki-67 in breast cancer or p16 in oral squamous cell carcinoma, are not without controversy [36, 37].

Whereas a prognostic marker is one that indicates overall outcome, regardless of therapy utilized, a predictive marker is one that provides information whether or not the therapeutic intervention is likely to be effective [38]. In addition, in the modern era, drug development has shifted to target individual molecular alterations; thus, genetic and molecular markers, which are often times the target of therapeutic intervention, are increasingly tested to guide precision medicine. In oncology, IHC-based predictive markers undoubtedly play a significant role in personalized treatment selection. Although we may think of molecularly guided treatment selection as something new, we have, in fact, been practicing precision medicine since the early 1970s with endocrine-based treatments of breast and prostate cancers [39, 40]. It was in the mid-1970s that an ER assay was introduced and later morphed into modern-day testing of estrogen receptor status by IHC, to predict responsiveness to endocrine therapy for breast cancer [40].

4.9 Targeted Therapy IHC Tests

The three most important properties of an ideal drug target are that the target is disease modifying, has proven function in the pathophysiology of disease, and be measurable [41]. Identification of drug targets for oncology can somewhat be an exercise of reverse engineering, i.e., identification of the molecular changes that "drive" cancer cells and develop therapies that intercept those molecular interactions that are required for cancer cell growth. Therefore, oncogenic events such as gene amplifications that lead to protein overexpression, kinase activation through activating mutations, and genomic translocations that lead to constitutive expression of oncogenic proteins are ideal candidates for drug targets [42].

Indeed, the past 20 years of drug development in oncology have produced therapies including monoclonal antibodies and small-molecule inhibitors that exploit these molecular addictions [43]. Certain molecular results are required to guide treatment options for advanced cancer patients, across various cancer types. Broad-based molecular profiling assays which include large NGS panels to identify mutation variants, amplification events, and fusion genes are now widely used, given abundant commercial options, falling costs, and increasing coverage by insurance carriers. Obtaining these results is highly dependent on specimen requirements, and unfortunately, some biopsies yield very small specimens that are highly unlikely to yield results from a standard NGS method. These instances are examples where IHC tests are ideal given they require only 1–2 slides for testing. In situations where targeted therapies require results for treatment options, development of antibodies that detect mutation variants provides a very practical and highly impactful approach for patient selection.

4.10 Oncogenic Up-Regulation of Proteins Due to Gene Amplification

One of the most well known and successful of these examples is the development of trastuzumab, a humanized monoclonal antibody that binds to the extracellular domain of HER2, a transmembrane receptor tyrosine kinase overexpressed (due to gene amplification) in 15–20% of breast cancers [44, 45]. After many prospective and randomized clinical trials, the benefit of trastuzumab has been confined to breast cancer patients whose tumors have gene amplification as detected by FISH (fluorescent in situ hybridization), which is tightly associated with protein expression levels as detected by IHC. HER2 IHC testing is now routine part of clinical workup for newly diagnosed breast cancer patients.

Given the hugely successful targeting of HER2-positive breast cancers with an assembly of HER2-directed therapies (e.g., trastuzumab, ado-trastuzumab, pertuzumab, lapatinib, neratinib), exploration of other cancer types where HER2 overexpression provides cancer cell's a survival advantage was inevitable. Expression levels of HER2 across cancer types have been explored, identifying cancers where HER2 expression is abundant and ranging between 10 and 30% including colon, bladder, bile duct, and gastric cancers [46, 47]. Many studies have been conducted to assess the therapeutic effect of trastuzumab in other HER2-driven cancers; however, to date the strong mechanistic association between HER2 and HER2-directed therapy has only been cleared for gastric adenocarcinomas [48]. Many case reports and series exist, and many clinical trials are still ongoing to evaluate the utility of HER2-directed therapies in other cancers in order to broaden its administration [49–52].

4.11 Oncogenic Overexpression of RTKs and/or Ligands Due to Gene Fusions

Another mechanism of oncogene activation in cancer is genomic translocation of two genes which can result in pathologic expression of a chimeric protein with potent oncogenic properties [53] or overexpression of a gene downstream of a new promoter. Gene fusions are common alterations in hematological malignancies whereby testing for fusions is used for diagnostic and/or theranostic purposes. With increasing utilization of broad-based molecular testing in clinical practice for all advanced malignancies, progress has also been made to identify fusion events in solid tumors that drive cancer growth [53] and testing for some of these fusions are necessary for the clinical management of patients.

4.12 ALK Fusions—ALK IHC

Detection of *ALK* gene fusions, which occur in about 3–4% of NSCLC, is part of the standard molecular workup for all newly diagnosed advanced lung cancers. Fusion with the echinoderm microtubule-associated protein-like 4 gene is the most common binding partner for *ALK* (*EML4-ALK*) and has emerged as the second most important driver oncogene in lung cancer and the first targetable fusion to be identified in lung adenocarcinomas [54]. The historical gold standard detection method of FISH with a dually labeled break-apart probe has been used to identify fusions which are visually detected as a "split" hybridization signal [55]. Reports indicate interpretation of these signals can be difficult or missed completely as they are often subtle differences, but also due to complex FISH patterns that may be misinterpreted [55, 56].

Furthermore, more recent technologies that detect fusion proteins such as DNA-based targeted hybrid capture-based next generation sequencing (NGS) and targeted RNA sequencing with multiplex PCR have also led to the identification of ALK-positive cases that were otherwise found to be negative by FISH testing [57, 58]. A recent report demonstrated in 31 cases identified as *ALK* fusion positive by NGS (4.4% ALK-positive rate), 35% (11/31) had discordant FISH results. Given limitations of FISH, IHC has become an attractive alternative given low specimen requirements, cost, and ease of testing [58]. Also favorable is the development of a high concordance antibody, D5F3, with a sensitivity and specificity exceeding 90%. Due to the high impact of identifying ALK-positive NSCLC with available treatments like crizotinib yielding response rates of approximately 74% and median progression-free survival of 10 months, compared to 45% and 7 months for chemotherapy, respectively, the ALK (D5F3) antibody has been recently fully cleared by the FDA as a companion diagnostic test for NSCLC [59–61].

Additional clinically impactful gene fusions following the discovery of *ALK* in lung cancer have also been identified, including *ROS1* [62], *RET* [63], and *NTRK* [64]. Current methodological strategies to identify these fusions (some of which are relevant across cancer types) depend on the availability of probes and antibodies for target of interest. Currently, FISH probes are available for *ROS1, RET,* and *NTRK*, and antibodies with good concordance to FISH and/or NGS technologies are available for ROS1 and NTRK [65–67]. Potential diagnostic utility for ROS1 IHC test for detection of *ROS1* gene rearrangements in NSCLC patients had been described [68, 69].

4.13 ROS1 Fusions—ROS1 IHC

Oncogenic *ROS1* gene fusion in NSCLC involves *CD74*, *SLC34A2*, *EZR*, *LRIG3*, *SDC4*, *TPM3*, *FIG*, *CCDC6*, and *KDELR2* and leads to expression of chimeric protein with a constitutive ROS1 kinase activity. *ROS1*-rearranged lung cancer comprises about 1% adenocarcinomas. Using D4D6 antibody, Yoshida et al. applied H-scoring to the series of *ROS1* rearranged and non-rearranged NSCLC and obtained optimal discrimination (94% sensitivity and 98% specificity) with H-score cutoff of ≥ 150 (e.g., 2+ intensity in 75% of cells) [70].

4.13.1 NTRK Fusions—Pan NTRK IHC

Targeted inhibitors of neurotropic tyrosine kinases are highly effective in selected patients (adults and children) with gene fusions involving *NTRK1, NTRK2,* or *NTRK3* [71, 72]. In a large prospective study, all three *NTRK* genes were involved in fusions with 13 different gene partners; *TPM3:NTRK1,* and *ETV6:NTRK3* were the most common (six cases each) [73]. These fusions are consistently detected in rare cancer types (e.g., secretory breast carcinoma, mammary analog secretory carcinoma, congenital mesoblastic nephroma, and congenital infantile fibrosarcoma) and in a small percentage of common cancers in adult patients (non-small cell lung cancer, salivary gland, colorectal, head and neck, thyroid, bladder cancers as well as malignant melanomas, soft tissue sarcomas, and CNS tumors/gliomas). In order to maximize the detection of patients with tumors carrying targetable NTRK fusions, recent studies have demonstrated that pan-Trk IHC testing with mAb EPR17341 may serve as an effective screening tool before highly sensitive, confirmatory molecular tests (FISH or NGS) were performed [67, 74].

4.14 NUTM1 Fusions—NUT IHC

NUTM1 is an example of diagnostic marker and emerging predictive biomarker for bromodomain and extra-terminal (BET) inhibitors.

NUT midline carcinoma (NMC) was originally defined as any malignant (epithelial) tumor with rearrangement of the nuclear protein in testis gene (*NUTM1*) [75]. Although immunohistochemical NUT detection appears to be highly sensitive for detection of the rearrangement (NUT is normally expressed only in testis) [50], it is important to identify specific *NUTM1* gene fusion in IHC-positive cases due to the effective, targeted therapy with BET inhibitors. In the majority of cases, *NUTM1* gene is fused to *BRD4* gene, forming the *BRD4-NUT* fusion. Remaining cases have *NUTM1* partnered with *BRD3* or other rare partners (e.g., *NSD3, MGA, MXD4*). The efficacy of targeted therapy with BET inhibitors in cases with these novel fusions is not known, and additional functional studies on various fusion partners are needed [76, 77].

4.15 Loss of Protein Expression Due to Epigenetic Silencing—MGMT Promoter Hypermethylation (Genetic Vs. IHC Assay [78])

MGMT (O6-methylguanine-DNA methyltransferase) promoter methylation has been established as a predictive biomarker in patients diagnosed with gliomas, for treatment with alkylating agent temozolomide (TMZ). Patients whose tumors had hyper-methylated MGMT promoter appear to benefit from TMZ. Expression of the MGMT gene is regulated by the methylation-dependent epigenetic silencing. Gliomas with inactivation of the MGMT gene are less capable of repairing DNA, which leads to increased sensitivity to alkylating chemotherapy. The use of IHC for the detection of MGMT protein has been described in a number of studies, with significant discordance between MGMT expression as detected by IHC and by MGMT DNA methylation, as well as discordance for survival. In patients with leiomyosarcomas, a trend toward higher response to TMZ was observed among patients whose tumors were lacking MGMT expression, as determined by IHC [79].

4.16 Expression of Mutated Genes

Immunohistochemical detection of specific epitopes in the protein derived from the expression of a mutated gene ("mutation-specific antibodies") has some advantages over DNA sequencing approaches including direct visualization of the heterogeneity in the distribution of targeted proteins (e.g., clonal effect in the tumor) and perhaps more importantly ability to detect mutations in a very limited sample and in a short testing turnaround time [80]. Activating mutations in receptor tyrosine kinases are cancer drivers where targeted therapies have been developed, including EGFR and BRAF, two of the most successful drug-target stories in modern precision oncology era. Multiple antibodies have been developed that detect these specific variants, with varying degrees of specificity and sensitivity. The significant clinical benefit of small-molecule tyrosine kinase inhibitors (TKIs) in patients with advanced NSCLC underscores the importance of accurately identifying patients that would benefit from appropriate treatment for each molecular subtype.

4.17 Mutation-Specific Antibodies

4.17.1 EGFR

Epidermal growth factor receptor (*EGFR*) mutations in NSCLC are frequent, and about 90% of these mutations occur in exons 19 (e.g., E746-A750 deletion) and 21 (leucine to arginine substitution at amino acid 858, L858R). The finding of an activating *EGFR* mutation in NSCLC is the best single predictor of efficacy using selective tyrosine kinase inhibitors (TKI) [81]. Mutation-specific antibodies that can detect E746_A750 deletion and L858R mutant EGFR proteins by IHC are available [82]. However, as reported by Seo et al., various forms of exon 19 deletions (except E746_A750) were rarely detected by the mutant-specific antibody. Therefore, IHC-negative cases require further molecular analysis to confirm the absence of *EGFR* mutations. Due to lower sensitivity and variable specificity, these assays are more likely to be reserved for situations of limited tissue (e.g., cytological samples contain only a few neoplastic cells) [83].

4.17.2 BRAF

Determination of the *BRAF* mutation status is of great importance in management of patients with cancer and is now especially relevant given its role in guiding options for precision medicine of solid tumors [84–86]. *BRAF* gene mutation analysis is routinely performed using various DNA-based molecular assays, but cost, expertise, and tissue requirements limit their widespread use. A BRAF p. V600E-specific antibody (VE1 antibody; Ventana Medical Systems) has been developed for use by IHC, and studies have shown good concordance, 100% sensitivity and 91% specificity with detection of the BRAF p.V600E (BRAF c.1799T > A) mutation (Fig. 4.2) [87]. Thus, IHC evaluation of BRAF p.V600E may serve as a candidate surrogate for detection of mutation particularly in tumor types with high proportion of *V600E* mutation (e.g., thyroid, melanoma, colon; Fig. 4.2) [88] or in malignancies where BRAF-mutated cells within the tumor are rare but clinically impactful (e.g., histiocytoses, GIST) [89, 90]. However, a number of non-c.1799T > A mutations in *BRAF* gene lead to activation of the protein (e.g., V600K) and are potentially targetable, but are not going to be detected using the V600E-specific antibody [87].

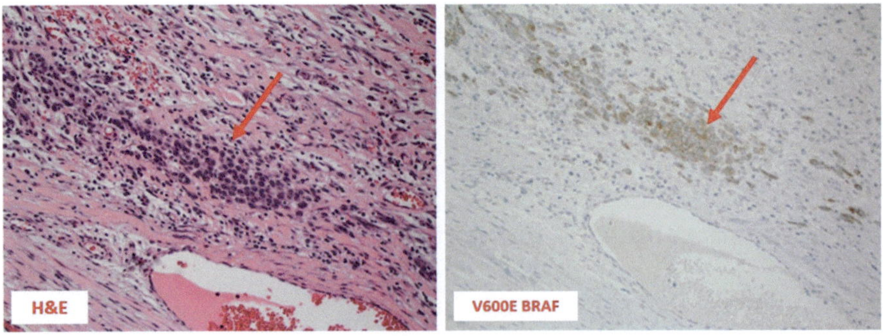

Fig. 4.2 BRAF V600E (c.1799_1800delinsAA) detection in limited sample of metastatic melanoma. A small cluster of cells within the stromal tissue (arrow in H&E stained slide, left image) may be too small for extraction of sufficient quantities of DNA/RNA for molecular (sequencing, RT-PCR) testing. In this situation, a reliable BRAF V600E IHC staining (brown cluster, right image) detects druggable target using a single tissue section

4.18 Detection of Antigens Relevant for the Antibody-Drug-Conjugated (ADC) Therapies

Antibody-drug conjugates (ADCs) are an emerging class of targeted therapies utilized in oncology. Instead of counteracting molecular interactions or processes within the cell, ADCs deliver a chemotherapy payload to a specific target on the cell [91]. The antibody component of the ADC is directed against an epitope enriched in the targeted cancer cells population. Several ADCs are in clinical use, such as trastuzumab emtansine for breast cancer (expressing Her2) and brentuximab vedotin for lymphoma (expressing CD30), and many more are in pharmaceutical development for cancer [46]. Patient selection relies on either (1) knowledge the target of interest is highly expressed in specific cancer types such as Trop2 in TNBC [92], or dependent on development of an antibody to test for expression in tumor tissues such as DLL3 in SCLC [93] and folate receptor alpha in ovarian cancer [94]. Due to the success of these therapies in many chemotherapy refractory diseases including TNBC, SCLC, and platinum-resistant ovarian cancer, their development and reliance on quality metrics for detection of the expression of the drug target make this class of agents a very active area of clinical research.

4.19 Chemotherapy-Predictive IHC Tests

Chemotherapy-based treatments are the backbone of standard cancer care. Most chemotherapies are cytotoxic; they modulate or interrupt cellular processes required for cell viability. By inducing unrepairable DNA damage (e.g., bulky adducts caused by platinum agents) or cellular instability that cannot be overcome (e.g., microtubule de-stabilization caused by taxanes), these toxic agents force both tumor and normal cells to die. Through our understanding of the cellular targets of chemotherapies (i.e., mechanism of action), many studies have investigated whether the presence or absence of certain molecules within tumor cells, which are often aberrantly expressed, may be used to predict response to cytotoxic chemotherapy. Some of the most extensively studied biomarkers as detected by IHC include ERCC1 for platinum in lung cancer and TOPO1 for irinotecan in colorectal cancer [95, 96]. Although these cellular targets are mechanistically sound, the multifactorial mechanisms of response/sensitivity and lack of reproducibility due to variances in antibodies and cutoffs may all contribute to these markers not being fully implemented clinically [97].

4.20 Immune Therapy

Targeted therapies that unblock immune checkpoint upregulation or immune checkpoint inhibitors are another emerging class of agents that are expanding quickly in oncology. These therapies have yielded impressive responses including lasting durable benefit in certain cancers, including NSCLC, melanoma, renal cell carcinoma, and others. Current predictive markers include (1) tumor mutation burden (TMB) often caused by long-term environmental exposures that result in extensive DNA damage, (2) microsatellite instability (MSI) in turn caused by deficiencies in mismatch repair mechanisms, and (3) expression of inhibitory signals of immune checkpoints like PD-L1 in tumor cells and/or infiltrating immune cells [98]. As a matter of fact, FDA approval of pembrolizumab is the first time the agency has approved a cancer treatment based on a common biomarker rather than the primary location in the body where the tumor originated. Two biomarkers, referred to as microsatellite instability-high (MSI-H, a DNA-based test) or mismatch repair deficient (dMMR, protein/IHC-based test), can be interchangeably used for assessment of the treatment eligibility.

4.21 Immune Therapy IHC Tests

4.21.1 PD-L1

The most commonly used test for the eligibility assessment for immune checkpoint inhibitors is expression of PD-L1 (CD274) on tumor cells (TC) or tumor-infiltrating immune cells (IC). Several different antibodies against PD-L1 are in use as companion diagnostics kits, complimentary diagnostics kits, or laboratory-developed tests (LDTs) (Table 4.3). Thresholds for positivity of expression of PD-L1 on tumor cells vary widely based on the intended use (e.g., in NSCLC pembrolizumab monotherapy for pretreated, metastatic NSCLC is for tumors with 1 to <50% cancer cells expression, while as a single agent, it is indicated for the first-line treatment of patients with metastatic non-small cell lung cancer (NSCLC) whose tumors have high PD-L1 expression [tumor proportion score (TPS) $\geq$ 50%]). Expression of PD-L1 on immune cells (IC) within the tumor is taken into calculation of combined positive score (CPS), which is the number of PD-L1 staining cells (tumor cells, lymphocytes, macrophages) divided by the total number of viable tumor cells, multiplied by 100. The specimen should be considered positive for PD-L1 expression if CPS $\geq$ 1 [99]. CPS is companion diagnostics approved for gastric/GEJ adenocarcinomas and cervical carcinomas for treatment with pembrolizumab.

A particular difficulty in interpretation of PD-L1 expression is encountered in tumors surrounded by a strong immune cells reaction and expression of PD-L1 (Fig. 4.3). In these tumors, LDTs with double immunohistochemistry (one for PD-L1 and the other for cancer lineage specific antigen) may offer advantage over a single PD-L1 staining (Fig. 4.3).

Table 4.3 Overview of the available PD-L1 antibodies and their FDA status in regard to different anti-PD-1/PD-L1 drugs

PD-L1 antibody IO therapy	SP142 (Ventana) Atezolizumab (Roche)	SP263 (Ventana) Durvalumab (Astrazeneca)	22c3 (Dako) Pembrolizumab (Merck)	28-8 (Dako) Nivolumab (BMS)	73-10 (Dako) Avelumab (Merck KGaA)
Non-small cell lung cancer (NSCLC)	Complementary status Threshold: ≥ 50% TC or ≥ 10% IC [106]		Companion status Threshold: TPS 1%; 50% [107, 108]	Complementary status Threshold: TC ≥ 1% (increasing benefit for 5 and 10%) [109]	
Bladder cancer	Companion status; Threshold: IC2/3 (≥ 5%) (TILs) [110]	Complementary status; Threshold(s): ≥ 25% TC (membranous) or ICP > 1% and IC + ≥ 25% or ICP = 1% and IC + = 100% [111, 112]	Companion status; Threshold: > 1%; (CPS) ≥ 10 [113]	Complementary status; Threshold: TC ≥ 1% [114]	Threshold: TC ≥ 5% [115]
Melanoma			Threshold: >1% [116]	Complementary status; Threshold: TC ≥ 5% [116]	
Head and neck squamous cell carcinoma (HNSCC)			Threshold: TC or stromal cells ≥ 1% [117]	Complementary status; Threshold: TC ≥ 1% [118]	
Kidney cancer				Threshold: TC ≥ 1% [119]	
Merkel cell carcinoma (MCC)					Threshold: TC ≥ 1% [120]
Gastric and gastroesophageal junction cancers (GE/GEJ)			Companion status; Threshold: CPS ≥ 1 [121]		
Cervical cancer			Companion status; Threshold: CPS ≥ 1 [122]		
Hepatocellular cancer (HCC)				Threshold: TC ≥ 1% [123]	

IO: Immuno-oncology; *IC:* immune cells; *TILs:* tumor-infiltrating lymphocytes; *TC:* tumor cells; *ICP:* immune cells present; *CPS:* combined positive score

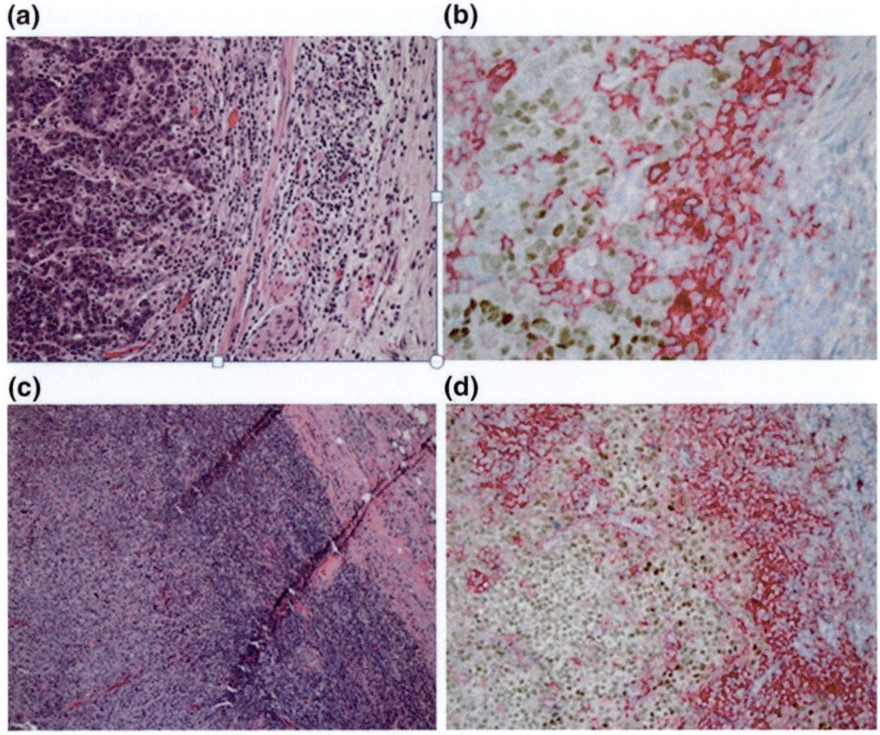

Fig. 4.3 Application of double IHC stains to interpretation of PD-L1 expression in the tumor. **a** and **b** colorectal carcinoma; **c** and **d** melanoma. PD-L1/CDX2 combination in case of metastatic colorectal carcinoma (**b**) and PD-L1/MiTF combination (**d**) in a case of metastatic melanoma. In both cases, PD-L1 expression (red membranous/cytoplasmic staining) is present at the interface between the metastatic malignancy and stromal immune cells (a mixture of lymphocytes, macrophages, and other cell types) and it is entirely restricted to the immune cells (negative for nuclear brown CDX2 staining in the case of CRC and negative for nuclear brown MiTF staining in the case of melanoma)

4.22 Conclusion and Future of IHC-Enabled Precision Medicine

4.22.1 Is There Space for IHC or Will Everything Be Gene (NGS) Based?

Like with every new method, early enthusiasm over a period of time gets tempered by its shortcomings. Without a doubt, sequencing of the human genome had opened an unprecedentedly large view of the genome role in development of cancer, but it is only a component of comprehensive system biology network at play in development of the disease. Protein expression is an integral part of the system biology and can be best investigated with IHC due to its ability to provide in situ morphologic correlation at the cellular or subcellular level.

4.22.2 How to Overcome Shortcoming of IHC?

Classical IHC approach using one antibody stain at the time may no more be suitable for the needs of clinical cancer care. Biopsy samples are frequently small and do not allow for numerous sections needed for consecutive staining. Using multiple antibodies on a single section can be greatly enhanced with the use of fluorescent labeling and image analysis to accurately interpret composition of the heterogeneous tumor sample.

4.22.3 Can a Functional Analysis of Biology Systems Using Phosphoprotein-Specific Antibodies Be Used in Clinical Applications?

The phosphoprotein levels provide insights into the activation/deactivation status of the components of cell signaling pathways, and quantification of their levels could have implications for prognosis and treatment in oncology. For example, phosphorylated forms of epidermal growth factor receptor (EGFR) or ERBB-2 (HER-2) have been found predictive of progression-free survival in patients with metastatic breast cancer treated with trastuzumab [100]. However, phosphoprotein levels are affected by a multitude of pre-analytical variables such as tissue handling (ischemia and time to fixation) and the method of fixation [101]. Furthermore, the levels of phosphoprotein may be affected even before resection resulting from the stress conditions during surgery itself. All this constitutes significant hurdles for the introduction of phosphoproteins as biomarkers in clinical practice.

4.22.4 Can Non-antibody-Based Techniques (Aptamers) for In Situ Detection of Protein Targets Be Used?

Aptamers, first reported in 1990, are single-stranded DNA or RNA sequences (as well as peptides) that can specifically bind to targets by folding into well-defined three-dimensional structures [102, 103]. They are promising recognition molecules that can specifically bind to target molecules and cells in tissue-based assays and can be detected using chromogenic methods similar to IHC [104]. Due to their excellent specificity and high affinity to targets, aptamers have attracted great attention in various fields in which selective recognition units are required. Recently, DNA aptamers were successfully employed in development of a poly-ligand profiling (PLP) that surveys phenotypic diversity underlying tumor progression and distinguishes breast cancer patients who did or did not derive benefit from trastuzumab [105].

References

1. Fitzgibbons PL et al (2015) Principles of analytic validation for immunohistochemical assays—guideline from the Pathology and Laboratory Quality Center. Arch Pathol Lab Med. Supplemental Digital Content Methodology (February 2015)
2. Torlakovic EE et al (2017) Evolution of quality assurance for clinical immunohistochemistry in the era of precision medicine–Part 2: Immunohistochemistry test performance characteristics. Appl Immunohistochem Mol Morphol 25(2):79–85
3. Administration, U.S.F.D. (2018) Companion diagnostics [cited 2018 05/29/2018]. Available from: https://www.fda.gov/MedicalDevices/ProductsandMedicalProcedures/InVitroDiagnostics/ucm407297.htm
4. Barr NJ, Taylor CR, Approach to the "unknown primary"–anaplastic tumors
5. Taylor CR, Cote RJ (1994) Immunomicroscopy: a diagnostic tool for the surgical pathologist, 2nd edn. W B Saunders Co. 452
6. Lin F, Liu H (2014) Immunohistochemistry in undifferentiated neoplasm/tumor of uncertain origin. Arch Pathol Lab Med 138(12):1583–1610
7. Fizazi K et al (2015) Cancers of unknown primary site: ESMO clinical practice guidelines for diagnosis treatment and follow-up. Ann Oncol 26(5):v133–v138
8. Gatalica Z et al (2018) Comprehensive analysis of cancers of unknown primary for the biomarkers of response to immune checkpoint blockade therapy. Eur J Cancer 94:179–186
9. Perou CM et al (2000) Molecular portraits of human breast tumours. Nature 406(6797): 747–752
10. Sorlie T et al (2001) Gene expression patterns of breast carcinomas distinguish tumor subclasses with clinical implications. Proc Natl Acad Sci USA 98(19):10869–10874
11. Sorlie T et al (2003) Repeated observation of breast tumor subtypes in independent gene expression data sets. Proc Natl Acad Sci USA 100(14):8418–8423
12. Reis-Filho JS, Pusztai L (2011) Gene expression profiling in breast cancer: classification, prognostication, and prediction. Lancet 378(9805):1812–1823
13. Goldhirsch A et al (2011) Strategies for subtypes—dealing with the diversity of breast cancer: highlights of the St. Gallen International Expert Consensus on the primary therapy of early breast cancer. Ann Oncol 22(8):1736–1747
14. Metzger-Filho O et al (2012) Dissecting the heterogeneity of triple-negative breast cancer. J Clin Oncol 30(15):1879–1887
15. Millis SZ et al (2015) Predictive biomarker profiling of >6000 breast cancer patients shows heterogeneity in TNBC with treatment implications. Clin Breast Cancer 15(6):473–481.e3
16. Traina TA et al (2018) Enzalutamide for the treatment of androgen receptor-expressing triple-negative breast cancer. J Clin Oncol 36(9):884–890
17. Jaspers HC et al (2011) Androgen receptor-positive salivary duct carcinoma: a disease entity with promising new treatment options. J Clin Oncol 29(16):e473–e476
18. Arce-Salinas C et al (2016) Complete response of metastatic androgen receptor-positive breast cancer to bicalutamide: case report and review of the literature. J Clin Oncol 34(4): e21–e24
19. Bhargava R, Dabbs DJ (2017) Magee equations and oncotype DX®—a perspective. Breast Cancer Res Treat 164(1):245–246
20. Klein ME et al (2013) Prediction of the oncotype DX recurrence score: use of pathology-generated equations derived by linear regression analysis. Mod Pathol 26(5): 658–664
21. McCart Reed AE et al (2015) Invasive lobular carcinoma of the breast: morphology, biomarkers and 'omics. Breast Cancer Res 17:12
22. Oberg K (2012) Neuroendocrine tumors of the digestive tract: impact of new classifications and new agents on therapeutic approaches. Curr Opin Oncol 24(4):433–440

23. Travis WD et al (2015) The 2015 world health organization classification of lung tumors: impact of genetic, clinical and radiologic advances since the 2004 classification. J Thorac Oncol 10(9):1243–1260
24. Miettinen M, Sarlomo-Rikala M, Lasota J (1999) Gastrointestinal stromal tumors: recent advances in understanding of their biology. Hum Pathol 30(10):1213–1220
25. Hornick JL, Fletcher CD (2002) Immunohistochemical staining for KIT (CD117) in soft tissue sarcomas is very limited in distribution. Am J Clin Pathol 117(2):188–193
26. Hirota S (1998) Gain-of-function mutations of C-KIT in human gastrointestinal stromal tumors. Science 279(5350):577–580
27. Joensuu H et al (2001) Effect of the tyrosine kinase inhibitor STI571 in a patient with a metastatic gastrointestinal stromal tumor. N Engl J Med 344(14):1052–1056
28. Demetri GD (2001) Targeting c-kit mutations in solid tumors: scientific rationale and novel therapeutic options. Semin Oncol 28(5 Suppl 17):19–26
29. Heinrich MC et al (2003) Kinase mutations and imatinib response in patients with metastatic gastrointestinal stromal tumor. J Clin Oncol 21(23):4342–4349
30. Wong SF (2005) Cetuximab: an epidermal growth factor receptor monoclonal antibody for the treatment of colorectal cancer. Clin Ther 27(6):684–694
31. Chung KY et al (2005) Cetuximab shows activity in colorectal cancer patients with tumors that do not express the epidermal growth factor receptor by immunohistochemistry. J Clin Oncol 23(9):1803–1810
32. De Roock W et al (2010) Effects of KRAS, BRAF, NRAS, and PIK3CA mutations on the efficacy of cetuximab plus chemotherapy in chemotherapy-refractory metastatic colorectal cancer: a retrospective consortium analysis. Lancet Oncol 11(8):753–762
33. Tejpar S et al (2012) Association of KRAS G13D tumor mutations with outcome in patients with metastatic colorectal cancer treated with first-line chemotherapy with or without cetuximab. J Clin Oncol 30(29):3570–3577
34. Shi W et al (2017) Pathway level alterations rather than mutations in single genes predict response to HER2-targeted therapies in the neo-ALTTO trial. Ann Oncol 28(1):128–135
35. Altman DG et al (2012) Reporting recommendations for tumor marker prognostic studies (remark): explanation and elaboration. PLOS Medicine 9(5):e1001216
36. Acs B et al (2017) Ki-67 as a controversial predictive and prognostic marker in breast cancer patients treated with neoadjuvant chemotherapy. Diagn Pathol 12(1):20
37. Misiukiewicz K et al (2014) Controversies and role of HPV16 in recurrent/metastatic squamous cell cancers of the head and neck. Ann Oncol 25(8):1667–1668
38. Oldenhuis CN et al (2008) Prognostic versus predictive value of biomarkers in oncology. Eur J Cancer 44(7):946–953
39. Pritchard KI (2013) Endocrine therapy: is the first generation of targeted drugs the last? J Int Med 274(2):144–152
40. Jordan VC (2009) A century of deciphering the control mechanisms of sex steroid action in breast and prostate cancer: the origins of targeted therapy and chemoprevention. Cancer Res 69(4):1243–1254
41. Gashaw I et al (2012) What makes a good drug target? Drug Discov Today 17(Suppl): S24–S30
42. Hanahan D, Weinberg RA (2011) Hallmarks of cancer: the next generation. Cell 144 (5):646–674
43. Baudino TA (2015) Targeted cancer therapy: the next generation of cancer treatment. Curr Drug Discov Technol 12(1):3–20
44. Harries M, Smith I (2002) The development and clinical use of trastuzumab (Herceptin). Endocr Relat Cancer 9(2):75–85
45. Wolff AC et al (2013) Recommendations for human epidermal growth factor receptor 2 testing in breast cancer: American Society of Clinical Oncology/College of American Pathologists clinical practice guideline update. J Clin Oncol 31(31):3997–4013

46. Parakh S et al (2017) Evolution of anti-HER2 therapies for cancer treatment. Cancer Treat Rev 59:1–21
47. Yan M et al (2015) HER2 expression status in diverse cancers: review of results from 37,992 patients. Cancer Metastasis Rev 34(1):157–164
48. Bang YJ et al (2010) Trastuzumab in combination with chemotherapy versus chemotherapy alone for treatment of HER2-positive advanced gastric or gastro-oesophageal junction cancer (ToGA): a phase 3, open-label, randomised controlled trial. Lancet 376(9742):687–697
49. Clamon G et al (2005) Lack of trastuzumab activity in nonsmall cell lung carcinoma with overexpression of erb-B2: 39810: a phase II trial of Cancer and Leukemia Group B. Cancer 103(8):1670–1675
50. Sartore-Bianchi A et al (2016) Dual-targeted therapy with trastuzumab and lapatinib in treatment-refractory, KRAS codon 12/13 wild-type, HER2-positive metastatic colorectal cancer (HERACLES): a proof-of-concept, multicentre, open-label, phase 2 trial. Lancet Oncol 17(6):738–746
51. Cabel L et al (2018) Efficacy of histology-agnostic and molecularly-driven HER2 inhibitors for refractory cancers. Oncotarget 9(11):9741–9750
52. Teplinsky E, Muggia F (2014) Targeting HER2 in ovarian and uterine cancers: challenges and future directions. Gynecol Oncol 135(2):364–370
53. Mertens F et al (2015) The emerging complexity of gene fusions in cancer. Nat Rev Cancer 15(6):371–381
54. Teixido C et al (2014) Concordance of IHC, FISH and RT-PCR for EML4-ALK rearrangements. Transl Lung Cancer Res 3(2):70–74
55. Martin V et al (2015) ALK testing in lung adenocarcinoma: technical aspects to improve FISH evaluation in daily practice. J Thorac Oncol 10(4):595–602
56. Horn L, Pao W (2009) EML4-ALK: honing in on a new target in non-small-cell lung cancer. J Clin Oncol 27(26):4232–4235
57. Ali SM et al (2016) Comprehensive genomic profiling identifies a subset of crizotinib-responsive ALK-rearranged non-small cell lung cancer not detected by fluorescence in situ hybridization. Oncologist 21(6):762–770
58. Dagogo-Jack I, Shaw AT (2016) Screening for ALK rearrangements in lung cancer: time for a new generation of diagnostics? Oncologist 21(6):662–663
59. van der Wekken AJ et al (2017) Dichotomous ALK-IHC is a better predictor for ALK inhibition outcome than traditional ALK-FISH in advanced non-small cell lung cancer. Clin Cancer Res 23(15):4251–4258
60. Conde E et al (2016) Profile of ventana ALK (D5F3) companion diagnostic assay for non-small-cell lung carcinomas. Expert Rev Mol Diagn 16(6):707–713
61. Thorne-Nuzzo T et al (2017) A sensitive ALK immunohistochemistry companion diagnostic test identifies patients eligible for treatment with crizotinib. J Thorac Oncol 12(5):804–813
62. Bergethon K et al (2012) ROS1 rearrangements define a unique molecular class of lung cancers. J Clin Oncol 30(8):863–870
63. Wang R et al (2012) RET fusions define a unique molecular and clinicopathologic subtype of non-small-cell lung cancer. J Clin Oncol 30(35):4352–4359
64. Amatu A, Sartore-Bianchi A, Siena S (2016) NTRK gene fusions as novel targets of cancer therapy across multiple tumour types. ESMO Open 1(2):e000023
65. Shan L et al (2015) Detection of ROS1 gene rearrangement in lung adenocarcinoma: comparison of IHC, FISH and real-time RT-PCR. PLoS ONE 10(3):e0120422
66. Zhang T et al (2015) An evaluation and recommendation of the optimal methodologies to detect RET gene rearrangements in papillary thyroid carcinoma. Genes Chromosom Cancer 54(3):168–176
67. Hechtman JF et al (2017) Pan-Trk immunohistochemistry is an efficient and reliable screen for the detection of NTRK fusions. Am J Surg Pathol 41(11):1547–1551
68. Sholl LM et al (2013) ROS1 immunohistochemistry for detection of ROS1-rearranged lung adenocarcinomas. Am J Surg Pathol 37(9):1441–1449

69. Cha YJ et al (2014) Screening of ROS1 rearrangements in lung adenocarcinoma by immunohistochemistry and comparison with ALK rearrangements. PLoS ONE 9(7): e103333
70. Yoshida A et al (2014) Immunohistochemical detection of ROS1 is useful for identifying ROS1 rearrangements in lung cancers. Mod Pathol 27(5):711–720
71. Drilon A et al (2018) Efficacy of larotrectinib in TRK fusion-positive cancers in adults and children. N Engl J Med 378(8):731–739
72. Smith KM et al (2018) Antitumor activity of entrectinib, a Pan-TRK, ROS1, and ALK inhibitor, in ETV6-NTRK3-positive acute myeloid leukemia. Mol Cancer Ther 17(2): 455–463
73. Gatalica Z et al (2019) Molecular characterization of cancers with NTRK gene fusions. Mod Pathol 32(1):147–153
74. Murphy DA et al (2017) Detecting gene rearrangements in patient populations through a 2-step diagnostic test comprised of rapid IHC enrichment followed by sensitive next-generation sequencing. Appl Immunohistochem Mol Morphol 25(7):513–523
75. French CA (2010) Demystified molecular pathology of NUT midline carcinomas. J Clin Pathol 63(6):492–496
76. French CA et al (2014) NSD3-NUT fusion oncoprotein in NUT midline carcinoma: implications for a novel oncogenic mechanism. Cancer Discov 4(8):928–941
77. Gatalica Z et al (2018) NUTM1 gene rearranged neoplasia. Mod Pathol 31(2. abst. 1944):698–699
78. Cankovic M et al (2013) The role of MGMT testing in clinical practice: a report of the association for molecular pathology. J Mol Diagn 15(5):539–555
79. Ferriss JS et al (2010) Temozolomide in advanced and recurrent uterine leiomyosarcoma and correlation with o6-methylguanine DNA methyltransferase expression: a case series. Int J Gynecol Cancer 20(1):120–125
80. Guo Z, Lloyd RV (2016) Use of monoclonal antibodies to detect specific mutations in formalin-fixed, paraffin-embedded tissue sections. Hum Pathol 53:168–177
81. Rossi G et al (2017) Does immunohistochemistry represent a robust alternative technique in determining drugable predictive gene alterations in non-small cell lung cancer? Curr Drug Targets 18(1):13–26
82. Seo AN et al (2014) Novel EGFR mutation-specific antibodies for lung adenocarcinoma: highly specific but not sensitive detection of an E746_A750 deletion in exon 19 and an L858R mutation in exon 21 by immunohistochemistry. Lung Cancer 83(3):316–323
83. Bellevicine C et al (2015) Performance of EGFR mutant-specific antibodies in different cytological preparations: a validation study. Cytopathology 26(2):99–105
84. Hyman DM et al (2015) Vemurafenib in multiple nonmelanoma cancers with BRAF V600 mutations. N Engl J Med 373(8):726–736
85. Diamond EL et al (2018) Vemurafenib for BRAF V600-mutant Erdheim-Chester disease and langerhans cell histiocytosis: analysis of data from the histology-independent, phase 2 open-label VE-BASKET study. JAMA Oncol 4(3):384–388
86. Falchook GS et al (2013) BRAF mutant gastrointestinal stromal tumor: first report of regression with BRAF inhibitor dabrafenib (GSK2118436) and whole exomic sequencing for analysis of acquired resistance. Oncotarget 4(2):310–315
87. Gatalica Z et al (2016) Concordance of anti-BRAF p. V600E immunohistochemistry with BRAF gene sequence in solid tumors carrying diverse BRAF mutations. Mod Pathol 29 (2):454A
88. Gatalica Z et al (2015) BRAF mutations are potentially targetable alterations in a wide variety of solid cancers. Eur J Cancer 51(Suppl. 3):S31
89. Gatalica Z et al (2015) Disseminated histiocytoses biomarkers beyond BRAFV600E: frequent expression of PD-L1. Oncotarget 6(23):19819–19825

90. Huss S et al (2017) Clinicopathological and molecular features of a large cohort of gastrointestinal stromal tumors (GISTs) and review of the literature: BRAF mutations in KIT/PDGFRA wild-type GISTs are rare events. Hum Pathol 62:206–214
91. Parslow AC et al (2016) Antibody-drug conjugates for cancer therapy. Biomedicines 4(3)
92. Bardia A et al (2017) Efficacy and safety of anti-trop-2 antibody drug conjugate sacituzumab govitecan (IMMU-132) in heavily pretreated patients with metastatic triple-negative breast cancer. J Clin Oncol 35(19):2141–2148
93. Rudin CM et al (2017) Rovalpituzumab tesirine, a DLL3-targeted antibody-drug conjugate, in recurrent small-cell lung cancer: a first-in-human, first-in-class, open-label, phase 1 study. Lancet Oncol 18(1):42–51
94. Martin LP et al (2017) Characterization of folate receptor alpha (FRalpha) expression in archival tumor and biopsy samples from relapsed epithelial ovarian cancer patients: a phase I expansion study of the FRalpha-targeting antibody-drug conjugate mirvetuximab soravtansine. Gynecol Oncol 147(2):402–407
95. Olaussen KA et al (2006) DNA repair by ERCC1 in non-small-cell lung cancer and cisplatin-based adjuvant chemotherapy. N Engl J Med 355(10):983–991
96. Braun MS et al (2008) Predictive biomarkers of chemotherapy efficacy in colorectal cancer: results from the UK MRC FOCUS trial. J Clin Oncol 26(16):2690–2698
97. Von Hoff DD et al (2010) Pilot study using molecular profiling of patients' tumors to find potential targets and select treatments for their refractory cancers. J Clin Oncol 28(33):4877–4883
98. Topalian SL et al (2016) Mechanism-driven biomarkers to guide immune checkpoint blockade in cancer therapy. Nat Rev Cancer 16(5):275–287
99. Agilent (2018) PD-L1 IHC 22C3 pharmDx testing for gastric or GEJ adenocarcinoma. pharmDx 2018 [cited 2018 05/29/2018]. Available from: https://www.agilent.com/en-us/products/pharmdx/pd-l1-ihc-22c3-pharmdx-testing-for-gastric-gej
100. Hudelist G et al (2006) Her-2/neu and EGFR tyrosine kinase activation predict the efficacy of trastuzumab-based therapy in patients with metastatic breast cancer. Int J Cancer 118(5):1126–1134
101. David K, Juhl H (2015) Immunohistochemical detection of phosphoproteins and cancer pathways. Handbook of practical immunohistochemistry. Springer, New York
102. Ellington AD, Szostak JW (1990) In vitro selection of RNA molecules that bind specific ligands. Nature 346(6287):818–822
103. Tuerk C, Gold L (1990) Systematic evolution of ligands by exponential enrichment: RNA ligands to bacteriophage T4 DNA polymerase. Science 249(4968):505–510
104. Wu X et al (2015) Aptamers: active targeting ligands for cancer diagnosis and therapy. Theranostics 5(4):322–344
105. Domenyuk V et al (2018) Poly-ligand profiling differentiates trastuzumab-treated breast cancer patients according to their outcomes. Nat Commun 9(1):1219
106. Rittmeyer A et al (2017) Atezolizumab versus docetaxel in patients with previously treated non-small-cell lung cancer (OAK): a phase 3, open-label, multicentre randomised controlled trial. Lancet 389(10066):255–265
107. Reck M et al (2016) Pembrolizumab versus chemotherapy for PD-L1-positive non-small-cell lung cancer. N Engl J Med 375(19):1823–1833
108. Herbst RS et al (2016) Pembrolizumab versus docetaxel for previously treated, PD-L1-positive, advanced non-small-cell lung cancer (KEYNOTE-010): a randomised controlled trial. Lancet 387(10027):1540–1550
109. Borghaei H et al (2015) Nivolumab versus docetaxel in advanced nonsquamous non-small-cell lung cancer. N Engl J Med 373(17):1627–1639
110. Rosenberg JE et al (2016) Atezolizumab in patients with locally advanced and metastatic urothelial carcinoma who have progressed following treatment with platinum-based chemotherapy: a single-arm, multicentre, phase 2 trial. Lancet 387(10031):1909–1920

111. Massard C et al (2016) Safety and efficacy of durvalumab (medi4736), an anti-programmed cell death ligand-1 immune checkpoint inhibitor, in patients with advanced urothelial bladder cancer. J Clin Oncol 34(26):3119–3125
112. Powles T et al (2017) Efficacy and safety of durvalumab in locally advanced or metastatic urothelial carcinoma: updated results from a phase 1/2 open-label study. JAMA Oncol 3(9): e172411
113. Bellmunt J et al (2017) Pembrolizumab as second-line therapy for advanced urothelial carcinoma. N Engl J Med 376(11):1015–1026
114. Sharma P et al (2017) Nivolumab in metastatic urothelial carcinoma after platinum therapy (CheckMate 275): a multicentre, single-arm, phase 2 trial. Lancet Oncol 18(3):312–322
115. Apolo AB et al (2017) Avelumab, an anti-programmed death-ligand 1 antibody, in patients with refractory metastatic urothelial carcinoma: results from a multicenter, phase Ib study. J Clin Oncol 35(19):2117–2124
116. Robert C et al (2015) Pembrolizumab versus ipilimumab in advanced melanoma. N Engl J Med 372(26):2521–2532
117. Seiwert TY et al (2016) Safety and clinical activity of pembrolizumab for treatment of recurrent or metastatic squamous cell carcinoma of the head and neck (KEYNOTE-012): an open-label, multicentre, phase 1b trial. Lancet Oncol 17(7):956–965
118. Ferris RL et al (2016) Nivolumab for recurrent squamous-cell carcinoma of the head and neck. N Engl J Med 375(19):1856–1867
119. Motzer RJ et al (2015) Nivolumab versus everolimus in advanced renal-cell carcinoma. N Engl J Med 373(19):1803–1813
120. Kaufman HL et al (2016) Avelumab in patients with chemotherapy-refractory metastatic Merkel cell carcinoma: a multicentre, single-group, open-label, phase 2 trial. Lancet Oncol 17(10):1374–1385
121. Fuchs CS et al (2018) Safety and efficacy of pembrolizumab monotherapy in patients with previously treated advanced gastric and gastroesophageal junction cancer: phase 2 clinical keynote-059 trial. JAMA Oncol 4(5):e180013
122. Schellens JHM et al (2018) Pembrolizumab for previously treated advanced cervical squamous cell cancer: preliminary results from the phase 2 KEYNOTE-158 study. J Clin Oncol 15:5514
123. El-Khoueiry AB et al (2017) Nivolumab in patients with advanced hepatocellular carcinoma (CheckMate 040): an open-label, non-comparative, phase 1/2 dose escalation and expansion trial. Lancet 389(10088):2492–2502

Genomics-Enabled Precision Medicine for Cancer

5

Alison Roos and Sara A. Byron

Contents

A. Roos · S. A. Byron (✉)
Integrated Cancer Genomics Division,
Translational Genomics Research Institute, Phoenix, AZ, USA
e-mail: sbyron@tgen.org

D. D. Von Hoff and H. Han (eds.), *Precision Medicine in Cancer Therapy*,
Cancer Treatment and Research 178, https://doi.org/10.1007/978-3-030-16391-4_5

5.1 Introduction

Next-generation sequencing (NGS) technologies have provided the unparalleled capacity to interrogate the genomic landscape of cancer. Large-scale research sequencing efforts, such as those undertaken by the Cancer Genome Atlas (TCGA) or the International Cancer Genome Consortium (ICGC) initiatives, have expanded the catalog of "driver" mutations and provided key insights into the genomic landscape of tumors, including identifying molecularly defined tumor subgroups and genomic features with potential clinical value [1–7].

Genomic information is increasingly being integrated into molecularly guided diagnosis, prognosis, and treatment of cancer. Genomic profiling is now included in the standard clinical management of various tumor types, including melanoma, glioma, sarcoma, lung cancer, breast cancer, ovarian cancer, colorectal cancer, and thyroid cancer. In addition to gene-centric variants (mutations, copy number events, and translocations/fusions), broader genomic features, such as mutational burden, are also being utilized to aid in clinical decision-making.

In this chapter, we aim to provide a general overview of the ways genomic information is being used to inform diagnosis, prognosis, and treatment of cancer.

5.2 Methods

A variety of DNA-based genomic tests are currently used in oncology, ranging from single gene tests to whole genome sequencing. Single-gene assays are widely used and focus on the detection of specific recurrent variants within key cancer genes, particularly genetic variants with well-characterized prognostic and predictive value. Clinically validated drug–gene relationships include the use of imatinib in Philadelphia chromosome–positive chronic myeloid leukemia, trastuzumab in *HER2*-amplified breast cancer, erlotinib and gefitinib in *EGFR*-mutated non-small cell lung cancer (NSCLC), crizotinib in *ALK*-positive NSCLC, vemurafenib in *BRAF*-mutated melanoma, and panitumumab in RAS wild-type colorectal cancer [8–13].

However, serial testing using single-gene assays can be time consuming and may deplete limited tumor tissue samples. Advancements in DNA sequencing technologies and data processing tools have enabled the detection of several types of genetic variation, including genomic mutations, amplifications, deletions, and translocations, from a single tumor biopsy [14]. NGS utilizes massively parallel sequencing to perform genomic analysis with a turnaround time and cost that are feasible for clinical application [15–17].

With the growing adoption of NGS in clinical laboratories, there is momentum toward using more comprehensive sequencing strategies, typically targeted cancer gene panels, though whole exome sequencing (WES) or whole genome sequencing (WGS) assays are also being leveraged [18]. These NGS assays allow the detection of a broader range of clinically relevant alterations and can aid in the identification of additional patients who may benefit from genomics-informed molecularly targeted therapy. NSCLC is a prime example, where the National Comprehensive Cancer Network (NCCN) recommends broad genomic profiling beyond single-gene *EGFR* and *ALK* testing, as the identification of rare driver alterations may also inform treatment, either with an approved agent or enrollment on a clinical trial [19].

Use of NGS approaches, including targeted sequencing panels, WES, and WGS, for genomics-enabled precision medicine in oncology is discussed and summarized in Table 5.1.

5.2.1 Targeted Panel Sequencing

Targeted sequencing panels represent the most common NGS-based strategy currently being used to inform the clinical management in oncology [20]. These targeted sequencing panels use a priori knowledge to select genes and genomic variants of clinical interest and utility for measurement. Targeted sequencing panels are customized, ranging from hotspot assays that detect specific, recurrent mutations in a handful of defined genes, to assays that measure the entire coding region of a larger set of selected genes. These sequencing panels can be designed to be tumor-type-specific measuring key alterations within a defined tumor-type, or tumor agnostic, measuring alterations more broadly relevant to cancer.

Various targeted sequencing panels are available within local hospital, university, or commercial Clinical Laboratory Improvements Amendments (CLIA) certified laboratories. In 2017, the US Food and Drug Administration (FDA) approved the first two NGS cancer gene panel diagnostic tests, the Memorial Sloan Kettering-Integrated Mutational Profiling of Actionable Cancer Targets (MSK-IMPACT) and the Foundation One CDx (F1CDx) tests. These approvals illustrate the growing shift toward more widespread and comprehensive genomic evaluation for clinical management in oncology, where in vitro diagnostic tests are used to measure multiple genomic variants in a single test rather than the traditional model of measuring single cancer biomarkers linked to individual therapies in separate assays. MSK-IMPACT is a 468-gene NGS assay that measures true somatic variants through tumor-normal paired sequencing analysis of formalin-fixed, paraffin-embedded (FFPE) tumor tissue for patients with solid malignancies [21]. The test reports information on somatic mutations, copy number alterations, and selected structural rearrangements, as well as mutational burden and microsatellite instability (MSI) status. This expanded exome panel has been used to

Table 5.1 Next-generation sequencing strategies

Assay type	Pros	Cons
Targeted panel sequencing	• Most common NGS platform used in oncology • High-throughput assay with deep coverage of targeted regions • Focuses on current clinically actionable alterations • Can be customized based on disease type or clinical interest • Various panels available through local institutions or commercial CLIA-certified laboratories	• Dependent on a priori knowledge to design the targeted panel • Alterations outside of the reportable target space will not be detected or reported • Can be tumor-only or paired tumor-normal for true somatic calls, depending on the assay • Limited opportunities for future research studies
Whole exome sequencing (WES)	• Covers the entire coding region of the genome allowing the assay to capture and report on rare variants in cancer genomics and on new biomarkers as they emerge, in addition to current clinically actionable alterations • Opportunities to evaluate genome-wide copy number variants • Available through local institutions or commercial CLIA-certified laboratories • Provides more comprehensive data for future research studies	• Not yet broadly adopted in the clinical setting • Typically utilizes a matched constitutional sample for true somatic variant calling • Requires computational resources, bioinformatics expertise, and clinical interpretation support
Whole genome sequencing (WGS)	• Most comprehensive and unbiased sequencing strategy, capturing coding and noncoding regions of the genome • Opportunities for the detection of translocations and noncoding events that may be missed by other approaches • Provides the most comprehensive data for future research studies	• Primarily used in the research setting, though examples of clinical WGS are emerging • Requires matched constitutional sample but allows for true somatic variant detection • Generally lower sequencing coverage compared to targeted panels or whole exome sequencing • Requires additional computational resources, bioinformatics expertise, and clinical interpretation support • Additional content included in the noncoding regions of the genome may not be well studied and thus may provide a limited immediate application for clinical care

NGS next-generation sequencing; *CLIA* Clinical Laboratory Improvements Amendments

guide patient treatment and enrollment on molecularly matched clinical trials. Indeed, prospective sequencing of over 10,000 patients with advanced cancer using the MSK-IMPACT test was recently reported to result in 11% of patients enrolling on a molecularly matched clinical trial [22]. F1CDx is a tumor-only NGS assay that measures mutations and copy number alterations in 324 genes, as well as selected gene rearrangements, MSI status, and tumor mutational burden from FFPE tumor samples. This assay is approved for use as a companion diagnostic test to identify patients with specific mutations that may benefit from selected FDA-approved therapies based on the approved drug labels. Seventeen on-label targeted therapies and associated genomic biomarkers are listed in the current companion diagnostic indications for this test. These include lung cancer patients that may benefit from EGFR or ALK inhibitors, melanoma patients that may benefit from BRAF and/or MEK inhibitors, breast cancer patients who may benefit from ERBB2 (HER2) inhibitors, colorectal cancer patients that may benefit from EGFR inhibitors, and ovarian cancer patients that may benefit from treatment with a PARP inhibitor. Various other targeted exome assays are also available to aid in clinical decision support. In addition to Foundation One, commercial testing is available from other companies, such as Caris Life Sciences or Tempus. The Caris Molecular Intelligence platform incorporates a targeted exome sequencing assay with immunohistochemistry and in situ hybridization assays [23, 24]. Tempus xO provides an expanded NGS-based sequencing panel, evaluating over 1700 cancer-related genes using paired tumor-normal analysis while also incorporating whole transcriptome RNA sequencing for unbiased fusion detection [25]. Institutions have also internally developed their own platforms [26] or implemented commercially available platforms, such as the Oncomine Dx Target assay [27], a 23-gene panel that is approved by the FDA as a companion diagnostic for NSCLC, or the Ion Torrent AmpliSeq cancer hotspot panels [28], both from Thermo Fisher Scientific (www.thermofisher.com). Local testing allows for customization of the gene panel content based on local needs, but also requires local expertise in bioinformatics and molecular diagnostics.

Exome panels provide for high-throughput, deep coverage measurement of clinically significant alterations, allowing for the detection of low allele frequency variants within heterogeneous or low tumor content samples. Panel characteristics should be considered, as a potentially actionable event may not be detected or reported if it is not within the defined gene list or reportable target space for the panel. More comprehensive profiling may be particularly valuable for patients that have failed the standard of care treatment and for whom the standard molecular testing is negative [29, 30].

5.2.2 Whole Exome Sequencing

Though not yet broadly adopted for clinical management, WES is increasingly being leveraged in precision medicine clinical trials and care for patients with advanced cancer [31]. WES utilizes a selection or enrichment step to capture the exome, or the coding region of the genome, for sequencing and is often performed as a paired analysis with a patient-specific non-malignant sample, such as peripheral blood [15, 32]. While the exome represents only ~1–2% of the human genome, it contains the majority of current clinically actionable variants. Indeed, the major genome sequencing efforts by ICGC and TCGA utilized WES to develop a catalog of genomic alterations across cancer [2, 7, 33], informing our understanding of the genomic basis of these diseases and revealing a landscape of potentially targetable alterations that is being leveraged in the modern practice of genomics-enabled medicine.

WES provides a broader view of the spectrum of genomic alterations within a tumor, capturing alterations across nearly the entire coding region of the genome, including the regions targeted on focused gene panel tests. This more comprehensive approach allows for the detection and reporting of rare variants in cancer, as well as the inclusion of new and emerging biomarkers without the need to validate a new test. However, the increased data generated with WES compared to targeted gene panel tests also requires increased bioinformatic and clinical interpretation support [34]. This may be particularly relevant for reporting variants of uncertain significance. WES provides an added potential benefit of more broadly contributing to the field of precision oncology research, with the potential to leverage these more comprehensive data in research studies to identify novel therapeutic targets and mechanisms of drug sensitivity or resistance [34]. However, WES may not capture alterations in noncoding regions of the genome, which can be particularly relevant for detecting breakpoints involved in clinically informative translocations. The inclusion of RNA sequencing can help overcome some of these challenges by providing an orthogonal measure to detect these clinically relevant gene fusion events [35]. RNA sequencing can also aid in variant prioritization by confirming that variants of potential interest are expressed in the RNA and by providing insight into allele-specific expression [36]. Several studies have reported the use of integrative clinical exome and RNA sequencing and demonstrated feasibility for this approach in the management of advanced pediatric and adult cancers [35, 37–42].

5.2.3 Whole Genome Sequencing

Whole genome sequencing allows for sequencing of the entire genome. While generally providing lower sequencing coverage, WGS can effectively detect most types of somatic variation. In addition to exome coverage, WGS also detects mutations in noncoding regions, including untranslated regions, introns, promoters, and noncoding RNAs, as well as large deletions, insertions, duplications, and translocations. Thus, WGS provides a more comprehensive view of the tumor genome [43].

WGS produces a large amount of sequencing information, which requires expansive computational and bioinformatics expertise and resources, and impacts cost and turnaround time for reporting results [44]. Furthermore, the limited understanding of noncoding regions of the genome raises questions as to the biological ramifications and current clinical utility of the additional alterations detected by WGS.

While WGS is leveraged primarily in the research setting, there are emerging reports applying clinical WGS in cancer. Laskin et al. performed CAP-accredited WGS for 100 patients with advanced cancer as part of a personalized oncogenomics study [45]. Of the 78 patients for which WGS testing was completed, 55 patients received actionable results and 23 patients (42%) were treated based on these results. Of note, 61% (14/23) of these patients showed clinical or radiographic improvement on the genomics-informed treatment regimen. Together, these results showed WGS is feasible for use in personalized medicine trials. Another recent study out of the UK reported results from eight advanced cancer patients enrolled on a clinical WGS study [46]. WGS analysis resulted in the identification of potential treatment options for all eight patients, clarification of a diagnosis for one patient, and de-escalation of therapy for one patient. Of note, the authors reported that clinical WGS resulted in the identification of more potentially actionable variants compared to typical targeted NGS, suggesting the potential for these more comprehensive sequencing assays to expand the catalog of variants detected to support clinical decision-making.

5.2.4 Additional Considerations and Applications

Clinical genomics applications can include various types of patient-derived input material, such as fresh tissue, FFPE tissue, bone marrow aspirate, fine-needle aspirates, and peripheral blood. The inclusion of a "normal" non-malignant constitutional DNA sample for paired tumor-normal analysis is important for the comprehensive WES and WGS assays, and is common for many large sequencing panels, allowing for the identification of true somatic variants.

NGS techniques are also being applied to the detection of cell-free tumor DNA (cfDNA) or RNA (cfRNA). These "liquid biopsy" applications provide a less invasive strategy for genomic analysis. These assays allow the detection of somatic genomic alterations in the circulation for tumors that are inaccessible for a tissue biopsy, and can also be used for monitoring disease burden, treatment response, and development of therapy resistance through serial sampling [47]. cfDNA assays can be targeted, measuring specific known mutations relevant to cancer care. In 2016, the FDA approved the first liquid biopsy test, cobas EGFR Mutation Test v2, which measures targeted *EGFR* mutations from plasma samples as a companion diagnostic test for lung cancer [48]. In addition to single gene testing, cfDNA can also be evaluated using multi-gene NGS panels [49]. In 2018, the FDA granted Breakthrough Device designation to multi-gene panels from Foundation Medicine and Personal Genome Diagnostics, and Expedited Access Pathway designation to Guardant Health's multi-gene Guardant360 liquid biopsy assay. These approvals represent promising initial steps toward broader clinical use of cfDNA measurements in oncology [50].

5.3 Genomics-Enabled Medicine for Cancer Diagnosis

In concert with anatomic pathology, molecular diagnostics, including genomic characterization of a tumor, can aid in clinical diagnosis. Genomic profiling can be used to identify molecular markers of malignancy and thus aid in disease

Table 5.2 Use of genomic profiling in cancer diagnosis, prognosis, and treatment

Diagnosis	Prognosis	Treatment
Genomic profiling can aid in cancer diagnosis • Adjunct test for indeterminant disease (distinguishing malignant from benign disease) • Detection of pathognomonic genomic alterations for accurate diagnosis, as well as for potential use in early cancer detection • Molecular subclassification of tumors, distinguishing disease subgroups with distinct clinical trajectories • Cancers of unknown primary	Genomic alterations for risk assessment and to identify which patients are most and least likely to benefit from more aggressive therapy • Transcriptome profiles • Single gene measures (*MYCN* amplification, *TP53* mutation, etc.) • Genomic features (17p deletion, dMMR) • Noncoding variants (*TERT* promoter mutations)	Detection of genomic alterations that can inform treatment strategies • Alterations in drug targets that confer drug sensitivity or resistance • Alterations in pathway modifiers that confer drug sensitivity or resistance • Alterations in genes that induce drug sensitivity through synthetic lethal interactions • Broader genomic features associated with drug response (MSI, dMMR, mutational burden) • Germline variants that influence drug pharmacokinetics or pharmacodynamics, including polymorphisms associated with drug toxicity and biomarkers of drug sensitivity

MYCN MYCN proto-oncogene, BHLH transcription factor; *TP53* tumor protein 53; *dMMR* mismatch repair deficiency; *TERT* telomerase reverse transcriptase; *MSI* microsatellite instability

classification and clinical decision-making (Table 5.2). For example, though thyroid nodules are common, less than 10% represent malignant tumors. Fine-needle aspiration cytology is a widely used diagnostic tool to identify patients at risk of malignancy that should undergo surgery. However, in 15–30% of cases the cytology results are indeterminant. Previously, these patients underwent diagnostic thyroid surgery, with a majority found to have benign disease. Molecular testing, together with clinical and ultrasound features, has shown promise in classifying these indeterminant nodules. By identifying common mutations associated with thyroid cancer, such as *BRAF* mutations, molecular testing can be used to stratify patients for surgery or surveillance [51]. For example, the ThyroSeq v3 assay uses DNA and RNA sequencing to measure mutations, copy number events, fusions, and gene expression changes that are together used to classify samples as malignant or benign [52]. Thus, genomic testing can be used as an adjunct test for clinical cancer diagnosis, particularly in the context of indeterminant malignant classifications, and may help identify patients with benign nodules that can circumvent surgery.

Understanding the genomic features of a tumor can also assist in cancer diagnosis through the identification of pathognomonic genomic alteration. Several tumor types, particularly rare tumors, are characterized by pathognomonic genomic events [53]. For example, Ewing's sarcoma is characterized by a pathognomonic reciprocal chromosomal translocation involving EWS and an ETS transcription factor, typically FLI1. The EWS-FLI1 fusion protein is found in more than 80% of Ewing's sarcoma tumors [54]. Additional examples of characteristic pathognomonic alterations include gastrointestinal stromal tumors (*KIT* or *PDGFRA* mutations) [55, 56], hairy cell leukemia (*BRAF* V600E mutation) [57], small cell carcinoma of the ovary hypercalcemic type (*SMARCA4* mutations) [58–60], and granulosa cell tumors of the ovary (*FOXL2* C134W mutation) [61].

Genomic features have also contributed to the ongoing refinement of the molecular classification of tumors. The 2016 World Health Organization (WHO) classification of central nervous system (CNS) tumors provides a prime example of the shift toward incorporating molecular features with tumor histology for disease classification and diagnosis. Here, molecular features including copy number state (i.e., codeletion of chromosomal arms 1p and 19q), mutation status (i.e., *IDH1*/*IDH2*, *TP53*, H3 K27M mutations), and fusion detection (i.e., RELA fusion positive) are used to molecularly classify CNS tumors [62]. Genomic features also provide value in molecularly classifying tumor subgroups, which can be clinically relevant for distinguishing subgroups with distinct disease trajectories and treatment approaches. In rhabdomyosarcoma (RMS), the identification of PAX-FOXO gene translocations led to the reclassification into fusion positive and fusion negative RMS, which have distinct clinical and histological profiles [63]. Genomic profiling also allows the identification and classification of tumors with shared characteristic genomic features. For example, mutations and deletions of members of the SWI/SNF chromatin remodeling complex (*SMARCA4*/*SMARCA2*/*SMARCB1*) have been identified in multiple tumor types [58–60, 64–68]. Efforts are underway to evaluate treatment approaches collectively within these "SWI/SNF-omas" [69].

Genomic profiling may also have diagnostic utility for metastatic carcinoma of unknown primary (CUP) site. Each year, more than 30,000 patients receive a CUP diagnosis [70]. The diagnostic workup for CUP leverages molecular testing, though this testing is typically focused on immunohistochemical (IHC) analysis [71, 72]. CUP is a difficult to treat malignancy that has historically been managed as a single disease, with patients typically treated using platinum-based chemotherapy. Potential applications for genomic profiling in CUP management are emerging, including growing interest in using genomic profiling to identify potential treatment options and improve outcomes for these patients [70, 73, 74]. A recent study used NGS to evaluate 236 cancer-related genes in 200 CUP tumor samples and found 85% of CUP tumors had at least one clinically actionable genomic alteration detected [70]. Similarly, Gatalica et al. reported results from a multi-platform study using sequencing, in situ hybridization, and IHC analysis for over 1800 CUP tumors, where a biomarker associated with potential drug response was identified in over 90% of tumors [75].

5.4 Genomics-Enabled Medicine for Cancer Prognosis

Prognostic biomarkers are used at the time of diagnosis to identify individuals at a higher risk of a future clinical event, including disease recurrence, tumor progression, and death, independent of therapy. Traditional prognostic biomarkers in oncology include features such as tumor size, lymph node positivity, and metastasis. Genomic information is increasingly being used, together with clinical and pathologic prognostic factors, to improve prognostication (Table 5.2).

Various molecular profiling assays have demonstrated clinical utility and are used in routine practice to provide prognostic information [76]. In breast cancer, multi-gene transcriptome assays are routinely used to identify patients who are most and least likely to benefit from adjuvant chemotherapy. For example, the Oncotype Dx 21-gene recurrence score has been prospectively validated to identify patients with lymph node-negative, hormone receptor-positive breast cancer with a favorable prognosis and low risk of recurrence, such that endocrine therapy alone is sufficient and chemotherapy is unlikely to provide additional clinical benefit [77]. In addition to the recurrence score, the American Society of Clinical Oncology has also recently supported the use of additional prognostic profiles in breast cancer, including EndoPredict, predictor analysis of microarray 50, and the Breast Cancer Index. Prognostic profiles are also being developed and used in other tumor types, including colorectal cancer, prostate cancer, lung cancer, and melanoma [78–81].

Individual genomic alterations can also be leveraged as prognostic biomarkers. For example, in neuroblastoma, molecular and cytogenetic features are used for risk assessment and to guide treatment recommendations. *MYCN* amplification is associated with poor prognosis and is used to identify patients with high-risk disease, irrespective of patient age or localized versus metastatic disease at diagnosis [82]. In addition to *MYCN* amplification, DNA ploidy and segmental chromosomal alterations (such as loss of heterozygosity on 11q) have also been incorporated into the International Neuroblastoma Risk Group classification system [82].

Broader genomic features can also serve as prognostic biomarkers. In localized colorectal cancer, mismatch repair (MMR) deficiency is associated with longer survival compared to MMR proficient tumors [83, 84]. MMR deficiency is associated with a high number of DNA replication errors and is characterized by high levels of microsatellite instability (MSI). MSI status is considered a clinically significant prognostic factor, and MSI or MMR deficiency evaluation is recommended during colorectal cancer staging [85].

The utility of genomic information for prognostication is well illustrated by its use in hematological malignancies. Genomic abnormalities are used to classify acute myeloid leukemia (AML) into distinct risk groups. *NPM1* mutations and biallelic *CEBPA* mutations are associated with favorable prognosis, whereas internal tandem duplication in *FLT3* (FLT3-ITD), or *RUNX1*, *ASXL1*, or *TP53* mutations is associated with adverse risk [86]. Molecular genetic testing is also routinely performed in chronic lymphocytic leukemia (CLL), where specific cytogenetic abnormalities are associated with favorable (del(13q) or trisomy 12) or unfavorable (del(17p) or del(11q)) prognosis [87]. Unmutated *IGHV* is associated with poor prognosis and worse survival outcomes in CLL, irrespective of disease stage [88, 89]. *TP53* mutation status and chromosome 17p deletions are also important prognostic markers in CLL, with *TP53* mutation and/or 17p deletion associated with more rapid disease progression and poor outcomes. Recent prognostic models, such as the CLL international prognostic index (CLL-IPI), are incorporating these genomic features with classical clinical parameters. In the CLL-IPI, *TP53* mutation and/or 17p deletion showed the greatest adverse association with overall survival [90]. Notably, though these patients historically demonstrated resistance to the standard fludarabine-based chemotherapy, recent clinical trials have shown that patients with *TP53* mutations or 17p deletion respond well to newer agents, including the B-cell receptor inhibitor, ibrutinib, and the BCL2 pathway inhibitor, venetoclax [91]. Ibrutinib and venetoclax are now FDA-approved for CLL patients with 17p deletions [92].

5.5 Genomics-Enabled Medicine for Cancer Treatment

Genomic profiling can also be used to identify key oncogenic drivers or genomic vulnerabilities that can be targeted with a therapeutic agent (Table 5.2). Genetically driven tumor dependencies have been identified and successfully targeted in various tumor types, including CML, melanoma, lung cancer, and breast cancer [8–11, 93–95]. In each of these examples, a specific genomic alteration has been associated with improved response to a molecularly targeted agent, and tests to detect these alterations have been developed as companion diagnostics for the FDA-approved therapy. The current FDA-approved companion diagnostic tests are listed on the FDA Web site (http://www.fda.gov/medicaldevices/productsandmedicalprocedures/invitrodiagnostics/ucm301431.htm). Together, the current companion diagnostic tests in oncology measure a broad spectrum of therapeutically informative genomic alteration types, including gene fusions, point mutations, and copy number events, as described in the examples below (Table 5.3).

5.5.1 Therapeutically Informative Translocations and Fusions

Structural rearrangements leading to gene fusions are a key area of focus in precision oncology. Targeting these constitutively active fusion proteins can lead to dramatic clinical responses and transform clinical management, as exemplified by targeting of BCR–ABL fusions in chronic myeloid leukemia (CML) [96]. BCR–ABL gene fusion results from a reciprocal translocation involving chromosomes 9 and 22 producing the Philadelphia chromosome. The BCR–ABL fusion is found in 95% of CML, and the introduction of agents that inhibit this gene fusion, such as imatinib and nilotinib, dramatically improved overall survival for patients with this

Table 5.3 Selected examples of genomic alterations used to inform cancer treatment

Types of genomic alterations	Examples of applications to inform cancer treatment		
	Alteration	Tumor type	Clinical use
Gene fusions	*BCR–ABL* fusion	Chronic myelogenous leukemia	Informs treatment with BCR–ABL inhibitors
	ALK fusions	Lung cancer	Informs treatment with ALK inhibitors
	ROS1 fusions	Lung cancer	Informs treatment with ROS1 inhibitors
	NTRK fusions	Tumor-type agnostic—solid tumors	Informs treatment with TRK inhibitor
Single-nucleotide variants	*EGFR* mutations (L858R, T790M, exon 19 deletions, etc.)	Lung cancer	Targeted companion diagnostic tests for tissue or liquid biopsies to detect sensitive or resistant mutations to inform treatment with EGFR inhibitor
	BRAF V600E	Melanoma	Informs treatment with a BRAF V600E inhibitor and MEK inhibitor
	KRAS or *NRAS* mutations (exons 2, 3, 4)	Colorectal cancer	RAS mutations are associated with resistance to EGFR inhibitors; RAS mutation status is typically measured in metastatic colorectal cancer patients for whom EGFR inhibitor treatment is being considered
	BRCA1 or *BRCA2* mutations	Ovarian cancer	Informs treatment with PARP inhibitors
Copy number alterations	*ERBB2*	Breast cancer, gastric adenocarcinoma, esophagogastric junction adenocarcinoma	Amplification of *ERBB2* (HER2) defines a subgroup of HER2-positive breast cancer and is used to guide treatment with ERBB2 inhibitors in this patient population
Other genomic features	Microsatellite instability	Tumor-type agnostic—solid tumors	Inform treatment with immune checkpoint inhibitors
	Mismatch repair deficiency	Tumor-type agnostic—solid tumors	Inform treatment with immune checkpoint inhibitors

disease such that life expectancy is now approaching that is seen in the non-CML population [96–100].

Building on the landmark success of inhibiting BCR–ABL in CML, chromosomal translocations and gene fusions have now been identified in a wide range of tumor types, including epithelial cancers, brain tumors, sarcomas, and hematological malignancies [101–103]. The catalog of potentially actionable gene fusions is growing, as is the evidence for clinical benefit from targeting these fusions [4, 104–106].

Several companion diagnostic tests have been approved for the detection of therapeutically relevant translocations and fusions. For example, translocations involving anaplastic lymphoma kinase (*ALK*) occur in 3–5% of NSCLC. EML4-ALK represents the most common *ALK* fusion in lung cancer, though several other fusion partners for *ALK* have been identified [107]. Current guidelines recommend *ALK* testing for patients with advanced NSCLC [108, 109]. ALK inhibitors, such as crizotinib, ceritinib, and alectinib, have demonstrated clinical activity in ALK-rearranged NSCLC and are considered first-line therapy in this setting [110, 111]. In addition, *ROS1* fusions are found in 1–2% of NSCLC [112], as well as in other tumor types (glioblastoma, cholangiocarcinoma, angiosarcoma, and others [113]). *ROS1* fusions result from a translocation between *ROS1* and an expanding roster of fusion partners, most commonly *CD74* [112, 113]. The ALK inhibitor, crizotinib, has shown clinical activity in ROS1-rearranged NSCLC [93] and was approved by the FDA in 2016 for use in this genomically defined patient population.

There is a growing movement toward treating fusion positive tumors with targeted inhibitors regardless of the tissue of origin. FGFR inhibitors have shown activity in various FGFR fusion positive tumors, including cholangiocarcinoma, bladder cancer, and gliomas [114]. Another emerging example is the detection of *NTRK* fusions, where one of the three NTRK genes (*NTRK1*, *NTRK2*, and *NTRK3*) is fused with one of over 50 different fusion partners [115]. NTRK fusions occur at low prevalence overall in cancer, but have been reported in multiple adult and pediatric tumor types. Inhibitors with activity against *NTRK* have shown promising results in clinical trials [116, 117]. Recent trials with larotrectinib, an NTRK1/2/3 inhibitor, reported an overall response rate of 75% in adults and children with NTRK fusion positive tumors [117]. Notably, 17 different tumor types were represented on the study, supporting a tumor agnostic approach to treating NTRK fusion tumors. Larotrectinib was recently approved by the FDA for use in NTRK fusion-positive solid tumors.

5.5.2 Therapeutically Informative Mutations

Single-nucleotide variants represent a common mechanism of genomic alteration in cancer. These alterations can contribute to a molecular context of the therapeutic vulnerability, either as direct targets for molecularly guided inhibitors or due to resulting pathway activation or synthetic lethal interactions. Specific examples are described below.

In lung cancer, multiple therapeutically informative biomarkers have been identified and validated and are now evaluated as part of standard clinical care to determine the therapeutic course. In addition to the *ALK* translocations described above, roughly 15–20% of NSCLCs in the USA contain activating mutations in *EGFR*, most frequently deletions in exon 19 or the L858R mutation in exon 21. Treatment with an EGFR tyrosine kinase inhibitor as first-line therapy, second-line therapy, or as maintenance therapy is associated with prolonged progression-free survival in NSCLC patients with *EGFR* mutations [118]. *EGFR* variants can be detected by various NGS tests, including companion diagnostic tests that detect specific *EGFR* mutations (L858R, T790M, exon 19 deletions) in tumor samples or in liquid biopsies, as well as broader NGS tests that measure across the coding region of *EGFR*.

BRAF is a serine/threonine protein kinase that activates the MAPK pathway. *BRAF* mutations are present in 40–60% of advanced cutaneous melanomas, with nearly 90% of these mutations representing the hotspot activating BRAF V600E mutation [119]. The BRAF V600E-targeted inhibitor, vemurafenib, was the first of several targeted agents to show improved survival for patients with *BRAF* V600E mutant metastatic melanoma [11, 120, 121]. Single-agent inhibition has largely been replaced by multi-targeted pathway inhibition, combining a BRAF inhibitor (vemurafenib, dabrafenib) and a downstream MEK inhibitor (trametinib, cobimetinib) to prolong disease control [121–124]. Though *BRAF* V600E is used as a biomarker for BRAF/MEK inhibitor response in melanoma, these agents have shown mixed responses in other *BRAF* V600E mutant tumor types [125], demonstrating the importance of considering genomic features in the context of the tumor type as well as the genomic landscape of the tumor.

Genomics features can also provide information about which treatments may not be effective for a patient. In colorectal cancer, *KRAS/NRAS* mutation status is routinely measured prior to treatment with the upstream EGFR monoclonal antibodies, cetuximab and panitumumab. Roughly one-third of metastatic colorectal tumors carry *KRAS* or *NRAS* mutations, and RAS mutations have been shown to confer resistance to EGFR inhibitors [126–128]. Current treatment guidelines recommend *KRAS* and *NRAS* testing (exons 2, 3, and 4) for patients being considered as candidates for EGFR inhibitors [129].

5.5.3 Therapeutically Informative Copy Number Alterations

Genomic amplifications and deletions can also be therapeutically informative. In breast cancer, *ERBB2* (HER2) amplification is seen in ~15–20% of breast cancers [130], and HER2 testing is recommended for all patients with invasive breast cancer [131]. Various ERBB inhibitors have now been approved for use in HER2-positive metastatic breast cancer, including monoclonal antibodies targeting ERBB2 (trastuzumab, pertuzumab), antibody-drug conjugates (trastuzumab emtansine), and tyrosine kinase inhibitors with activity against ERBB2 (lapatinib, neratinib). Dual ERBB2 inhibitor treatment has shown increased efficacy in recent clinical trials in

HER2-positive metastatic breast cancer [132]. Trastuzumab has also been approved for use in patients with HER2-positive metastatic gastric or esophagogastric junction adenocarcinomas and, in combination with chemotherapy, is considered the standard first-line treatment for HER2-positive advanced esophagogastric cancer [133].

5.5.4 Other Genomic Features

5.5.4.1 Noncoding Variants

Noncoding variants are alterations in regions outside the coding exons of the genome. These noncoding elements include intronic regions and regulatory regions, such as gene enhancers, promoters, and untranslated regions (UTRs). The landscape of noncoding variants in cancer is less well characterized compared to protein-coding variants. However, the identification and characterization of clinically relevant noncoding alterations are emerging.

One of the most well-characterized noncoding driver alterations in cancer is a recurrent mutation in the *TERT* promoter. *TERT* encodes the catalytic subunit of telomerase, an enzyme involved in maintaining telomere length of chromosomes. Telomerase activation is a hallmark of cancer [134]. Recurrent hotspot mutations in the *TERT* promoter (C228T, C250T) have been shown to modulate TERT activity by increasing TERT expression via the creation of novel ETS family transcription factor binding sites [135]. Originally reported as a causal germline variant in a large melanoma pedigree, somatic *TERT* promoter mutations have also been reported in 71% of cutaneous melanomas [136] and in over 40 other cancer types [22, 137], including frequent mutations in glioblastoma, bladder cancer, and thyroid cancer [138–141]. *TERT* promoter mutations have been associated with more aggressive disease and worse outcome in various tumor types [142–146]. *TERT* promoter mutations can be identified using next-generation sequencing assays, including targeted *TERT* promoter sequencing analysis, exome panels and whole exome sequencing assays covering the *TERT* promoter region, and whole genome sequencing assays. TERT promoter analysis is included on several clinically available targeted exome panels. In the largest pan-cancer analysis of *TERT* promoter mutations to date, Zehir et al. recently reported the detection of *TERT* promoter mutations in 43 different tumor types based on prospective clinical exome panel sequencing of over 10,000 advanced cancer patients using the MSK-IMPACT panel [22]. Bladder cancer, glioma, thyroid cancer, and melanoma showed the highest frequency of *TERT* promoter mutations, with a trend for shorter survival for patients with *TERT* mutant tumors.

Additional clinically informative noncoding variants are likely to emerge with ongoing efforts by the research community to identify and characterize the functional implications of changes in the noncoding regions of the genome.

5.5.4.2 Microsatellite Instability Status

Microsatellite instability (MSI) is a hypermutability phenotype characterized by increased or decreased length of short nucleotide (microsatellite) repeats that result from defects in DNA mismatch repair activity. The failure to repair errors leads to a high number of somatic mutations, particularly in repetitive sequences. MSI is frequently seen in tumors associated with Lynch syndrome, a cancer predisposition disorder characterized by germline alterations in mismatch repair genes.

Importantly, MSI status has demonstrated utility as a predictive biomarker for anti-programmed cell death (PD-1) monoclonal antibody immune checkpoint inhibitor response [147–149]. In 2017, the FDA granted tumor agnostic approval for use of the anti-PD-1 immune checkpoint inhibitor, pembrolizumab, in treatment of pediatric or adult patients with unresectable or metastatic solid tumors that are MSI-high or DNA mismatch repair deficient. This approval was a historical advancement as it represented the first approval for a cancer treatment that was not based on tumor type, but instead was based on the presence of a unifying genomic biomarker [150]. Notably, pembrolizumab had previously received approval for use in multiple tumor types, including melanoma, NSCLC, head and neck squamous cell carcinoma, and urothelial carcinoma.

Traditionally, MSI status is determined by immunohistochemistry to evaluate MMR protein expression or using polymerase chain reaction (PCR) analysis of a panel of five core microsatellite markers, where tumors are classified as MSI-high if two or more markers show instability [151]. Given the clinical importance of identifying MSI-high tumors for potential immune checkpoint inhibitor treatment, there has been strong interest in reporting MSI status from genomic sequencing results. Vanderwalde et al. retrospectively analyzed over 2000 tumors with MSI testing performed by exome panel sequencing and by the standard PCR methods. The authors reported a high concordance with PCR-based results [152]. Current clinical guidelines have recommended MSI testing for colon and endometrial cancer patients. With tumor agnostic approval of pembrolizumab for MSI-high tumors, there is a growing move toward providing MSI testing for all patients with advanced solid tumors that lack treatment options. The ability to measure MSI status from exome-based sequencing assays provides a promising avenue for clinicians to access this information without a need for extra tumor tissue or molecular testing. Indeed, the catalog of tumor types impacted by MSI is expanding, with several recent large-scale profiling studies suggesting MSI is a more generalized cancer phenotype that has been detected in more than 20 different tumor types [22, 153, 154].

5.5.4.3 Mutational Burden

Mutational burden is a quantitative measure representing the total number of mutations detected within the coding area of the tumor genome, typically expressed as mutations per megabase (mut/Mb). Elevated mutational burden can reflect an underlying DNA repair defect in the tumor. Germline or somatic mutations in DNA mismatch repair genes (*MSH2*, *MSH6*, *PMS2*) as well as DNA replication genes (*POLE*, *POLD1*) have been associated with tumor hypermutation [155–159].

Mutational burden can be measured from targeted exome, whole exome, or whole genome platforms. The Cancer Genome Atlas (TCGA) project measured tumor mutational burden using whole exome sequencing data from $\sim$30 tumor types and found a range of mutational burdens both within and across tumor types [5]. Tumor types associated with mutagen exposure, such as melanoma and lung cancer, showed the highest median number of somatic mutations, whereas pediatric tumors, such as pilocytic astrocytoma and medulloblastoma, showed the lowest number of somatic mutations. Notably, hypermutated tumors, defined as those with >10 mut/Mb, were identified in a majority of tumor types. Chalmers et al. also recently reported mutational burden analysis from targeted exome panel data across >100,000 tumors representing 167 tumor types [160]. In addition to identifying additional tumor types with the high mutational burden, their analysis found individual tumors with high mutational burden in nearly all tumor types evaluated. Thirty-eight different tumor types were identified where more than 5% of patients had high mutational burden tumors. A hypermutated genotype can also arise due to treatment-induced changes, as has been reported for a subset of temozolomide-treated glioblastomas [161]. The emergence of this genomic feature during a patient's treatment course provides a rationale for repeat genomic testing of the tumor at recurrence/relapse when possible.

High mutational burden has been associated with improved response to immune checkpoint inhibitors in multiple tumor types, including melanoma, lung cancer, and mismatch repair deficient tumors [33, 147, 148, 162, 163]. The FDA recently provided tumor agnostic approval for pembrolizumab in pediatric and adult tumors with mismatch repair deficiency [150].

5.5.5 Emerging Applications

In addition to validated genomic biomarkers used in companion diagnostics, genomic information may be useful for identifying potential treatment options beyond the standard of care, either as an off-label use of an FDA-approved agent or for informing eligibility for a clinical trial (www.clinicaltrials.gov). The Bisgrove study provided an initial proof of principle that molecular profiling could improve patient outcomes. This prospective clinical trial used immunohistochemistry and gene expression profiling to inform treatment selection for 66 patients with advanced, treatment-refractory cancers. By comparing the time to progression on the molecularly guided treatment to the time to progression on the patient's previous therapy, the authors demonstrated that 27% of the patients benefited from the molecularly informed treatment (measured as a PFS ratio greater than or equal to 1.3) [164]. In 2012, the MD Anderson Cancer Center reported results from a phase 1 program using molecular profiling to guide treatment selection, where they found that advanced cancer patients treated with a molecularly guided therapy had higher response rates, longer time-to-treatment failure, and longer survival than patients who were not treated with a matched therapy [165]. Additional non-randomized studies have also shown increased response rates for patients enrolled on genomics-guided clinical trials [166]. In contrast, the SHIVA trial found no benefit for molecularly matched therapy compared to physician's choice in a prospective, randomized phase 2 study in heavily pretreated advanced cancer patients [167], though only three molecular pathways were used to assign patients to treatment with one of ten targeted agents.

Various clinical trials are underway testing the efficacy of more broadly using genomics to inform treatment. The recent MOSCATO 01 trial showed that genomics-guided therapy can improve patient outcome when the biomarker–drug pairs are well characterized and supported by strong clinical or preclinical evidence [168]. This prospective clinical trial used next-generation sequencing (including WES) and RNA sequencing to profile more than 800 patients with advanced cancer. Nearly half of the patients had an actionable alteration identified, with one-third of patients showing improved progression-free survival with the genomics-informed therapy compared to prior treatment. Several additional large-scale clinical trials are underway that aim to evaluate the utility of genomic profiling for adult and pediatric cancer patients (e.g., NCI-MATCH, ASCO TAPUR, INFORM2, ESMART) [169]. For example, the NCI Molecular Analysis for Therapeutic Choice (NCI-MATCH) trial is a basket trial that matches patients with recurrent or refractory solid tumors to a selected subset of molecularly targeted agents based on pre-defined drug–target pairs, regardless of the tumor type [170]. Reports from exceptional responders, as well as non-responders, can also be used to identify potential genomic alterations that are associated with treatment response and can guide future clinical trial designs [31, 171–175]. The US National Cancer Institute (NCI) launched an Exceptional Responders Initiative to retrospectively perform whole exome and RNA sequencing analysis to evaluate genomic markers in patients with exceptional, durable responses to therapy [176]. This study has met its accrual goal of 100 patients, and molecular analysis is ongoing (https://www.cancer.gov/about-cancer/treatment/research/exceptional-responders-initiative-qa).

One of the challenges with more widespread adoption of genomic profiling to guide patient treatment is the need for consistent interpretation of genomic variants and potential therapeutic associations, particularly for the many variants of uncertain significance that are detected with more comprehensive genomic profiling strategies [177, 178]. Expert curation of evidence for variant pathogenicity and variant–drug associations is needed. While many groups have developed their own internal frameworks and databases for variant reporting, a consensus on actionability does not currently exist [177], and there is a need for harmonized effort and agreement for consistent reporting in the clinical context. Ongoing efforts are focused on developing resources and guidelines for variant interpretation and variant–drug associations [179].

5.6 Germline Considerations

5.6.1 Clinically Actionable Germline Variants

Large-scale sequencing studies suggest the presence of pathogenic, cancer-associated germline variants in ~7–10% of pediatric and adult cancer patients [6, 180–182]. Germline genetic testing is recommended for high-risk individuals where the results will impact the patient's medical management, with genetic counseling recommended both prior to and after genetic testing. This includes patients with a family history that is multi-generational or early onset, or in cases informed by the clinical presentation, such as the presence of multiple tumor types in the same patient or of bilateral disease. However, testing based on current guidelines may miss the evaluation of clinically informative germline variants in an additional subset of patients. Interrogation of existing tumor-normal paired sequencing data for patients with advanced cancer revealed informative germline variants in 17.5% of patients (182/1040), where over half of these patients (101/182, 55%) would not have had germline testing performed based on guidelines [183]. Results such as these encourage continued discussion around the utility and challenges of expanding germline testing in oncology.

Importantly, in addition to cancer risk, germline variants can also inform treatment options. The pinnacle example of this association is the link between pathogenic germline *BRCA1/2* mutations and increased sensitivity to PARP inhibitors [184]. PARP inhibitors are FDA-approved for use in germline BRCA-mutated advanced ovarian cancers and breast cancers [185–187] and are being evaluated for use in other solid tumors [188].

There are also emerging examples of germline variants in DNA repair genes associated with increased response to immune checkpoint inhibitors. For example, two siblings with germline biallelic mismatch repair deficiency (BMMRD), a pediatric cancer syndrome associated with hypermutated tumors, developed recurrent glioblastoma tumors and showed clinical responses to the anti-PD1 immune checkpoint inhibitor, nivolumab [155]. *POLE* mutations have also been associated with increased response to immune checkpoint inhibitors. *POLE* is a DNA polymerase involved in DNA replication and repair. Germline and somatic mutations in the exonuclease domain of *POLE* have been reported in various tumor types and associated with a hypermutant genotype [189, 190]. There are a growing number of reports demonstrating response to PD1 inhibitors in patients with germline *POLE* mutations and hypermutated tumors, including in colorectal cancer, glioblastoma, and endometrial cancer [156–159].

5.6.2 Germline Pharmacogenomics in Oncology

Germline variants can also provide valuable pharmacogenomic information that can be leveraged to avoid or minimize treatment toxicity. Single-nucleotide polymorphisms in drug-metabolizing enzymes have been identified that are associated with increased risk for toxicity with the standard drug dosing. In oncology, several agents have germline pharmacogenomics recommendations included in their drug labels, including capecitabine, fluorouracil, irinotecan, 6-mercaptopurine, and thioguanine. The Clinical Pharmacogenetics Implementation Consortium (CPIC) has also released guidelines for fluoropyrimidines (capecitabine/5-fluorouracil), mercaptopurine/thioguanine, and tamoxifen [191–193]. Selected examples are discussed below.

It is estimated that 3–5% of Caucasians carry non-functional variants of *DYPD*, a gene that encodes the dihydropyrimidine dehydrogenase (DPD) enzyme involved in the rate-limiting step in fluoropyrimidine metabolism. These individuals are at increased risk for capecitabine/5-fluorouracil toxicity. The CPIC recommends genomics-informed dosing, with dose reduction for patients with partial DPD activity, and alternative therapy for those considered poor metabolizers [191]. Irinotecan represents another potential application for pharmacogenomics testing in oncology. Clearance of irinotecan involves metabolite inactivation by UDP-glucuronosyltransferase 1A1 (UGT1A1)-mediated glucuronidation. Individuals that are homozygous for the reduced function UGT1A1 polymorphism, UGT1A1*28, are at an increased risk for life-threatening neutropenia at the standard doses of irinotecan. Irinotecan should be used with caution in these patients with reduced UGT1A1 activity. Similarly, 6-mercaptopurine and thioguanine are inactivated by the enzyme thiopurine methyltransferase (TPMT). Individuals with very low TPMT activity due to reduced function polymorphisms can experience severe bone marrow toxicity on the standard doses of 6-mercaptopurine or thioguanine therapy. TPMT testing is recommended for individuals being treated with these agents, as individuals can be offered reduced dosing based on the presence of one or two non-functional TPMT alleles [192]. Additional pharmacogenomics markers for oncology agents are also being explored [194].

Despite genotype-driven dosing guidelines, upfront pharmacogenomic screening is not universally performed prior to starting these treatments. Further effort is needed to explore more widespread adoption of these tests and to evaluate opportunities to incorporate relevant pharmacogenomic profiling and reporting into current NGS platforms.

5.7 Conclusions

Cancer genomic testing has become more widely available in community hospitals and academic cancer centers and through commercial testing laboratories. The expanding knowledge and application of genomic profiling are anticipated to improve cancer diagnosis, risk stratification, and treatment selection. While early studies have focused on patients with rare tumors that lack standard of care treatment options and patients with advanced cancer that have failed standard of care treatments, responses seen in these patient populations have opened up opportunities to apply this information earlier in the treatment course, as exemplified by the current clinical management of NSCLC. It is anticipated that continued advances in the era of modern genomics-enabled medicine will expand its application to a broader spectrum on oncology patients.

Acknowledgements We thank the Ben and Catherine Ivy Foundation and the Dell Inc. Powering the Possible Program for support.

References

1. Vogelstein B, Papadopoulos N, Velculescu VE, Zhou S, Diaz LA Jr, Kinzler KW (2013) Cancer genome landscapes. Science 339(6127):1546–1558. https://doi.org/10.1126/science.1235122
2. Kandoth C, McLellan MD, Vandin F, Ye K, Niu B, Lu C et al (2013) Mutational landscape and significance across 12 major cancer types. Nature 502(7471):333–339. https://doi.org/10.1038/nature12634
3. Bailey MH, Tokheim C, Porta-Pardo E, Sengupta S, Bertrand D, Weerasinghe A et al (2018) Comprehensive characterization of cancer driver genes and mutations. Cell 173(2):371–385 e18. https://doi.org/10.1016/j.cell.2018.02.060
4. Gao Q, Liang WW, Foltz SM, Mutharasu G, Jayasinghe RG, Cao S et al (2018) Driver fusions and their implications in the development and treatment of human cancers. Cell Rep 23(1):227–238 e3. https://doi.org/10.1016/j.celrep.2018.03.050
5. Alexandrov LB, Nik-Zainal S, Wedge DC, Aparicio SA, Behjati S, Biankin AV et al (2013) Signatures of mutational processes in human cancer. Nature 500(7463):415–421. https://doi.org/10.1038/nature12477
6. Grobner SN, Worst BC, Weischenfeldt J, Buchhalter I, Kleinheinz K, Rudneva VA et al (2018) The landscape of genomic alterations across childhood cancers. Nature 555(7696):321–327. https://doi.org/10.1038/nature25480
7. International Cancer Genome Consortium, Hudson TJ, Anderson W, Artez A, Barker AD, Bell C et al (2010) International network of cancer genome projects. Nature 464(7291):993–998. https://doi.org/10.1038/nature08987
8. Druker BJ, Sawyers CL, Kantarjian H, Resta DJ, Reese SF, Ford JM et al (2001) Activity of a specific inhibitor of the BCR-ABL tyrosine kinase in the blast crisis of chronic myeloid leukemia and acute lymphoblastic leukemia with the Philadelphia chromosome. N Engl J Med 344(14):1038–1042. https://doi.org/10.1056/nejm200104053441402
9. Slamon DJ, Leyland-Jones B, Shak S, Fuchs H, Paton V, Bajamonde A et al (2001) Use of chemotherapy plus a monoclonal antibody against HER2 for metastatic breast cancer that overexpresses HER2. N Engl J Med 344(11):783–792. https://doi.org/10.1056/nejm200103153441101
10. Lynch TJ, Bell DW, Sordella R, Gurubhagavatula S, Okimoto RA, Brannigan BW et al (2004) Activating mutations in the epidermal growth factor receptor underlying responsiveness of non-small-cell lung cancer to gefitinib. N Engl J Med 350(21):2129–2139. https://doi.org/10.1056/nejmoa040938
11. Chapman PB, Hauschild A, Robert C, Haanen JB, Ascierto P, Larkin J et al (2011) Improved survival with vemurafenib in melanoma with BRAF V600E mutation. N Engl J Med 364(26):2507–2516. https://doi.org/10.1056/nejmoa1103782
12. Shaw AT, Kim DW, Nakagawa K, Seto T, Crino L, Ahn MJ et al (2013) Crizotinib versus chemotherapy in advanced ALK-positive lung cancer. N Engl J Med 368(25):2385–2394. https://doi.org/10.1056/nejmoa1214886
13. Douillard JY, Oliner KS, Siena S, Tabernero J, Burkes R, Barugel M et al (2013) Panitumumab-FOLFOX4 treatment and RAS mutations in colorectal cancer. N Engl J Med 369(11):1023–1034. https://doi.org/10.1056/nejmoa1305275
14. Berger MF, Mardis ER (2018) The emerging clinical relevance of genomics in cancer medicine. Nat Rev Clin Oncol 15(6):353–365. https://doi.org/10.1038/s41571-018-0002-6
15. Mardis ER (2017) DNA sequencing technologies: 2006–2016. Nat Protoc 12(2):213–218. https://doi.org/10.1038/nprot.2016.182

16. Gong J, Pan K, Fakih M, Pal S, Salgia R (2018) Value-based genomics. Oncotarget 9(21):15792–15815. https://doi.org/10.18632/oncotarget.24353
17. Hynes SO, Pang B, James JA, Maxwell P, Salto-Tellez M (2017) Tissue-based next generation sequencing: application in a universal healthcare system. Br J Cancer 116(5): 553–560. https://doi.org/10.1038/bjc.2016.452
18. Shen T, Pajaro-Van de Stadt SH, Yeat NC, Lin JC (2015) Clinical applications of next generation sequencing in cancer: from panels, to exomes, to genomes. Front Genet 6:215. https://doi.org/10.3389/fgene.2015.00215
19. Ettinger DS, Wood DE, Akerley W, Bazhenova LA, Borghaei H, Camidge DR et al (2015) Non-small cell lung cancer, version 6.2015. J Natl Compr Cancer Netw JNCCN 13(5):515–524
20. Nagarajan R, Bartley AN, Bridge JA, Jennings LJ, Kamel-Reid S, Kim A et al (2017) A window into clinical next-generation sequencing-based oncology testing practices. Arch Pathol Lab Med 141(12):1679–1685. https://doi.org/10.5858/arpa.2016-0542-cp
21. Cheng DT, Mitchell TN, Zehir A, Shah RH, Benayed R, Syed A et al (2015) Memorial Sloan Kettering-Integrated Mutation Profiling of Actionable Cancer Targets (MSK-IMPACT): a hybridization capture-based next-generation sequencing clinical assay for solid tumor molecular oncology. J Mol Diagn JMD 17(3):251–264. https://doi.org/10.1016/j.jmoldx.2014.12.006
22. Zehir A, Benayed R, Shah RH, Syed A, Middha S, Kim HR et al (2017) Mutational landscape of metastatic cancer revealed from prospective clinical sequencing of 10,000 patients. Nat Med 23(6):703–713. https://doi.org/10.1038/nm.4333
23. Seeber A, Gastl G, Ensinger C, Spizzo G, Willenbacher W, Kocher F et al (2016) Treatment of patients with refractory metastatic cancer according to molecular profiling on tumor tissue in the clinical routine: an interim-analysis of the ONCO-T-PROFILE project. Genes Cancer 7(9–10):301–308. https://doi.org/10.18632/genesandcancer.121
24. Herzog TJ, Spetzler D, Xiao N, Burnett K, Maney T, Voss A et al (2016) Impact of molecular profiling on overall survival of patients with advanced ovarian cancer. Oncotarget 7(15):19840–19849. https://doi.org/10.18632/oncotarget.7835
25. Beaubier N, Tell R, Huether R, Bontrager M, Bush S, Parsons J et al (2018) Clinical validation of the Tempus xO assay. Oncotarget 9(40):25826–25832. https://doi.org/10.18632/oncotarget.25381
26. Wagle N, Berger MF, Davis MJ, Blumenstiel B, Defelice M, Pochanard P et al (2012) High-throughput detection of actionable genomic alterations in clinical tumor samples by targeted, massively parallel sequencing. Cancer Discov 2(1):82–93. https://doi.org/10.1158/2159-8290.cd-11-0184
27. Hamblin A, Wordsworth S, Fermont JM, Page S, Kaur K, Camps C et al (2017) Clinical applicability and cost of a 46-gene panel for genomic analysis of solid tumours: retrospective validation and prospective audit in the UK National Health Service. PLoS Med 14(2): e1002230. https://doi.org/10.1371/journal.pmed.1002230
28. Lee A, Lee SH, Jung CK, Park G, Lee KY, Choi HJ et al (2018) Use of the Ion AmpliSeq Cancer Hotspot Panel in clinical molecular pathology laboratories for analysis of solid tumours: with emphasis on validation with relevant single molecular pathology tests and the Oncomine Focus Assay. Pathol Res Pract 214(5):713–719. https://doi.org/10.1016/j.prp.2018.03.009
29. Lim SM, Kim EY, Kim HR, Ali SM, Greenbowe JR, Shim HS et al (2016) Genomic profiling of lung adenocarcinoma patients reveals therapeutic targets and confers clinical benefit when standard molecular testing is negative. Oncotarget 7(17):24172–24178. https://doi.org/10.18632/oncotarget.8138
30. Suh JH, Johnson A, Albacker L, Wang K, Chmielecki J, Frampton G et al (2016) Comprehensive genomic profiling facilitates implementation of the National Comprehensive Cancer Network guidelines for lung cancer biomarker testing and identifies patients who may benefit from enrollment in mechanism-driven clinical trials. Oncologist 21(6):684–691. https://doi.org/10.1634/theoncologist.2016-0030

31. Beltran H, Eng K, Mosquera JM, Sigaras A, Romanel A, Rennert H et al (2015) Whole-exome sequencing of metastatic cancer and biomarkers of treatment response. JAMA Oncol 1(4):466–474. https://doi.org/10.1001/jamaoncol.2015.1313
32. Teer JK, Mullikin JC (2010) Exome sequencing: the sweet spot before whole genomes. Hum Mol Genet 19(R2):R145–R151. https://doi.org/10.1093/hmg/ddq333
33. Panda A, Betigeri A, Subramanian K, Ross JS, Pavlick DC, Ali S et al (2017) Identifying a clinically applicable mutational burden threshold as a potential biomarker of response to immune checkpoint therapy in solid tumors. JCO Precis Oncol 2017. https://doi.org/10.1200/po.17.00146
34. Horak P, Frohling S, Glimm H (2016) Integrating next-generation sequencing into clinical oncology: strategies, promises and pitfalls. ESMO Open 1(5):e000094. https://doi.org/10.1136/esmoopen-2016-000094
35. Robinson DR, Wu YM, Lonigro RJ, Vats P, Cobain E, Everett J et al (2017) Integrative clinical genomics of metastatic cancer. Nature 548(7667):297–303. https://doi.org/10.1038/nature23306
36. Byron SA, Van Keuren-Jensen KR, Engelthaler DM, Carpten JD, Craig DW (2016) Translating RNA sequencing into clinical diagnostics: opportunities and challenges. Nat Rev Genet 17(5):257–271. https://doi.org/10.1038/nrg.2016.10
37. Mody RJ, Wu YM, Lonigro RJ, Cao X, Roychowdhury S, Vats P et al (2015) Integrative clinical sequencing in the management of refractory or relapsed cancer in youth. JAMA 314(9):913–925. https://doi.org/10.1001/jama.2015.10080
38. Byron SA, Tran NL, Halperin RF, Phillips JJ, Kuhn JG, de Groot JF et al (2018) Prospective feasibility trial for genomics-informed treatment in recurrent and progressive glioblastoma. Clin Cancer Res 24(2):295–305. https://doi.org/10.1158/1078-0432.ccr-17-0963
39. Uzilov AV, Ding W, Fink MY, Antipin Y, Brohl AS, Davis C et al (2016) Development and clinical application of an integrative genomic approach to personalized cancer therapy. Genome Med 8(1):62. https://doi.org/10.1186/s13073-016-0313-0
40. Borad MJ, Egan JB, Condjella RM, Liang WS, Fonseca R, Ritacca NR et al (2016) Clinical implementation of integrated genomic profiling in patients with advanced cancers. Sci Rep 6(1):25. https://doi.org/10.1038/s41598-016-0021-4
41. Aguirre AJ, Nowak JA, Camarda ND, Moffitt RA, Ghazani AA, Hazar-Rethinam M et al (2018) Real-time genomic characterization of advanced pancreatic cancer to enable precision medicine. Cancer Discov. https://doi.org/10.1158/2159-8290.cd-18-0275
42. Roychowdhury S, Iyer MK, Robinson DR, Lonigro RJ, Wu YM, Cao X et al (2011) Personalized oncology through integrative high-throughput sequencing: a pilot study. Sci Transl Med 3(111):111ra21. https://doi.org/10.1126/scitranslmed.3003161
43. Nakagawa H, Wardell CP, Furuta M, Taniguchi H, Fujimoto A (2015) Cancer whole-genome sequencing: present and future. Oncogene 34(49):5943–5950. https://doi.org/10.1038/onc.2015.90
44. Weymann D, Laskin J, Roscoe R, Schrader KA, Chia S, Yip S et al (2017) The cost and cost trajectory of whole-genome analysis guiding treatment of patients with advanced cancers. Mol Genet Genomic Med 5(3):251–260. https://doi.org/10.1002/mgg3.281
45. Laskin J, Jones S, Aparicio S, Chia S, Ch'ng C, Deyell R et al (2015) Lessons learned from the application of whole-genome analysis to the treatment of patients with advanced cancers. Cold Spring Harb Mol Case Stud 1(1):a000570. https://doi.org/10.1101/mcs.a000570
46. Schuh A, Dreau H, Knight SJL, Ridout K, Mizani T, Vavoulis D et al (2018)Clinically actionable mutation profiles in patients with cancer identified by whole-genome sequencing. Cold Spring Harb Mol Case Stud 4(2). https://doi.org/10.1101/mcs.a002279
47. Wan JCM, Massie C, Garcia-Corbacho J, Mouliere F, Brenton JD, Caldas C et al (2017) Liquid biopsies come of age: towards implementation of circulating tumour DNA. Nat Rev Cancer 17(4):223–238. https://doi.org/10.1038/nrc.2017.7

48. Kwapisz D (2017) The first liquid biopsy test approved. Is it a new era of mutation testing for non-small cell lung cancer? Ann Transl Med 5(3):46. https://doi.org/10.21037/atm.2017.01.32
49. Schwaederle M, Chattopadhyay R, Kato S, Fanta PT, Banks KC, Choi IS et al (2017) Genomic alterations in circulating tumor DNA from diverse cancer patients identified by next-generation sequencing. Can Res 77(19):5419–5427. https://doi.org/10.1158/0008-5472.can-17-0885
50. Stewart CM, Kothari PD, Mouliere F, Mair R, Somnay S, Benayed R et al (2018) The value of cell-free DNA for molecular pathology. J Pathol 244(5):616–627. https://doi.org/10.1002/path.5048
51. Haugen BR, Alexander EK, Bible KC, Doherty GM, Mandel SJ, Nikiforov YE et al (2016) 2015 American Thyroid Association management guidelines for adult patients with thyroid nodules and differentiated thyroid cancer: the American Thyroid Association guidelines task force on thyroid nodules and differentiated thyroid cancer. Thyroid 26(1):1–133. https://doi.org/10.1089/thy.2015.0020
52. Nikiforova MN, Mercurio S, Wald AI, Barbi de Moura M, Callenberg K, Santana-Santos L et al (2018) Analytical performance of the ThyroSeq v3 genomic classifier for cancer diagnosis in thyroid nodules. Cancer 124(8):1682–1690. https://doi.org/10.1002/cncr.31245
53. Boyd N, Dancey JE, Gilks CB, Huntsman DG (2016) Rare cancers: a sea of opportunity. Lancet Oncol 17(2):e52–e61. https://doi.org/10.1016/S1470-2045(15)00386-1
54. Turc-Carel C, Aurias A, Mugneret F, Lizard S, Sidaner I, Volk C et al (1988) Chromosomes in Ewing's sarcoma. I. An evaluation of 85 cases and remarkable consistency of t (11; 22) (q24; q12). Cancer Genet Cytogenet 32(2):229–238
55. Hirota S, Isozaki K, Moriyama Y, Hashimoto K, Nishida T, Ishiguro S et al (1998) Gain-of-function mutations of c-kit in human gastrointestinal stromal tumors. Science 279 (5350):577–580
56. Hirota S, Ohashi A, Nishida T, Isozaki K, Kinoshita K, Shinomura Y et al (2003) Gain-of-function mutations of platelet-derived growth factor receptor alpha gene in gastrointestinal stromal tumors. Gastroenterology 125(3):660–667
57. Tiacci E, Trifonov V, Schiavoni G, Holmes A, Kern W, Martelli MP et al (2011) BRAF mutations in hairy-cell leukemia. N Engl J Med 364(24):2305–2315. https://doi.org/10.1056/nejmoa1014209
58. Jelinic P, Mueller JJ, Olvera N, Dao F, Scott SN, Shah R et al (2014) Recurrent SMARCA4 mutations in small cell carcinoma of the ovary. Nat Genet 46(5):424–426. https://doi.org/10.1038/ng.2922
59. Ramos P, Karnezis AN, Craig DW, Sekulic A, Russell ML, Hendricks WP et al (2014) Small cell carcinoma of the ovary, hypercalcemic type, displays frequent inactivating germline and somatic mutations in SMARCA4. Nat Genet 46(5):427–429. https://doi.org/10.1038/ng.2928
60. Witkowski L, Carrot-Zhang J, Albrecht S, Fahiminiya S, Hamel N, Tomiak E et al (2014) Germline and somatic SMARCA4 mutations characterize small cell carcinoma of the ovary, hypercalcemic type. Nat Genet 46(5):438–443. https://doi.org/10.1038/ng.2931
61. Shah SP, Kobel M, Senz J, Morin RD, Clarke BA, Wiegand KC et al (2009) Mutation of FOXL2 in granulosa-cell tumors of the ovary. N Engl J Med 360(26):2719–2729. https://doi.org/10.1056/nejmoa0902542
62. Louis DN, Perry A, Reifenberger G, von Deimling A, Figarella-Branger D, Cavenee WK et al (2016) The 2016 World Health Organization classification of tumors of the central nervous system: a summary. Acta Neuropathol 131(6):803–820. https://doi.org/10.1007/s00401-016-1545-1
63. Shern JF, Chen L, Chmielecki J, Wei JS, Patidar R, Rosenberg M et al (2014) Comprehensive genomic analysis of rhabdomyosarcoma reveals a landscape of alterations affecting a common genetic axis in fusion-positive and fusion-negative tumors. Cancer Discov 4(2):216–231. https://doi.org/10.1158/2159-8290.cd-13-0639

64. Hollmann TJ, Hornick JL (2011) INI1-deficient tumors: diagnostic features and molecular genetics. Am J Surg Pathol 35(10):e47–e63. https://doi.org/10.1097/pas.0b013e31822b325b
65. Le Loarer F, Watson S, Pierron G, de Montpreville VT, Ballet S, Firmin N et al (2015) SMARCA4 inactivation defines a group of undifferentiated thoracic malignancies transcriptionally related to BAF-deficient sarcomas. Nat Genet 47(10):1200–1205. https://doi.org/10.1038/ng.3399
66. Versteege I, Sevenet N, Lange J, Rousseau-Merck MF, Ambros P, Handgretinger R et al (1998) Truncating mutations of hSNF5/INI1 in aggressive paediatric cancer. Nature 394(6689):203–206. https://doi.org/10.1038/28212
67. Sevenet N, Sheridan E, Amram D, Schneider P, Handgretinger R, Delattre O (1999) Constitutional mutations of the hSNF5/INI1 gene predispose to a variety of cancers. Am J Hum Genet 65(5):1342–1348. https://doi.org/10.1086/302639
68. Kadoch C, Hargreaves DC, Hodges C, Elias L, Ho L, Ranish J et al (2013) Proteomic and bioinformatic analysis of mammalian SWI/SNF complexes identifies extensive roles in human malignancy. Nat Genet 45(6):592–601. https://doi.org/10.1038/ng.2628
69. Lang JD, Hendricks WPD, Orlando KA, Yin H, Kiefer J, Ramos P et al (2018) Ponatinib shows potent antitumor activity in small cell carcinoma of the ovary hypercalcemic type (SCCOHT) through multikinase inhibition. Clin Cancer Res 24(8):1932–1943. https://doi.org/10.1158/1078-0432.ccr-17-1928
70. Ross JS, Wang K, Gay L, Otto GA, White E, Iwanik K et al (2015) Comprehensive genomic profiling of carcinoma of unknown primary site: new routes to targeted therapies. JAMA Oncol 1(1):40–49. https://doi.org/10.1001/jamaoncol.2014.216
71. Kandalaft PL, Gown AM (2016) Practical applications in immunohistochemistry: carcinomas of unknown primary site. Arch Pathol Lab Med 140(6):508–523. https://doi.org/10.5858/arpa.2015-0173-cp
72. Losa F, Soler G, Casado A, Estival A, Fernandez I, Gimenez S et al (2018) SEOM clinical guideline on unknown primary cancer (2017). Clin Transl Oncol 20(1):89–96. https://doi.org/10.1007/s12094-017-1807-y
73. Benderra MA, Ilie M, Hofman P, Massard C (2016) Standard of care of carcinomas on cancer of unknown primary site in 2016. Bull Cancer 103(7–8):697–705. https://doi.org/10.1016/j.bulcan.2016.05.003
74. Economopoulou P, Mountzios G, Pavlidis N, Pentheroudakis G (2015) Cancer of unknown primary origin in the genomic era: elucidating the dark box of cancer. Cancer Treat Rev 41(7):598–604. https://doi.org/10.1016/j.ctrv.2015.05.010
75. Gatalica Z, Millis SZ, Vranic S, Bender R, Basu GD, Voss A et al (2014) Comprehensive tumor profiling identifies numerous biomarkers of drug response in cancers of unknown primary site: analysis of 1806 cases. Oncotarget 5(23):12440–12447. https://doi.org/10.18632/oncotarget.2574
76. Harris LN, Ismaila N, McShane LM, Andre F, Collyar DE, Gonzalez-Angulo AM et al (2016) Use of biomarkers to guide decisions on adjuvant systemic therapy for women with early-stage invasive breast cancer: American Society of Clinical Oncology clinical practice guideline. J Clin Oncol 34(10):1134–1150. https://doi.org/10.1200/jco.2015.65.2289
77. Sparano JA, Gray RJ, Makower DF, Pritchard KI, Albain KS, Hayes DF et al (2015) Prospective validation of a 21-gene expression assay in breast cancer. N Engl J Med 373(21):2005–2014. https://doi.org/10.1056/nejmoa1510764
78. Yamanaka T, Oki E, Yamazaki K, Yamaguchi K, Muro K, Uetake H et al (2016) 12-gene recurrence score assay stratifies the recurrence risk in stage II/III colon cancer with surgery alone: the SUNRISE study. J Clin Oncol 34(24):2906–2913. https://doi.org/10.1200/jco.2016.67.0414
79. Mahar AL, Compton C, Halabi S, Hess KR, Weiser MR, Groome PA (2017) Personalizing prognosis in colorectal cancer: a systematic review of the quality and nature of clinical prognostic tools for survival outcomes. J Surg Oncol 116(8):969–982. https://doi.org/10.1002/jso.24774

80. Klein EA, Cooperberg MR, Magi-Galluzzi C, Simko JP, Falzarano SM, Maddala T et al (2014) A 17-gene assay to predict prostate cancer aggressiveness in the context of Gleason grade heterogeneity, tumor multifocality, and biopsy undersampling. Eur Urol 66(3):550–560. https://doi.org/10.1016/j.eururo.2014.05.004
81. Eure G, Germany R, Given R, Lu R, Shindel AW, Rothney M et al (2017) Use of a 17-gene prognostic assay in contemporary urologic practice: results of an interim analysis in an observational cohort. Urology 107:67–75. https://doi.org/10.1016/j.urology.2017.02.052
82. Monclair T, Brodeur GM, Ambros PF, Brisse HJ, Cecchetto G, Holmes K et al (2009) The international neuroblastoma risk group (INRG) staging system: an INRG task force report. J Clin Oncol 27(2):298–303. https://doi.org/10.1200/jco.2008.16.6876
83. Popat S, Hubner R, Houlston RS (2005) Systematic review of microsatellite instability and colorectal cancer prognosis. J Clin Oncol 23(3):609–618. https://doi.org/10.1200/jco.2005.01.086
84. Roth AD, Delorenzi M, Tejpar S, Yan P, Klingbiel D, Fiocca R et al (2012) Integrated analysis of molecular and clinical prognostic factors in stage II/III colon cancer. J Natl Cancer Inst 104(21):1635–1646. https://doi.org/10.1093/jnci/djs427
85. Kawakami H, Zaanan A, Sinicrope FA (2015) Microsatellite instability testing and its role in the management of colorectal cancer. Curr Treat Options Oncol 16(7):30. https://doi.org/10.1007/s11864-015-0348-2
86. Dohner H, Estey E, Grimwade D, Amadori S, Appelbaum FR, Buchner T et al (2017) Diagnosis and management of AML in adults: 2017 ELN recommendations from an international expert panel. Blood 129(4):424–447. https://doi.org/10.1182/blood-2016-08-733196
87. Dohner H, Stilgenbauer S, Benner A, Leupolt E, Krober A, Bullinger L et al (2000) Genomic aberrations and survival in chronic lymphocytic leukemia. N Engl J Med 343(26):1910–1916. https://doi.org/10.1056/nejm200012283432602
88. Damle RN, Wasil T, Fais F, Ghiotto F, Valetto A, Allen SL et al (1999) Ig V gene mutation status and CD38 expression as novel prognostic indicators in chronic lymphocytic leukemia. Blood 94(6):1840–1847
89. Hamblin TJ, Davis Z, Gardiner A, Oscier DG, Stevenson FK (1999) Unmutated Ig V(H) genes are associated with a more aggressive form of chronic lymphocytic leukemia. Blood 94(6):1848–1854
90. International CLL-IPI Working Group (2016) An international prognostic index for patients with chronic lymphocytic leukaemia (CLL-IPI): a meta-analysis of individual patient data. Lancet Oncol 17(6):779–790. https://doi.org/10.1016/s1470-2045(16)30029-8
91. Stilgenbauer S, Eichhorst B, Schetelig J, Coutre S, Seymour JF, Munir T et al (2016) Venetoclax in relapsed or refractory chronic lymphocytic leukaemia with 17p deletion: a multicentre, open-label, phase 2 study. Lancet Oncol 17(6):768–778. https://doi.org/10.1016/s1470-2045(16)30019-5
92. Edelmann J, Gribben JG (2017) Managing patients with TP53-deficient chronic lymphocytic leukemia. J Oncol Pract 13(6):371–377. https://doi.org/10.1200/jop.2017.023291
93. Shaw AT, Ou SH, Bang YJ, Camidge DR, Solomon BJ, Salgia R et al (2014) Crizotinib in ROS1-rearranged non-small-cell lung cancer. N Engl J Med 371(21):1963–1971. https://doi.org/10.1056/nejmoa1406766
94. Paez JG, Janne PA, Lee JC, Tracy S, Greulich H, Gabriel S et al (2004) EGFR mutations in lung cancer: correlation with clinical response to gefitinib therapy. Science 304(5676):1497–1500. https://doi.org/10.1126/science.1099314
95. Pao W, Miller V, Zakowski M, Doherty J, Politi K, Sarkaria I et al (2004) EGF receptor gene mutations are common in lung cancers from “never smokers” and are associated with sensitivity of tumors to gefitinib and erlotinib. Proc Natl Acad Sci USA 101(36):13306–13311. https://doi.org/10.1073/pnas.0405220101

96. Druker BJ, Guilhot F, O'Brien SG, Gathmann I, Kantarjian H, Gattermann N et al (2006) Five-year follow-up of patients receiving imatinib for chronic myeloid leukemia. N Engl J Med 355(23):2408–2417. https://doi.org/10.1056/nejmoa062867
97. Hochhaus A, Saglio G, Hughes TP, Larson RA, Kim DW, Issaragrisil S et al (2016) Long-term benefits and risks of frontline nilotinib vs imatinib for chronic myeloid leukemia in chronic phase: 5-year update of the randomized ENESTnd trial. Leukemia 30(5):1044–1054. https://doi.org/10.1038/leu.2016.5
98. Hochhaus A, Larson RA, Guilhot F, Radich JP, Branford S, Hughes TP et al (2017) Long-term outcomes of imatinib treatment for chronic myeloid leukemia. N Engl J Med 376(10):917–927. https://doi.org/10.1056/nejmoa1609324
99. Kantarjian H, O'Brien S, Jabbour E, Garcia-Manero G, Quintas-Cardama A, Shan J et al (2012) Improved survival in chronic myeloid leukemia since the introduction of imatinib therapy: a single-institution historical experience. Blood 119(9):1981–1987. https://doi.org/10.1182/blood-2011-08-358135
100. Bower H, Bjorkholm M, Dickman PW, Hoglund M, Lambert PC, Andersson TM (2016) Life expectancy of patients with chronic myeloid leukemia approaches the life expectancy of the general population. J Clin Oncol 34(24):2851–2857. https://doi.org/10.1200/jco.2015.66.2866
101. Kumar-Sinha C, Kalyana-Sundaram S, Chinnaiyan AM (2015) Landscape of gene fusions in epithelial cancers: seq and ye shall find. Genome Med 7:129. https://doi.org/10.1186/s13073-015-0252-1
102. Brastianos PK, Ippen FM, Hafeez U, Gan HK (2018) Emerging gene fusion drivers in primary and metastatic central nervous system malignancies: a review of available evidence for systemic targeted therapies. Oncologist. https://doi.org/10.1634/theoncologist.2017-0614
103. Mertens F, Antonescu CR, Mitelman F (2016) Gene fusions in soft tissue tumors: recurrent and overlapping pathogenetic themes. Genes Chromosom Cancer 55(4):291–310. https://doi.org/10.1002/gcc.22335
104. Stransky N, Cerami E, Schalm S, Kim JL, Lengauer C (2014) The landscape of kinase fusions in cancer. Nat Commun 5:4846. https://doi.org/10.1038/ncomms5846
105. Yoshihara K, Wang Q, Torres-Garcia W, Zheng S, Vegesna R, Kim H et al (2015) The landscape and therapeutic relevance of cancer-associated transcript fusions. Oncogene 34(37):4845–4854. https://doi.org/10.1038/onc.2014.406
106. Schram AM, Chang MT, Jonsson P, Drilon A (2017) Fusions in solid tumours: diagnostic strategies, targeted therapy, and acquired resistance. Nat Rev Clin Oncol 14(12):735–748. https://doi.org/10.1038/nrclinonc.2017.127
107. Katayama R, Lovly CM, Shaw AT (2015) Therapeutic targeting of anaplastic lymphoma kinase in lung cancer: a paradigm for precision cancer medicine. Clin Cancer Res 21(10): 2227–2235. https://doi.org/10.1158/1078-0432.ccr-14-2791
108. Lindeman NI, Cagle PT, Beasley MB, Chitale DA, Dacic S, Giaccone G et al (2013) Molecular testing guideline for selection of lung cancer patients for EGFR and ALK tyrosine kinase inhibitors: guideline from the College of American Pathologists, International Association for the Study of Lung Cancer, and Association for Molecular Pathology. Arch Pathol Lab Med 137(6):828–860. https://doi.org/10.5858/arpa.2012-0720-oa
109. Leighl NB, Rekhtman N, Biermann WA, Huang J, Mino-Kenudson M, Ramalingam SS et al (2014) Molecular testing for selection of patients with lung cancer for epidermal growth factor receptor and anaplastic lymphoma kinase tyrosine kinase inhibitors: American Society of Clinical Oncology endorsement of the College of American Pathologists/International Association for the study of lung cancer/association for molecular pathology guideline. J Clin Oncol 32(32):3673–3679. https://doi.org/10.1200/jco.2014.57.3055
110. Solomon BJ, Mok T, Kim DW, Wu YL, Nakagawa K, Mekhail T et al (2014) First-line crizotinib versus chemotherapy in ALK-positive lung cancer. N Engl J Med 371(23):2167–2177. https://doi.org/10.1056/nejmoa1408440

111. Soria JC, Tan DSW, Chiari R, Wu YL, Paz-Ares L, Wolf J et al (2017) First-line ceritinib versus platinum-based chemotherapy in advanced ALK-rearranged non-small-cell lung cancer (ASCEND-4): a randomised, open-label, phase 3 study. Lancet 389(10072):917–929. https://doi.org/10.1016/s0140-6736(17)30123-x
112. Bergethon K, Shaw AT, Ou SH, Katayama R, Lovly CM, McDonald NT et al (2012) ROS1 rearrangements define a unique molecular class of lung cancers. J Clin Oncol 30(8):863–870. https://doi.org/10.1200/jco.2011.35.6345
113. Lin JJ, Shaw AT (2017) Recent advances in targeting ROS1 in lung cancer. J Thorac Oncol 12(11):1611–1625. https://doi.org/10.1016/j.jtho.2017.08.002
114. Tabernero J, Bahleda R, Dienstmann R, Infante JR, Mita A, Italiano A et al (2015) Phase I dose-escalation study of JNJ-42756493, an oral pan-fibroblast growth factor receptor inhibitor, in patients with advanced solid tumors. J Clin Oncol 33(30):3401–3408. https://doi.org/10.1200/jco.2014.60.7341
115. Kheder ES, Hong DS (2018) Emerging targeted therapy for tumors with NTRK fusion proteins. Clin Cancer Res. https://doi.org/10.1158/1078-0432.ccr-18-1156
116. Drilon A, Siena S, Ou SI, Patel M, Ahn MJ, Lee J et al (2017) Safety and antitumor activity of the multitargeted pan-TRK, ROS1, and ALK inhibitor entrectinib: combined results from two phase I trials (ALKA-372-001 and STARTRK-1). Cancer Discov 7(4):400–409. https://doi.org/10.1158/2159-8290.cd-16-1237
117. Drilon A, Laetsch TW, Kummar S, DuBois SG, Lassen UN, Demetri GD et al (2018) Efficacy of larotrectinib in TRK fusion-positive cancers in adults and children. N Engl J Med 378(8):731–739. https://doi.org/10.1056/nejmoa1714448
118. Lee CK, Brown C, Gralla RJ, Hirsh V, Thongprasert S, Tsai CM et al (2013) Impact of EGFR inhibitor in non-small cell lung cancer on progression-free and overall survival: a meta-analysis. J Natl Cancer Inst 105(9):595–605. https://doi.org/10.1093/jnci/djt072
119. Cheng L, Lopez-Beltran A, Massari F, MacLennan GT, Montironi R (2018) Molecular testing for BRAF mutations to inform melanoma treatment decisions: a move toward precision medicine. Mod Pathol 31(1):24–38. https://doi.org/10.1038/modpathol.2017.104
120. Hauschild A, Grob JJ, Demidov LV, Jouary T, Gutzmer R, Millward M et al (2012) Dabrafenib in BRAF-mutated metastatic melanoma: a multicentre, open-label, phase 3 randomised controlled trial. Lancet 380(9839):358–365. https://doi.org/10.1016/s0140-6736(12)60868-x
121. Flaherty KT, Robert C, Hersey P, Nathan P, Garbe C, Milhem M et al (2012) Improved survival with MEK inhibition in BRAF-mutated melanoma. N Engl J Med 367(2):107–114. https://doi.org/10.1056/nejmoa1203421
122. Flaherty KT, Infante JR, Daud A, Gonzalez R, Kefford RF, Sosman J et al (2012) Combined BRAF and MEK inhibition in melanoma with BRAF V600 mutations. N Engl J Med 367(18):1694–1703. https://doi.org/10.1056/nejmoa1210093
123. Long GV, Stroyakovskiy D, Gogas H, Levchenko E, de Braud F, Larkin J et al (2014) Combined BRAF and MEK inhibition versus BRAF inhibition alone in melanoma. N Engl J Med 371(20):1877–1888. https://doi.org/10.1056/nejmoa1406037
124. Larkin J, Ascierto PA, Dreno B, Atkinson V, Liszkay G, Maio M et al (2014) Combined vemurafenib and cobimetinib in BRAF-mutated melanoma. N Engl J Med 371(20):1867–1876. https://doi.org/10.1056/nejmoa1408868
125. Hyman DM, Puzanov I, Subbiah V, Faris JE, Chau I, Blay JY et al (2015) Vemurafenib in multiple nonmelanoma cancers with BRAF V600 mutations. N Engl J Med 373(8):726–736. https://doi.org/10.1056/nejmoa1502309
126. Karapetis CS, Khambata-Ford S, Jonker DJ, O'Callaghan CJ, Tu D, Tebbutt NC et al (2008) K-ras mutations and benefit from cetuximab in advanced colorectal cancer. N Engl J Med 359(17):1757–1765. https://doi.org/10.1056/nejmoa0804385
127. Douillard JY, Siena S, Cassidy J, Tabernero J, Burkes R, Barugel M et al (2014) Final results from PRIME: randomized phase III study of panitumumab with FOLFOX4 for first-line

treatment of metastatic colorectal cancer. Ann Oncol 25(7):1346–1355. https://doi.org/10.1093/annonc/mdu141
128. Van Cutsem E, Lenz HJ, Kohne CH, Heinemann V, Tejpar S, Melezinek I et al (2015) Fluorouracil, leucovorin, and irinotecan plus cetuximab treatment and RAS mutations in colorectal cancer. J Clin Oncol 33(7):692–700. https://doi.org/10.1200/jco.2014.59.4812
129. Allegra CJ, Rumble RB, Hamilton SR, Mangu PB, Roach N, Hantel A et al (2016) Extended RAS gene mutation testing in metastatic colorectal carcinoma to predict response to anti-epidermal growth factor receptor monoclonal antibody therapy: American Society of Clinical Oncology provisional clinical opinion update 2015. J Clin Oncol 34(2):179–185. https://doi.org/10.1200/jco.2015.63.9674
130. King CR, Kraus MH, Aaronson SA (1985) Amplification of a novel v-erbB-related gene in a human mammary carcinoma. Science 229(4717):974–976
131. Wolff AC, Hammond ME, Hicks DG, Dowsett M, McShane LM, Allison KH et al (2013) Recommendations for human epidermal growth factor receptor 2 testing in breast cancer: American Society of Clinical Oncology/College of American Pathologists clinical practice guideline update. J Clin Oncol 31(31):3997–4013. https://doi.org/10.1200/jco.2013.50.9984
132. Swain SM, Baselga J, Kim SB, Ro J, Semiglazov V, Campone M et al (2015) Pertuzumab, trastuzumab, and docetaxel in HER2-positive metastatic breast cancer. N Engl J Med 372 (8):724–734. https://doi.org/10.1056/nejmoa1413513
133. Bang YJ, Van Cutsem E, Feyereislova A, Chung HC, Shen L, Sawaki A et al (2010) Trastuzumab in combination with chemotherapy versus chemotherapy alone for treatment of HER2-positive advanced gastric or gastro-oesophageal junction cancer (ToGA): a phase 3, open-label, randomised controlled trial. Lancet 376(9742):687–697. https://doi.org/10.1016/s0140-6736(10)61121-x
134. Hanahan D, Weinberg RA (2011) Hallmarks of cancer: the next generation. Cell 144(5): 646–674. https://doi.org/10.1016/j.cell.2011.02.013
135. Huang FW, Hodis E, Xu MJ, Kryukov GV, Chin L, Garraway LA (2013) Highly recurrent TERT promoter mutations in human melanoma. Science 339(6122):957–959. https://doi.org/10.1126/science.1229259
136. Horn S, Figl A, Rachakonda PS, Fischer C, Sucker A, Gast A et al (2013) TERT promoter mutations in familial and sporadic melanoma. Science 339(6122):959–961. https://doi.org/10.1126/science.1230062
137. Bell RJ, Rube HT, Xavier-Magalhaes A, Costa BM, Mancini A, Song JS et al (2016) Understanding TERT promoter mutations: a common path to immortality. Mol Cancer Res MCR 14(4):315–323. https://doi.org/10.1158/1541-7786.mcr-16-0003
138. Vinagre J, Almeida A, Populo H, Batista R, Lyra J, Pinto V et al (2013) Frequency of TERT promoter mutations in human cancers. Nat Commun 4:2185. https://doi.org/10.1038/ncomms3185
139. Killela PJ, Reitman ZJ, Jiao Y, Bettegowda C, Agrawal N, Diaz LA Jr et al (2013) TERT promoter mutations occur frequently in gliomas and a subset of tumors derived from cells with low rates of self-renewal. Proc Natl Acad Sci USA 110(15):6021–6026. https://doi.org/10.1073/pnas.1303607110
140. Liu X, Bishop J, Shan Y, Pai S, Liu D, Murugan AK et al (2013) Highly prevalent TERT promoter mutations in aggressive thyroid cancers. Endocr Relat Cancer 20(4):603–610. https://doi.org/10.1530/erc-13-0210
141. Landa I, Ganly I, Chan TA, Mitsutake N, Matsuse M, Ibrahimpasic T et al (2013) Frequent somatic TERT promoter mutations in thyroid cancer: higher prevalence in advanced forms of the disease. J Clin Endocrinol Metab 98(9):E1562–E1566. https://doi.org/10.1210/jc.2013-2383
142. Simon M, Hosen I, Gousias K, Rachakonda S, Heidenreich B, Gessi M et al (2015) TERT promoter mutations: a novel independent prognostic factor in primary glioblastomas. Neuro-Oncology 17(1):45–52. https://doi.org/10.1093/neuonc/nou158

143. Eckel-Passow JE, Lachance DH, Molinaro AM, Walsh KM, Decker PA, Sicotte H et al (2015) Glioma groups based on 1p/19q, IDH, and TERT promoter mutations in tumors. N Engl J Med 372(26):2499–2508. https://doi.org/10.1056/nejmoa1407279
144. Arita H, Yamasaki K, Matsushita Y, Nakamura T, Shimokawa A, Takami H et al (2016) A combination of TERT promoter mutation and MGMT methylation status predicts clinically relevant subgroups of newly diagnosed glioblastomas. Acta Neuropathol Commun 4(1):79. https://doi.org/10.1186/s40478-016-0351-2
145. Heidenreich B, Nagore E, Rachakonda PS, Garcia-Casado Z, Requena C, Traves V et al (2014) Telomerase reverse transcriptase promoter mutations in primary cutaneous melanoma. Nat Commun 5:3401. https://doi.org/10.1038/ncomms4401
146. Liu X, Qu S, Liu R, Sheng C, Shi X, Zhu G et al (2014) TERT promoter mutations and their association with BRAF V600E mutation and aggressive clinicopathological characteristics of thyroid cancer. J Clin Endocrinol Metab 99(6):E1130–E1136. https://doi.org/10.1210/jc.2013-4048
147. Le DT, Durham JN, Smith KN, Wang H, Bartlett BR, Aulakh LK et al (2017) Mismatch repair deficiency predicts response of solid tumors to PD-1 blockade. Science 357(6349):409–413. https://doi.org/10.1126/science.aan6733
148. Le DT, Uram JN, Wang H, Bartlett BR, Kemberling H, Eyring AD et al (2015) PD-1 blockade in tumors with mismatch-repair deficiency. N Engl J Med 372(26):2509–2520. https://doi.org/10.1056/nejmoa1500596
149. Lee V, Murphy A, Le DT, Diaz LA Jr (2016) Mismatch repair deficiency and response to immune checkpoint blockade. Oncologist 21(10):1200–1211. https://doi.org/10.1634/theoncologist.2016-0046
150. Lemery S, Keegan P, Pazdur R (2017) First FDA approval agnostic of cancer site—when a biomarker defines the indication. N Engl J Med 377(15):1409–1412. https://doi.org/10.1056/nejmp1709968
151. Vilar E, Gruber SB (2010) Microsatellite instability in colorectal cancer—the stable evidence. Nat Rev Clin Oncol 7(3):153–162. https://doi.org/10.1038/nrclinonc.2009.237
152. Vanderwalde A, Spetzler D, Xiao N, Gatalica Z, Marshall J (2018) Microsatellite instability status determined by next-generation sequencing and compared with PD-L1 and tumor mutational burden in 11,348 patients. Cancer Med 7(3):746–756. https://doi.org/10.1002/cam4.1372
153. Hause RJ, Pritchard CC, Shendure J, Salipante SJ (2016) Classification and characterization of microsatellite instability across 18 cancer types. Nat Med 22(11):1342–1350. https://doi.org/10.1038/nm.4191
154. Cortes-Ciriano I, Lee S, Park WY, Kim TM, Park PJ (2017) A molecular portrait of microsatellite instability across multiple cancers. Nat Commun 8:15180. https://doi.org/10.1038/ncomms15180
155. Bouffet E, Larouche V, Campbell BB, Merico D, de Borja R, Aronson M et al (2016) Immune checkpoint inhibition for hypermutant glioblastoma multiforme resulting from germline biallelic mismatch repair deficiency. J Clin Oncol 34(19):2206–2211. https://doi.org/10.1200/jco.2016.66.6552
156. Mehnert JM, Panda A, Zhong H, Hirshfield K, Damare S, Lane K et al (2016) Immune activation and response to pembrolizumab in POLE-mutant endometrial cancer. J Clin Investig 126(6):2334–2340. https://doi.org/10.1172/JCI84940
157. Bhangoo MS, Boasberg P, Mehta P, Elvin JA, Ali SM, Wu W et al (2018) Tumor mutational burden guides therapy in a treatment refractory POLE-mutant uterine carcinosarcoma. Oncologist 23(5):518–523. https://doi.org/10.1634/theoncologist.2017-0342
158. Gong J, Wang C, Lee PP, Chu P, Fakih M (2017) Response to PD-1 blockade in microsatellite stable metastatic colorectal cancer harboring a POLE mutation. J Natl Compr Cancer Netw JNCCN 15(2):142–147

159. Johanns TM, Miller CA, Dorward IG, Tsien C, Chang E, Perry A et al (2016) Immunogenomics of hypermutated glioblastoma: a patient with germline POLE deficiency treated with checkpoint blockade immunotherapy. Cancer Discov 6(11):1230–1236. https://doi.org/10.1158/2159-8290.cd-16-0575
160. Chalmers ZR, Connelly CF, Fabrizio D, Gay L, Ali SM, Ennis R et al (2017) Analysis of 100,000 human cancer genomes reveals the landscape of tumor mutational burden. Genome Med 9(1):34. https://doi.org/10.1186/s13073-017-0424-2
161. Hunter C, Smith R, Cahill DP, Stephens P, Stevens C, Teague J et al (2006) A hypermutation phenotype and somatic MSH6 mutations in recurrent human malignant gliomas after alkylator chemotherapy. Can Res 66(8):3987–3991. https://doi.org/10.1158/0008-5472.can-06-0127
162. Rizvi NA, Hellmann MD, Snyder A, Kvistborg P, Makarov V, Havel JJ et al (2015) Cancer immunology. Mutational landscape determines sensitivity to PD-1 blockade in non-small cell lung cancer. Science 348(6230):124–128. https://doi.org/10.1126/science.aaa1348
163. Goodman AM, Kato S, Bazhenova L, Patel SP, Frampton GM, Miller V et al (2017) Tumor mutational burden as an independent predictor of response to immunotherapy in diverse cancers. Mol Cancer Ther 16(11):2598–2608. https://doi.org/10.1158/1535-7163.mct-17-0386
164. Von Hoff DD, Stephenson JJ Jr, Rosen P, Loesch DM, Borad MJ, Anthony S et al (2010) Pilot study using molecular profiling of patients' tumors to find potential targets and select treatments for their refractory cancers. J Clin Oncol 28(33):4877–4883. https://doi.org/10.1200/jco.2009.26.5983
165. Tsimberidou AM, Iskander NG, Hong DS, Wheler JJ, Falchook GS, Fu S et al (2012) Personalized medicine in a phase I clinical trials program: the MD Anderson Cancer Center initiative. Clin Cancer Res 18(22):6373–6383. https://doi.org/10.1158/1078-0432.ccr-12-1627
166. Stockley TL, Oza AM, Berman HK, Leighl NB, Knox JJ, Shepherd FA et al (2016) Molecular profiling of advanced solid tumors and patient outcomes with genotype-matched clinical trials: the Princess Margaret IMPACT/COMPACT trial. Genome Med 8(1):109. https://doi.org/10.1186/s13073-016-0364-2
167. Le Tourneau C, Delord JP, Goncalves A, Gavoille C, Dubot C, Isambert N et al (2015) Molecularly targeted therapy based on tumour molecular profiling versus conventional therapy for advanced cancer (SHIVA): a multicentre, open-label, proof-of-concept, randomised, controlled phase 2 trial. Lancet Oncol 16(13):1324–1334. https://doi.org/10.1016/s1470-2045(15)00188-6
168. Massard C, Michiels S, Ferte C, Le Deley MC, Lacroix L, Hollebecque A et al (2017) High-throughput genomics and clinical outcome in hard-to-treat advanced cancers: results of the MOSCATO 01 trial. Cancer Discov 7(6):586–595. https://doi.org/10.1158/2159-8290.cd-16-1396
169. Forrest SJ, Geoerger B, Janeway KA (2018) Precision medicine in pediatric oncology. Curr Opin Pediatr 30(1):17–24. https://doi.org/10.1097/mop.0000000000000570
170. McNeil C (2015) NCI-MATCH launch highlights new trial design in precision-medicine era. J Natl Cancer Inst 107(7). https://doi.org/10.1093/jnci/djv193
171. Iyer G, Hanrahan AJ, Milowsky MI, Al-Ahmadie H, Scott SN, Janakiraman M et al (2012) Genome sequencing identifies a basis for everolimus sensitivity. Science 338(6104):221. https://doi.org/10.1126/science.1226344
172. Chau NG, Lorch JH (2015) Exceptional responders inspire change: lessons for drug development from the bedside to the bench and back. Oncologist 20(7):699–701. https://doi.org/10.1634/theoncologist.2014-0476
173. Rodriguez-Moreno JF, Apellaniz-Ruiz M, Roldan-Romero JM, Duran I, Beltran L, Montero-Conde C et al (2017) Exceptional response to temsirolimus in a metastatic clear cell renal cell carcinoma with an early novel mTOR-activating mutation. J Natl Compr Cancer Netw JNCCN 15(11):1310–1315. https://doi.org/10.6004/jnccn.2017.7018

174. Lim SM, Park HS, Kim S, Kim S, Ali SM, Greenbowe JR et al (2016) Next-generation sequencing reveals somatic mutations that confer exceptional response to everolimus. Oncotarget 7(9):10547–10556. https://doi.org/10.18632/oncotarget.7234
175. Drilon A, Somwar R, Mangatt BP, Edgren H, Desmeules P, Ruusulehto A et al (2018) Response to ERBB3-directed targeted therapy in NRG1-rearranged cancers. Cancer Discov 8(6):686–695. https://doi.org/10.1158/2159-8290.cd-17-1004
176. Do K, O'Sullivan Coyne G, Chen AP (2015) An overview of the NCI precision medicine trials-NCI MATCH and MPACT. Chin Clin Oncol 4(3):31. https://doi.org/10.3978/j.issn.2304-3865.2015.08.01
177. Prawira A, Pugh TJ, Stockley TL, Siu LL (2017) Data resources for the identification and interpretation of actionable mutations by clinicians. Ann Oncol 28(5):946–957. https://doi.org/10.1093/annonc/mdx023
178. Brusco LL, Wathoo C, Mills Shaw KR, Holla VR, Bailey AM, Johnson AM et al (2018) Physician interpretation of genomic test results and treatment selection. Cancer 124(5):966–972. https://doi.org/10.1002/cncr.31112
179. Tsang H, Addepalli K, Davis SR (2017) Resources for interpreting variants in precision genomic oncology applications. Front Oncol 7:214. https://doi.org/10.3389/fonc.2017.00214
180. Huang KL, Mashl RJ, Wu Y, Ritter DI, Wang J, Oh C et al (2018) Pathogenic germline variants in 10,389 adult cancers. Cell 173(2):355–370 e14. https://doi.org/10.1016/j.cell.2018.03.039
181. Zhang J, Walsh MF, Wu G, Edmonson MN, Gruber TA, Easton J et al (2015) Germline mutations in predisposition genes in pediatric cancer. N Engl J Med 373(24):2336–2346. https://doi.org/10.1056/nejmoa1508054
182. Parsons DW, Roy A, Yang Y, Wang T, Scollon S, Bergstrom K et al (2016) Diagnostic yield of clinical tumor and germline whole-exome sequencing for children with solid tumors. JAMA Oncol. https://doi.org/10.1001/jamaoncol.2015.5699
183. Mandelker D, Zhang L, Kemel Y, Stadler ZK, Joseph V, Zehir A et al (2017) Mutation detection in patients with advanced cancer by universal sequencing of cancer-related genes in tumor and normal DNA vs guideline-based germline testing. JAMA 318(9):825–835. https://doi.org/10.1001/jama.2017.11137
184. Fong PC, Boss DS, Yap TA, Tutt A, Wu P, Mergui-Roelvink M et al (2009) Inhibition of poly(ADP-ribose) polymerase in tumors from BRCA mutation carriers. N Engl J Med 361(2):123–134. https://doi.org/10.1056/nejmoa0900212
185. Kim G, Ison G, McKee AE, Zhang H, Tang S, Gwise T et al (2015) FDA approval summary: olaparib monotherapy in patients with deleterious germline BRCA-mutated advanced ovarian cancer treated with three or more lines of chemotherapy. Clin Cancer Res 21(19):4257–4261. https://doi.org/10.1158/1078-0432.ccr-15-0887
186. Balasubramaniam S, Beaver JA, Horton S, Fernandes LL, Tang S, Horne HN et al (2017) FDA approval summary: rucaparib for the treatment of patients with deleterious BRCA mutation-associated advanced ovarian cancer. Clin Cancer Res 23(23):7165–7170. https://doi.org/10.1158/1078-0432.ccr-17-1337
187. Robson M, Im SA, Senkus E, Xu B, Domchek SM, Masuda N et al (2017) Olaparib for metastatic breast cancer in patients with a germline BRCA mutation. N Engl J Med 377(6):523–533. https://doi.org/10.1056/nejmoa1706450
188. Kamel D, Gray C, Walia JS, Kumar V (2018) PARP inhibitor drugs in the treatment of breast, ovarian, prostate and pancreatic cancers: an update of clinical trials. Curr Drug Targets 19(1):21–37. https://doi.org/10.2174/1389450118666170711151518
189. Campbell BB, Light N, Fabrizio D, Zatzman M, Fuligni F, de Borja R et al (2017) Comprehensive analysis of hypermutation in human cancer. Cell 171(5):1042–1056 e10. https://doi.org/10.1016/j.cell.2017.09.048

190. Ahn SM, Ansari AA, Kim J, Kim D, Chun SM, Kim J et al (2016) The somatic POLE P286R mutation defines a unique subclass of colorectal cancer featuring hypermutation, representing a potential genomic biomarker for immunotherapy. Oncotarget 7(42):68638–68649. https://doi.org/10.18632/oncotarget.11862
191. Amstutz U, Henricks LM, Offer SM, Barbarino J, Schellens JHM, Swen JJ et al (2018) Clinical pharmacogenetics implementation consortium (CPIC) guideline for dihydropyrimidine dehydrogenase genotype and fluoropyrimidine dosing: 2017 update. Clin Pharmacol Ther 103(2):210–216. https://doi.org/10.1002/cpt.911
192. Relling MV, Gardner EE, Sandborn WJ, Schmiegelow K, Pui CH, Yee SW et al (2013) Clinical pharmacogenetics implementation consortium guidelines for thiopurine methyltransferase genotype and thiopurine dosing: 2013 update. Clin Pharmacol Ther 93(4):324–325. https://doi.org/10.1038/clpt.2013.4
193. Goetz MP, Sangkuhl K, Guchelaar HJ, Schwab M, Province M, Whirl-Carrillo M et al (2018) Clinical pharmacogenetics implementation consortium (CPIC) guideline for CYP2D6 and tamoxifen therapy. Clin Pharmacol Ther 103(5):770–777. https://doi.org/10.1002/cpt.1007
194. Wellmann R, Borden BA, Danahey K, Nanda R, Polite BN, Stadler WM et al (2018) Analyzing the clinical actionability of germline pharmacogenomic findings in oncology. Cancer. https://doi.org/10.1002/cncr.31382

Utilization of Proteomic Technologies for Precision Oncology Applications

6

Mariaelena Pierobon, Julie Wulfkuhle, Lance A. Liotta and Emanuel F. Petricoin III

Contents

M. Pierobon · J. Wulfkuhle · L. A. Liotta · E. F. Petricoin III (✉)
Center for Applied Proteomics and Molecular Medicine,
George Mason University, 20110 Manassas, VA, USA
e-mail: epetrico@gmu.edu

D. D. Von Hoff and H. Han (eds.), *Precision Medicine in Cancer Therapy*,
Cancer Treatment and Research 178, https://doi.org/10.1007/978-3-030-16391-4_6

6.1 Introduction

One of the major pillars of precision oncology is that a tumor-based molecular profile serves as the rationale for patient-tailored and targeted therapy selection. Currently, this molecularly based treatment matching has largely been based on genomics-centered analysis using either targeted exome panels, whole genome sequencing, and/or RNA sequencing comprising the molecular landscape considered. Certainly stratification and selection of patients for certain targeted therapies based on genomics analysis has certainly been successful with FDA-approved companion diagnostic assays and therapies such as for non-small cell lung cancer (NSCLC) where EGFR gene mutations [1], ROS/ALK gene translocations [2], HER2 amplification in breast cancer [3], and BRAFV600E mutations in melanoma [4] are highly predictive for therapeutic response.

However, these genomics-based approaches are imperfect and often times show little to no predictive value [5, 6], and of course not every NSCLC patient that harbors an EGFR mutation responds to EGFR-directed therapy, not every HER2+ breast cancer responds to Herceptin™. Genomic analysis alone is unable to completely explain all targeted therapeutic response even in an enriched population and misses patients who respond to a targeted therapy without the genomic alteration. Cancer is certainly causally determined by specific genomic derangements, but in fact cancer is a proteomic disease. More practically, the mechanism of action of many targeted precision therapies works by binding to and modulating protein enzymatic level (e.g., kinase inhibitors). Consequently, there is a growing and urgent need to develop new methodologies that measure not just the amount of a protein drug target but its "in-use" or activated state.

6.2 Cancer Is a Disease of the Protein "Circuitry"

Dysfunctional protein signaling networks play a central role in tumorigenesis and metastatic progression [7–14]. However, it is not necessarily the total expression levels of a protein that may control key biochemical processes but the posttranslational modifications such as phosphorylation that often play the dominant role in orchestrating and regulating cell signaling processes and those deranged in the tumorigenic processes.

Protein phosphorylation controls protein signaling largely through SH2 and SH3 protein–protein interactions [13–27] with the majority of protein phosphorylation occurring on serine and threonine residues with the remainder (approximately 10%) occurring on tyrosine residues. A large number of receptor tyrosine kinases (RTK) are the targets for clinically used anticancer therapeutics (e.g., EGFR, VEGFR, ROS, HER2 MET, KIT, PDGFR, ALK) that are themselves kinase enzymes. Upon ligand binding, the protein receptor becomes conformationally altered, which then changes intracellular protein interactions on its intracellular domain and signaling commences. RTKs can also become activated due to stochastic events such as genomic duplications/amplifications overexpressed due to genomic amplification, the receptors hetero- or homodimerize, trans-phosphorylate, which then form new binding sites for downstream scaffolding and protein kinase interactions [13–27]. Consequently, phosphoprotein-based biomarkers represent an emerging and critical new category of companion diagnostic markers for precision oncology applications [4, 8–10]. While activating EGFR mutations can identify NSCLC patients that respond to EGFR-directed therapy, recent studies reveal that EGFR phosphorylation associated with response to EGFR-targeted therapy [17], even in EGFR wild-type NSCLC patients [18]. mRNA expression has not been effectively able to predict and correlate with ongoing protein signaling/ phosphoprotein levels and act as an effective molecular surrogate for protein and phosphoprotein levels [11, 12]. Moreover, measurement of total protein expression levels often does not correlate with the phosphorylation levels of a given protein since protein signaling works by rapid phosphorylation of a large substrate pool, and total levels of a protein often do not predict therapy response, whereas the phosphorylation level carries the weight of response prediction [10, 17, 18, 21, 28]. Therefore, technologies that can directly measure and quantify the levels and amount of phosphorylation of proteins that represent the direct drug targets of many of the FDA-approved and experimental inhibitors are critically needed.

6.3 Phospho-Specific Flow Cytometry

Phospho-specific flow cytometry or phospho-flow (PF) is a high-throughput technology that allows multiplexed measurement of the phosphorylation levels of numerous cellular proteins mostly in non-solid tumors. Solid tumor analysis requires complex tissue disaggregation techniques that are only possible with fresh tissue. Each analyte is recognized by a phosphoepitope-specific fluorescent-labeled antibody [29], and quantification is achieved using standard flow cytometry instrumentation. The introduction of fluorescent cell barcoding systems (FCB) has allowed PF technology to become a more high-throughput multiplex platform [30]. Use of FCBs notably reduces inter-experiment variability since all samples are concomitantly incubated with the same phospho-specific antibodies and data are acquired simultaneously across samples.

Using PF, some recent investigators [31] analyzed whether time-dependent changes in the phosphorylation of S6 ribosomal protein (S6RP) associated with response to therapy in acute myeloid leukemia (AML) patients treated with the mTOR inhibitor Sirolimus in combination with a standard treatment regimen (mitoxantrone, etoposide, and cytarabine). Phosphorylation/activation of S6RP, an mTOR downstream substrate, was used as a direct readout of mTOR activity. Based on the changes in the phosphorylation level of S6RP after 4 d of treatment, patients were classified into three groups: sensitive, resistant, and unmodified. A total of 60% (3/5) patients with high levels of S6RP phosphorylation had at least 75% reduction in pS6RP compared to the baseline levels and had either complete or partial remission after therapy. Using a similar PF workflow, Irish and colleagues

[22] evaluated AML samples using PF with a comprehensive panel of antibodies targeting different phosphoproteins with baseline whole blood samples treated ex vivo with GM-CSF, G-SCF, IL3, FLT3, and INFγ ligands. The investigators sought to determine whether ligand-induced changes in the blood cell phosphoproteome were significantly associated with patient response to standard treatment [23]. The results indicated that a substantial number of patients presenting with resistant disease showed increased p-STAT3 and p-STAT5 myeloid signaling after stimulation with INFγ, indicating that the ex vivo obtained phosphoprotein signaling architecture of the patient blood cells could have prognostic value in identifying patients that most likely will respond to therapy.

6.4 Automated Quantitative Analysis (AQUA)

Traditional immunohistochemical (IHC) analyses represent gold-standard, FDA-approved methodologies for a number of important predictive and prognostic cancer biomarkers in the precision oncology space, such as PD-L1, HER2, and estrogen receptor measurement. These pathology-based CLIA/CAP accredited assays are highly standardized but are low-throughput and fraught with operator dependency, subjectivity in cut point determination, and underpinned by subtle differences in staining or subcellular localization interpretation that could have potential clinical relevance. To address some of the issues surrounding high-throughput IHC analyses, Rimm and colleagues developed a series of algorithms that provide automated, rapid, and quantitative analysis called automated quantitative analysis (AQUA) [32, 33]. AQUA analysis is comprised of algorithms that utilize fluorescent tags to differentiate tumor and stroma cellular localization, define specific subcellular compartments, and improve the assignment of pixels to particular subcellular localizations. The cellular distribution and localization of a given analyte of interest, e.g., HER2, are then quantitatively assessed according to its co-localization with these tags [32]. A major advantage of AQUA technology is that it allows a non-subjective continuous measurement of a target, expressed as an AQUA score that is a “pixel intensity/pixel area” value. The technology compares favorably with pathologist-based analysis of tissue microarrays, and Camp et al. demonstrated that the technology could determine and reproducibly differentiate subtle staining differences for nuclear β-catenin at the upper and lower extremes of the dynamic range that significantly impacted outcome predictions in a cohort of over 300 colon cancers compared to pathologist-based nominal classifications.

Assessment of phosphoprotein expression in clinical tissues by IHC has been generally restricted to research-based correlative studies, largely due to antigen retrieval issues of the phosphoepitope from FFPE material and questions surrounding the effective preservation of these posttranslational modifications during formalin fixation of tissues. Despite these issues, several studies have been published using AQUA or a combination of AQUA and IHC to evaluate phosphoprotein expression and its correlation with various clinical parameters. Analyzing two cohorts of ovarian cancer tumors, Faratian et al. used AQUA to measure the activation state of a number of druggable pathways, including AKT, MAPK, B-catenin, among others, in an effort to establish associations with clinical parameters and potentially identify treatment groups for targeted therapies and predictive markers for therapeutic response [34]. Their analysis identified four distinct groups of tumors based on phosphoprotein expression profiles in both cohorts of tumors but found no association of these clusters with response to standard chemotherapy. There was some association of individual phosphoproteins with traditional tumor histopathological subtype, but overall, the phosphoprotein expression profiles revealed new molecular subgroups that might facilitate new approaches to selecting molecular-targeted therapies for these patients and provide a rationale for testing them in prospective clinical trials [34].

6.5 Phosphoprotein Analysis by Mass Spectrometry

Recent technical advances in proteomics have made quantitative analysis of phosphoproteins in human clinical tissue specimens feasible. While a large number of proteins are ubiquitously phosphorylated to some extent, the levels of phosphorylation of key drug target signaling molecules are present at extremely low levels and thus require some form of enrichment prior to analysis by mass spectrometry. A number of affinity-based enrichment techniques have been developed to isolate phosphopeptides from complex cellular lysates. One example is the use of antibodies specific for phosphorylated amino acids such as phosphotyrosine, phosphoserine, and phospho-threonine which can be coupled to beads or other matrices and used in column form or directly incubated with lysates and retrieved by centrifugation. Other examples include immobilized metal affinity chromatography (IMAC), metal oxide affinity chromatography (MOAC), metal oxide coated bead-based enrichment, and more recently small-molecule kinase inhibitor-coupled beads. These enrichment strategies are often used in conjunction with pre-fractionation strategies such as strong cation or anion exchange chromatography to achieve reliably detectable amounts of phosphopeptides [35]. Phosphopeptide quantification from human tissues often incorporates various forms of protein labeling such as isobaric tags for relative and absolute quantitation (iTRAQ), dimethyl labeling, isobaric peptide terminal labeling (IPTL), and non-isobaric isotope-coded protein labeling (ICPL), but label-free quantitation strategies have also been employed [35]. Newer, highly sensitive mass spectrometry techniques such as selective and multiple reaction monitoring (SRM and MRM) are also being utilized to identify low-abundance phosphoprotein biomarkers in human tissues.

A number of recent publications have used the aforementioned techniques to focus on the measurement of signaling molecules and phosphoproteins in human tissues. Geiger et al. reported the development and use of a super-SILAC mix of cell lines as an internal standard for MS analysis of human breast cancer tissues

[36]. The investigators were able to measure more than 100 protein kinases such as ERBB2, EGFR, AKT, and members of the MAPK signaling cascade, as well as approximately 100 phosphopeptides without any additional enrichment strategies. The investigators were also able to detect and quantify a number of known and novel differences between ductal and lobular breast carcinoma tissues [36] Another recent study employed large-scale phosphoproteomic quantitation of human breast cancer tissues using IMAC enrichment and iTRAQ labeling for LC-MS/MS analysis coupled with validation using SRM/MRM to identify potential biomarkers differentiating high- and low-risk recurrence groups [37]. They identified many thousands of unique phosphoproteins and 133 phosphopeptides (131 phosphoproteins) were differentially expressed between high- and low-risk recurrence groups predicted by the MammaPrint gene expression assay. Nineteen of the candidate phosphopeptides were verified by SRM using stable isotope peptides, and 15 underwent successful SRM-based quantitation. These results suggest that large-scale phosphoproteome quantification coupled with SRM-based validation is a powerful tool for biomarker discovery using clinical samples.

6.6 Multiplex Immunoassays

Multiplex immunoassays (MI) are sandwich-based immunoassays that can provide a high-throughput approach to quantitatively measure a large number of analytes from a limited amount of biological material. In this type of assay, the analyte of interest is initially recognized by an antibody either immobilized into a solid substrate (planar array-based assay) or conjugated to a bead (microbead assays). A second antibody targeting a different epitope of the same protein is used to quantify the amount of analyte in a biological sample. Meso Scale Discovery (MSD), A2 protein microarray system, and FAST Quant are examples of the planar array-based assay, while Luminex and FlowCytomix are two examples of microbead-based assays.

Although all these platforms have been routinely used to monitor changes in the expression level of cytokines, chemokines, and their receptors after administration of bio- and chemotherapeutic agents [38], these technologies show great potential in monitoring changes in phosphorylation of drug targets and/or their downstream effectors. The high sensitivity of the MSD platform is attributable to combination of the high binding capacity of the carbon substrate on which antibodies are immobilized and the unique electrochemiluminescence detection system developed by MSD [38]. A variable number of carbon electrodes (up to 10 per well) are immobilized at the bottom of each well. Each electrode is then coated with one specific antibody targeting the analyte of interest. After the phosphoprotein analyte has been captured by the electrodes, it is recognized by a second ruthenium-conjugated antibody targeting a different epitope of the same protein. By applying an electroluminescent stimulation to the plate the ruthenium emits a signal that is proportional to the amount of analyte present in the analytical sample [38].

In a recent publication that described results from a phase II clinical trial testing the efficacy of Sorafenib in metastatic prostate cancer patients [39], the investigators used the MSD technology to interrogate phosphoprotein-based drug-related changes in the cellular signaling architecture from bone marrow cells. Sorafenib interferes with cell proliferation by modulating the MAPK pathway through inhibition of the Raf kinase and with angiogenesis by inhibiting the VEGFR and PDGFR signaling. The investigators collected pre- and on-therapy bone marrow aspirates from twenty-two androgen-independent prostate cancer patients with secondary bone and/or soft tissue lesions and investigated whether modulation of the phosphorylation level of ERK, the major downstream substrate of Raf, could be used as a predictive biomarker to determine the efficacy of Sorafenib in this group of patients. Although no complete or partial response was observed in this cohort, one of the two patients that showed radiological improvement of the metastatic lesion revealed a significant decrease in the phosphorylation of ERK while receiving Sorafenib, indicating that monitoring changes in the phosphorylation of kinase substrates of key drug targets during therapy might have some potential value in predicting patients' response to therapy. The same platform was used by Yap and colleagues [40] in monitoring changes in the phosphorylation level of AKT after administration of the oral pan-AKT inhibitor MK-2206 in patients affected by different types of solid tumors [40]. The authors collected matched pre- and on-treatment biopsies from a subgroup of nine subjects. All samples showed significant decrease in the phosphorylation level of AKT S473 after 15 d of treatment (median reduction of 88%) confirming that MK-2206 is a chemical compound capable of modulating AKT activity in vivo.

The Luminex technology uses polystyrene microspheres coupled with antibodies, oligonucleotides, peptides, or receptors capable of recognizing specific molecular targets [38]. The bead core is covered with a mixture of red and infrared fluorophores. Microspheres are prepared by combining different ratios of the two fluorophores, and each batch of beads is then coupled with one specific antibody able to recognize the analyte of interest [38]. By modulating the concentrations of the fluorophores and coupling each batch with a unique and specific antibody, dozens to hundreds of beads can be analyzed simultaneously. Once the microspheres have bound to the analyte of interest, a second fluorescent R-phycoerythrin-labeled antibody recognizing a different epitope of the same analyte is added to the mixture for the quantification of the protein of interest in the solution [38].

Detection of the signal and protein quantification is achieved using flow cytometry principles where individual microspheres are excited with a double laser system in a series of detection chambers [41]. This platform presents with several unique advantages. High accuracy/reproducibility, requirement of small amount of biological material (low detection range: lower pico-molar range), timely delivery multiplex results, and the possibility of creating customized platforms are all unique trademarks of the Luminex technology [41].

Perkins and colleagues [42] utilized the microbead-based platform to investigate whether the phosphorylation levels of a variety of EGFR kinase downstream substrates (MEK1; ERK1-2; AKT; P70S6K; and GSK3β) correlate with response to treatment with EGFR inhibitors in colorectal cancer patients. Forty-two metastatic colorectal cancer patients were included in the study and had been predetermined as EGFR positive by IHC. Patients were treated either with cetuximab or panitumumab as a single agent or in combination with standard of care. The investigators found a significant inverse association between p70S6K phosphorylation levels and response to therapy, indicating that highly activated p70S6K (a key member of the mTOR pro-survival pathway) prevented the targeted drug from inhibiting tumor growth and progression.

A phase I clinical trial recently conducted by Baselga and colleagues [43] investigated the safety and tolerability of Saracatinib, a Src inhibitor, in patients affected by solid tumors refractory to standard of care. One of the secondary objectives of this study was to evaluate changes in the Src-mediated activity after 21 d of treatment. Twenty-one matched pre- and post-therapy biopsies were collected from a subgroup of patients enrolled in the study. The investigators measured the expression and activation levels of Paxillin and FAK, two proteins known to directly indicate Src kinase activity [43], were quantified using the Luminex platform. Although no complete or partial response was achieved in this cohort of patients, this study showed significant dose-dependent reduction in the activation of Src downstream substrates after 21 d of treatment. Moreover, the authors reported that patients presenting with high activation levels of Src downstream effectors at baseline showed the greatest reduction in phosphorylation after the administration of Saracatinib indicating that pre-treatment selection of patients based on baseline Src activation might increase drug efficacy.

6.7 Reverse Phase Protein Microarrays as a Tool for Personalized Cancer Therapy

Based on the need to effectively measure the functional activated protein signaling architecture for targeted therapy applications, our laboratory developed a planar array-based technology that can quantitatively measure the phosphorylation/activation state of dozens to hundreds of signaling proteins concomitantly. This technology called the reverse phase protein microarray (RPPA) is proving to be a key enabling technology for the analysis of clinical material [44–50]. Unlike a forward phase array format (e.g., antibody array) where the analyte detecting molecule is immobilized, with the RPPA format, cellular or tissue lysates (or even body fluids) from individual samples are printed directly and immobilized on a planar surface such that an. Depending on the size of the pin used to print the samples, it is possible to print a few hundred to several thousand spots on each slide. Since each printing deposits as little as 1–5 nl, it is possible to as many as 100 slides from a lysate of only a few thousand cells [47]. The most widely used substrate is nitrocellulose, which has the aggregate attributes of low cost, high binding capacity, and low relative background. With the RPPA format, each slide is incubated with one specific primary antibody, and a single analyte endpoint is measured and directly compared across multiple samples on each slide. Each array is printed with a series of high and low controls and calibrator samples that contain predetermined and varying amounts of the target analyte that span the expected linear dynamic range of the analyte. The RPPA, when used as a calibrated immunoassay, provides a straightforward means of quantifying any input by interpolation or extrapolation to the printed calibrator. While the RPPA was initially designed for colorimetric detection, fluorescent detection using near-infrared dye coupled reagents [49] has become popular due to the dramatically increased within spot dynamic range of the assay (Fig. 6.1).

The RPPA is capable of extremely sensitive analyte detection, for example, with reported levels of a few hundred molecules per spot and a CV of less than 10% [47]. Overall analytical sensitivity is ultimately dependent on analyte concentration, antibody affinity, and avidity, and however, the general sensitivity of detection for the RPPA is such even extremely low-abundance phosphorylated signaling proteins can be measured from a lysate containing less than 10 cell equivalents [47]. The ability to generate a quantitative linear signal from such small amounts of material, and do so in high multiplex, is the unique attribute of the RPPA that distinguishes it from every other proteomic technique. This attribute becomes extremely important for clinical applications where often the starting input material is only a few hundred cells from a needle biopsy or fine needle aspirate specimen. Like a clinical immunoassay, the RPPA has been transitioned to a calibrated assay format that allows for cut point determination and extension of results into a CAP/CLIA setting

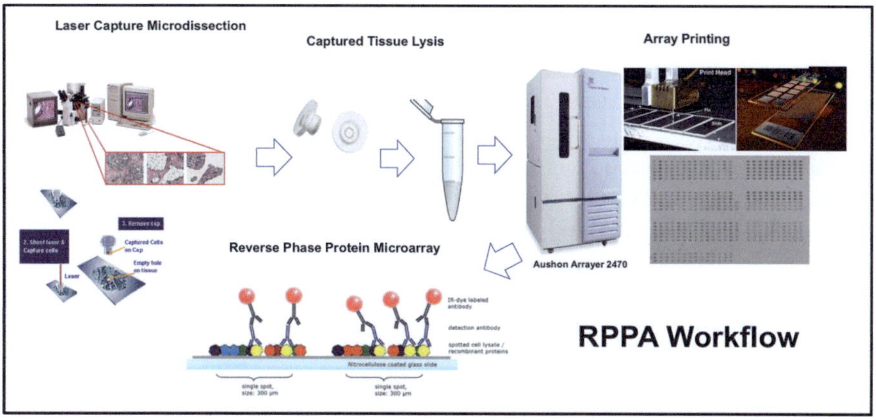

Fig. 6.1 Laser capture microdissection–reverse phase protein microarray workflow. Clinical tissue samples are subjected to laser capture microdissection to procure highly enriched and purified cell populations that are then lysed and printed on nitrocellulose slides. Each slide is then exposed to a specific primary antibody and secondary antibodies that amplify the analyte concentration within each spot to produce a colorimetric or fluorescent signal that is captured by the appropriate detector type and analyzed

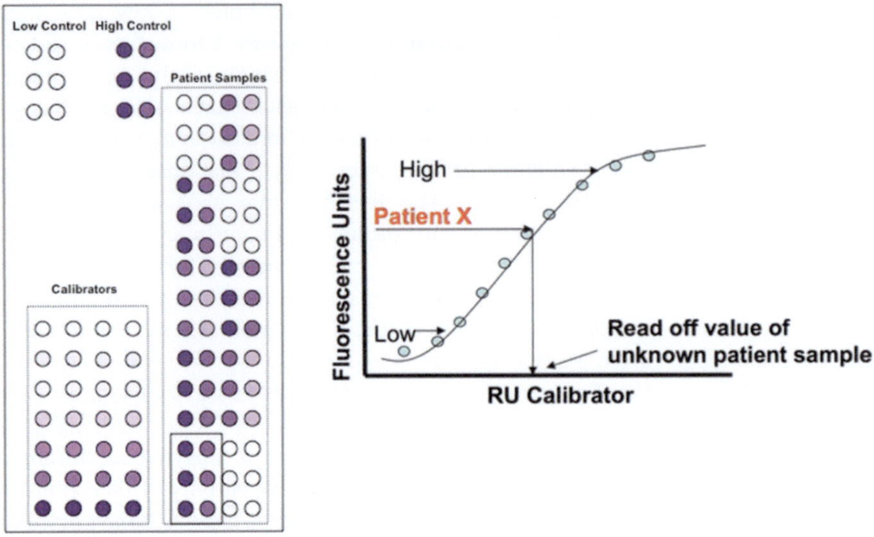

Fig. 6.2 Calibrated RPPA format for clinical use. Denatured cellular lysates, obtained from clinical isolates, laser capture microdissected material, etc., are spotted directly onto a nitrocellulose-coated slide and multiple samples are simultaneously probed with the same antibody. Each sample may be printed in a step-wise dilution curve (shown) or as a single replicate spot (not shown) with colorimetric or fluorescent detection, respectively. Similar to an ELISA or immunoassay, high and low controls and calibrators are printed on every slide with the RPPA format to ensure inter and intra-assay reproducibility, process QA/QC and fidelity of data generated. The final values for any patient sample can be interpolated to the reference calibrator printed on every array

(Fig. 6.2). RPPA, like immunohistochemistry, is dependent on the availability of high quality, specific antibodies, particularly those specific for posttranslational modifications or active states of proteins, and is a major limiting factor for the successful implementation of any immunoassay-type platforms. Up-front rigorous validation of each antibody is essential in order to be confident that the signal generated on the array is a result of the specific analyte being detected. Most RPPA workflows include background subtraction from arrays that have been exposed to the secondary antibody alone as well as local intra-array background subtraction. In addition, normalization of the signal itself is usually obtained by measuring the total amount of protein printed on the array, although newer techniques that normalize by DNA content of the lysate can be extremely helpful in instances where the sample is contaminated by exogenous proteins such as blood [50].

Key technological components of the RPPA offer several advantages over other array-based platforms. The RPPA can employ denatured lysates, so that antigen retrieval of sterically hindered phosphorylated epitopes, a significant limitation for tissue arrays, antibody arrays, and immunohistochemistry technologies, is not an issue. Kinase profiling efforts require maintenance of cellular/tissue kinase activity, yet maintaining that activity to reflect only what had occurred in the patient and not influenced by exogenous tissue processing artifact is extremely difficult. RPPAs only require a single class of antibody per analyte protein and do not require direct tagging of the protein as readout for the assay. Other technologies, such as suspension bead array platforms, have significant limitations in the portfolio of analytes that can be measured, even in multiplex, because of the requirement of a two-site assay. Moreover, since the RPPA platform can measure the activation state of so many individual signaling molecules at once, broad-scale analysis of the signaling architecture on a pathway basis can provide a detailed understanding of the interconnections within the cellular circuitry even though a single snapshot in time (e.g., biopsy) is the input for analysis.

RPPA technology was first described by our group over a decade ago wherein LCM-RPPA workflow (Fig. 6.2) revealed that AKT signaling is activated at the invasion front during prostate cancer progression with a number of those AKT pathway members activated in early stage prostatic intra-epithelial neoplasia [44]. In another study, a phosphoprotein-based signature comprised of multiple members of the AKT-mTOR pathway was found to be systematically activated in rhabdomyosarcoma tumors from children who did not respond to chemotherapy and progressed rapidly [48].

Since cancer is often diagnosed at later stages, many treatments center on management of metastatic disease. As metastasis is the lethal aspect of the disease, then analyzing the signaling profile of the metastatic lesion may be a critical requirement for the correct selection of targeted agents since there is a distinct possibility that the signaling architecture of the metastatic tumor cells will differ significantly from those of the primary tumor cells. In fact, recent analysis of patient-matched primary colorectal cancer lesions and liver metastases suggested that signaling in metastatic hepatic lesions differed considerably from that in the matched primary lesions [45].

Uncovering mechanisms of the development of resistance to targeted agents is another important area where the RPPA technology can have significant impact. In fact, RPPA analysis was used to identify protein markers predictive for therapeutic response or resistance in a number of different types of cancers [51–56]. Studies in ovarian cancer and colon cancer cell lines identified pathway markers involved in nucleotide excision repair that were associated with chemotherapy drug activity [51]. Pathway analysis of melanoma cell lines and patient samples revealed that phosphorylation of 4E-BP1 was increased in melanoma cell lines carrying mutations in BRAF and PTEN compared to cells with wild-type RAS/RAF/PTEN and was associated with worse overall and post-recurrence survival [52]. Analysis of breast cancer cell lines found that distinct patterns of signaling were present in groups representing different molecular subtypes of breast cancer that were not obvious from gene transcription profiling [53]. In this study, the investigators found that treatment of basal-type cells with MEK inhibitors resulted in AKT signaling activation, which could have implications for treatment response to other therapeutic agents. RPPA analysis of the signaling architecture of cells being evaluated for response and resistance to the PI3K inhibitors found that mutations in the genes for PI3K and loss of PTEN activity were potential predictors of sensitivity to these inhibitors [54]. Interestingly, Ras mutations (so prevalent in pancreatic cancers) were a major resistance marker in this study, even in the presence of PI3K mutations and measurements of phosphorylated AKT (S473). Moreover, expression of c-Myc and cyclin B, which are downstream targets of Ras, were up-regulated in PI3K inhibitor resistant cell lines in vivo and were also negatively associated with response to the drug in vivo.

Drugs targeting the EGFR and HER family signaling pathway are some of the most intensely studied in the field of molecular-targeted therapies. A recent study by Xia et al. identified an entirely novel mechanism of lapatinib resistance, a small-molecule inhibitor of EGFR and HER2, in breast cancer [55]. Using a series of isogenic lapatinib sensitive cell lines and those with acquired resistance and broad-scale RPPA-based pathway activation mapping of hundreds of key signaling proteins, the investigators found that resistance was due to the "leaky" nature of lapatinib whereby incomplete inhibition of EGFR phosphorylation by lapatinib supplied effective selective pressure to cause the cells to increase the production of the heregulin ligand and switch from HER2 to HER3 signaling to heregulin-driven EGFR-HER3 signaling. Investigators utilized RPPA-based pathway activation mapping to study mechanisms of estrogen resistance in breast cancer also using matched resistant/sensitive cell lines and found that several pathways involved in cell proliferation and survival were activated in tamoxifen-resistant lines [55]. Most recently [56], we utilized the RPPA platform to measure the activation/phosphorylation state of HER family proteins (e.g., HER2, EGFR, and HER3) in HER2+ and triple negative stage II/III breast cancer patients treated with the targeted therapeutic neratinib in the I-SPY2 TRIAL. Based on the mechanism of action of neratinib as a HER2 and EGFR dual kinase inhibitor, we postulated that the pre-treatment phosphorylation levels of these 2 protein targets would predict response (pathological complete response or pCR) in this cohort. Indeed, and intriguingly, phosphorylated EGFR (Y1173) and HER2 (Y1248) both highly correlated with response and were able to predict response to the drug in both the HER2+ and HER2− subgroups. Neither the total levels of HER2, EGFR nor the mRNA expression levels of these genes predicted response—only the phosphoprotein analyte.

6.8 Pre-analytical Factors Influence Phosphoprotein Pathway Activation Mapping

Clinical and preclinical tissues are most often a heterogeneous mixture of interacting cell populations, such as fat cells, nerve cells, endothelial vessel cells, muscle cells, fibroblasts, epithelial cells, and immune cells as well as acellular material such as collagen and serum. Workflows where whole tissue is lysed and analyzed as a whole may generate inaccurate measurements of signaling activation or deactivation since most signaling molecules are ubiquitously expressed in different cell populations. The use of laser capture microdissection (LCM) combined with RPPA provides a facile means of detailed molecular analysis of discrete cell populations within a clinical biopsy specimen. The impact of uncontrolled cellular heterogeneity on phosphoprotein measurements was recently described whereby pathway activation mapping was performed on patient-matched undissected and LCM procured glioblastoma, ovarian, and breast cancer tumor epithelium and revealed significant and numerous differences in pathway activation portraits between the two [57, 58] with most patient pairs not revealing any overarching similarity. Additionally, when comparing molecular correlations between expected relationships in PTEN protein and phosphoprotein expression and PTEN loss of heterozygosity and mutation status as well as EGFR activation and EGFR mutation status, only data obtained from the LCM material produced the expected results [57]. Moreover, despite the dramatic differences seen between LCM and undissected cells, these past studies utilized studies wherein many of the cases contained over 50% tumor, which would represent a relatively high upper end of what would normally be seen in a large clinical trial setting (where an average of approximately 20–30% tumor content is seen in a core needle biopsy.

Even if the impact of uncontrolled cellular heterogeneity is minimized by cellular enrichment techniques such as LCM, proteins and phosphoproteins are inherently labile and are acutely affected by pre-analytical variables such as post-excision delay, time of the tissue on the pathologist bench prior to fixation, etc. Recent results have found that within 15–30 min after a tissue specimen is removed from the body, many phosphoproteins become both activated and deactivated as the still-living tissue undergoes hypoxic and acidotic changes ex vivo and activate survival signaling [59, 60]. Obviously, treatment decisions cannot be based on molecular changes that occur because of how long the tissue sat on the pathologist's table. Since formalin fixation of tissue occurs so slowly ($\sim$1 mm/h), simply dropping a piece of tissue into formalin does not solve the issue of preserving the in vivo signaling portraits of a tissue sample. The development of next-generation rapid penetrating fixatives or tissue processing methods that can preserve the labile phosphoprotein signaling architecture while maintaining formalin-equivalent histomorphology is of critical importance, and such reagents and methods are being developed [61].

6.9 A View to the Near Future: Impact of Proteomics on Precision Oncology

As new classes of multiplexed proteomic technologies such as the RPPA establish themselves as necessary components of the tissue molecular work up and the use of phosphoprotein-based biomarkers for drug response prediction and patient selection accelerates, we can visualize a future where these approaches coexist with genomic analysis for a systems-level view of tumor biology. Such a multi-omic view will invariably provide a more detailed and accurate view of the druggable landscape of an individual patient tumor as well as help to more fully elucidate true driver molecular alterations that are causally important for tumorigenesis. Based on the current drug development pipeline, in less than 5 years there may be hundreds of targeted therapies cleared for use by the FDA, with as many or more protein companion diagnostic markers being offered. Consequently, it will not be possible to measure 50–75 phosphoproteins at once from a single biopsy specimen using standard IHC, ELISA, etc. technologies. At this time, new classes of multiplexed proteomic formats such as the RPPA are uniquely positioned to produce a quantitative readout of the activation state of dozens to hundreds of drug targets at once. In addition, as combination therapies tailored to each patient's tumor architecture begin to become part of routine pathological workup, the need to effectively measure the activated protein "circuitry" will be central to this effort. Indeed, one can envision a future vision for cancer patients whereby a "wiring diagram" of each patient's tumor biopsy is produced by these technologies and provided to the treating oncologist as part of a pathology report, providing a circuit view of the actionable/druggable landscape and a molecular rationale for patient-tailored therapy. These new opportunities are destined to change the landscape of precision oncology in the near future.

References

1. Lee CK, Brown C, Gralla RJ, Hirsh V, Thongprasert S et al (2013) Impact of EGFR inhibitor in non-small cell lung cancer on progression-free and overall survival: a meta-analysis. J Natl Cancer Inst 105(9):595–605
2. Rothschild SI, Gautschi O (2013) Crizotinib in the treatment of non-small-cell lung cancer. Clin Lung Cancer. 14(5):473–480
3. Rexer BN, Arteaga CL (2013) Optimal targeting of HER2-PI3K signaling in breast cancer: mechanistic insights and clinical implications. Cancer Res 73(13):3817–3820
4. Cheng S, Koch WH, Wu L (2012) Co-development of a companion diagnostic for targeted cancer therapy. N Biotechnol 29(6):682–688
5. Janku F, Broaddus R, Bakkar R, Hong DS, Stepanek V et al (2012) PTEN assessment and PI3K/mTOR inhibitors: importance of simultaneous assessment of MAPK pathway aberrations. In: ASCO annual meeting, Abstract 10510, presented 5 June 2012
6. Ganesan P, Janku F, Naing A, Hong DS, Tsimberidou AM et al (2013) Target-based therapeutic matching in early-phase clinical trials in patients with advanced colorectal cancer and PIK3CA mutations. Mol Cancer Ther
7. Faivre S, Djelloul S, Raymond E (2006) New paradigms in anticancer therapy: targeting multiple signaling pathways with kinase inhibitors. Semin Oncol 33(4):407–420
8. Huang PH, Mukasa A, Bonavia R, Flynn RA, Brewer ZE et al (2007) Quantitative analysis of EGFRvIII cellular signaling networks reveals a combinatorial therapeutic strategy for glioblastoma. Proc Natl Acad Sci USA 104(31):12867–12872
9. Engelman JA, Zejnullahu K, Mitsudomi T, Song Y, Hyland C et al (2007) MET amplification leads to gefitinib resistance in lung cancer by activating ERBB3 signaling. Science 316 (5827):1039–1043
10. Sawyers CL (2008) The cancer biomarker problem. Nature 452(7187):548
11. Parsons DW, Jones S, Zhang X, Lin JC, Leary RJ et al (2008) An integrated genomic analysis of human glioblastoma multiforme. Science 321(5897):1807–1812

12. Jones S, Zhang X, Parsons DW, Lin JC, Leary RJ et al (2008) Core signaling pathways in human pancreatic cancers revealed by global genomic analyses. Science 321(5897):1801–1806
13. Wood LD, Parsons DW, Jones S, Lin J, Sjöblom T et al (2007) The genomic landscapes of human breast and colorectal cancers. Science 318(5853):1108–1113
14. Liotta LA, Kohn EC, Petricoin EF (2001) Clinical proteomics: personalized molecular medicine. JAMA 286(18):2211–2214
15. Petricoin EF III, Bichsel VE, Calvert VS, Espina V, Winters M et al (2005) Mapping molecular networks using proteomics: a vision for patient-tailored combination therapy. J Clin Oncol 23:3614–3621
16. Wulfkuhle JD, Edmiston KH, Liotta LA, Petricoin EF (2006) Technology insight: pharmacoproteomics for cancer-promises of patient-tailored medicine using protein microarrays. Nat Clin Pract Oncol 3(5):256–268
17. Emery IF, Battelli C, Auclair PL, Carrier K, Hayes DM (2009) Response to gefitinib and erlotinib in non-small cell lung cancer: a retrospective study. BMC Cancer 9:333
18. Wang F, Wang S, Wang Z, Duan J, An T et al (2012) Phosphorylated EGFR expression may predict outcome of EGFR-TKIs therapy for the advanced NSCLC patients with wild-type EGFR. J Exp Clin Cancer Res 18(31):65
19. Anderson L, Seilhamer J (1997) A comparison of selected mRNA and protein abundances in human liver. Electrophoresis 18(3–4):533–537
20. Gygi SP, Rochon Y, Franza BR, Aebersold R (1999) Correlation between protein and mRNA abundance in yeast. Mol Cell Biol 19(3):1720–1730
21. Quaranta V, Tyson DR (2013) What lies beneath: looking beyond tumor genetics shows the complexity of signaling networks underlying drug sensitivity. Sci Signal 6(294)
22. Irish JM, Hovland R, Krutzik PO, Perez OD, Bruserud Ø, Gjertsen BT et al (2004) Single cell profiling of potentiated phospho-protein networks in cancer cells. Cell 118(2):217–228
23. Irish JM, Anensen N, Hovland R, Skavland J, Børresen-Dale AL et al (2007) Flt3 Y591 duplication and Bcl-2 overexpression are detected in acute myeloid leukemia cells with high levels of phosphorylated wild-type p53. Blood 109(6):2589–2596
24. Stern DF (2005) Phosphoproteomics for oncology discovery and treatment. Expert Opin Ther Targets 9(4):851–860
25. Moran MF, Tong J, Taylor P, Ewing RM (2006) Emerging applications for phospho-proteomics in cancer molecular therapeutics. Biochim Biophys Acta 1766(2):230–241
26. Hunter T (2000) Signaling-2000 and beyond. Cell 100:113–127
27. Figlin RA (2008) Mechanisms of disease: survival benefit of temsirolimus validates a role for mTOR in the management of advanced RCC. Nat Clin Pract Oncol 5(10):601–609
28. Ramić S, Asić K, Balja MP, Paić F, Benković V, Knežević F (2013) Correlation of phosphorylated HER2 with clinicopathological characteristics and efficacy of trastuzumab treatment for breast cancer. Anticancer Res 33(6):2509–2515
29. Krutzik PO, Trejo A, Schulz KR, Nolan GP (2011) Phospho flow cytometry methods for the analysis of kinase signaling in cell lines and primary human blood samples. Methods Mol Biol 699:179–202
30. Krutzik PO, Clutter MR, Trejo A, Nolan GP (2011) Fluorescent cell barcoding for multiplex flow cytometry. Curr Protoc Cytom (Chapter 6, Unit 6.31)
31. Perl AE, Kasner MT, Shank D, Luger SM, Carroll M (2012) Single-cell pharmacodynamic monitoring of S6 ribosomal protein phosphorylation in AML blasts during a clinical trial combining the mTOR inhibitor sirolimus and intensive chemotherapy. Clin Cancer Res 18 (6):1716–1725
32. Camp RL, Chung GG, Rimm DL (2002) Automated subcellular localization and quantification of protein expression in tissue microarrays. Nature Med 8:1323–1327
33. Camp RL, Neumeister V, Rimm DL (2008) A decade of tissue microarrays: progress in the discovery and validation of cancer biomarkers. J Clin Oncol 26:5630–5637

34. Faratian D, Um IH, Wilson DS, Mullen P, Langdon SP, Harrison DJ (2011) Phosphoprotein pathway profiling of ovarian carcinoma for the identification of potential new targets for therapy. Eur J Cancer 47:1420–1431
35. Stasyk T, Huber LA (2012) Mapping in vivo signal transduction defects by phosphoproteomics. Trends Mol Med 18:43–51
36. Geiger T, Cox J, Ostasiewicz P, Wisniewski JR, Mann M (2010) Super-SILAC mix for proteomics of human tumor tissue. Nat Methods 7:383–385
37. Narumi R, Murakami T, Kuga T, Adachi J, Shriomizu T, Muraoka S et al (2012) A strategy of large-scale phosphoproteomics and SRM-based validation of human breast cancer tissue samples. J Proteome Res 11:5311–5322
38. Chowdhury F, Williams A, Johnson P (2009) Validation and comparison of two multiplex technologies, Luminex and Mesoscale Discovery, for human cytokine profiling. J Immunol Methods 340(1):55–64. https://doi.org/10.1016/j.jim.2008.10.002
39. Dahut WL, Scripture C, Posadas E, Jain L, Gulley JL, Arlen PM, Wright JJ, Yu Y, Cao L, Steinberg SM, Aragon-Ching JB, Venitz J, Jones E, Chen CC, Figg WD (2008) A phase II clinical trial of sorafenib in androgen-independent prostate cancer. Clin Cancer Res 14 (1):209–214
40. Yap TA, Yan L, Patnaik A, Fearen I, Olmos D, Papadopoulos K, Baird RD, Delgado L, Taylor A, Lupinacci L, Riisnaes R, Pope LL, Heaton SP, Thomas G, Garrett MD, Sullivan DM, de Bono JS, Tolcher AW (2011) First-in-man clinical trial of the oral pan-AKT inhibitor MK-2206 in patients with advanced solid tumors. J Clin Oncol 29(35):4688–4695
41. Schwenk JM, Nilsson P (2011) Antibody suspension bead arrays. Methods Mol Biol 723:29–36
42. Perkins G, Lièvre A, Ramacci C, Méatchi T, de Reynies A, Emile JF, Boige V, Tomasic G, Bachet JB, Bibeau F, Bouché O, Penault-Llorca F, Merlin JL, Laurent-Puig P (2010) Additional value of EGFR downstream signaling phosphoprotein expression to KRAS status for response to anti-EGFR antibodies in colorectal cancer. Int J Cancer 127(6):1321–1331
43. Baselga J, Cervantes A, Martinelli E, Chirivella I, Hoekman K, Hurwitz HI, Jodrell DI, Hamberg P, Casado E, Elvin P, Swaisland A, Iacona R, Tabernero J (2010) Phase I safety, pharmacokinetics, and inhibition of SRC activity study of saracatinib in patients with solid tumors. Clin Cancer Res 16(19):4876–4883
44. Paweletz CP, Charboneau L, Roth MJ, Bichsel VE, Simone NL, Chen T et al (2001) Reverse phase proteomic microarrays which capture disease progression show activation of pro-survival pathways at the cancer invasion front. Oncogene 20(16):1981–1989
45. Pierobon M, Calvert V, Belluco C, Garaci E, Deng J, Lise M et al (2009) Multiplexed cell signaling analysis of metastatic and nonmetastatic colorectal cancer reveals COX2-EGFR signaling activation as a potential prognostic pathway biomarker. Clin Colorectal Cancer 8 (2):110–117
46. Vanmeter AJ, Rodriguez AS, Bowman ED, Harris CC, Deng J, Calvert VS et al (2008) LCM and protein microarray analysis of human NSCLC: differential EGFR phosphorylation events associated with mutated EGFR compared to wild type. Mol Cell Proteomics 7(10):1902–1924
47. Rapkiewicz A, Espina V, Zujewski JA, Lebowitz PF, Filie A, Wulfkuhle J et al (2007) The needle in the haystack: application of breast fine-needle aspirate samples to quantitative protein microarray technology. Cancer 111(3):173–184
48. Petricoin EF, Espina V, Araujo RP, Midura B, Yeung C, Wan X et al (2007) Phosphoprotein signal pathway mapping: Akt/mTOR pathway activation association with childhood rhabdomyosarcoma survival. Cancer Res 67(7):3431–3434
49. Calvert VS, Tang Y, Boveia V, Wulfkuhle J, Schutz-Geschwender Olive DM et al (2004) Development of multiplexed protein profiling and detection using near infrared detection of reverse-phase protein microarrays. Clin Proteomics 1(1):81–90
50. Chiechi A, Mueller C, Boehm KM, Romano A, Benassi MS, Picci P, Liotta LA, Espina V (2012) Improved data normalization methods for reverse phase protein microarray analysis of complex biological samples. Biotechniques, 1–7

51. Stevens EV, Nishizuka S, Antony S et al (2008) Predicting cisplatin and trabectedin drug sensitivity in ovarian and colon cancers. Mol Cancer Ther 7:10–18
52. O'Reilly KE, Warycha M, Davies MA et al (2009) Phosphorylated 4E-BP1 is associated with poor survival in melanoma. Clin Cancer Res 15:2872–2878
53. Boyd ZS, Wu QJ, O'Brien C et al (2008) Proteomic analysis of breast cancer molecular subtypes and biomarkers of response to targeted kinase inhibitors using reverse-phase protein microarrays. Mol Cancer Ther 7:3695–3706
54. Ihle NT, Lemos R, Wipf P et al (2009) Mutations I the phosphatidylinositol-3-kinase pathway predict for antitumor activity of the inhibitor PX-866 while oncogenic Ras is a dominant predictor for resistance. Cancer Res 69:143–150
55. Xia W, Petricoin EF 3rd, Zhao S, Liu L, Osada T, Cheng Q, Wulfkuhle JD, Gwin WR, Yang X, Gallagher RI, Bacus S, Lyerly HK, Spector NL (2013) An heregulin-EGFR-HER3 autocrine signaling axis can mediate acquired lapatinib resistance in HER2+ breast cancer models. Breast Cancer Res 15(5):R85
56. Wulfkuhle JD, Yau C, Wolf DM, Vis DJ, Gallagher RI, Brown-Swigart L, Hirst G, Voest EE, DeMichele A, Hylton H, Symmans F, Yee DT, Esserman L, Berry D, Liu M, Park JW, Wessels L, van't Veer L, Petricoin III EF (2018) Evaluation of the HER/PI3K/AKT family signaling network as a predictive biomarker of pathologic complete response for patients with breast cancer treated with neratinib in the I-SPY 2 TRIAL JCO precision oncology (2):1–20
57. Mueller C, Decarvalho AC, Mikkelsen T, Lehman NL, Calvert V, Espina V, Liotta LA, Petricoin EF 3rd (2014) Glioblastoma cell enrichment is critical for analysis of phosphorylated drug targets and proteomic-genomic correlations. Cancer Res 74(3):818–828
58. Baldelli E, Haura EB, Crinò L, Cress WD, Ludovini V, Schabath MB, Liotta LA, Petricoin EF, Pierobon M (2015) Impact of upfront cellular enrichment by laser capture microdissection on protein and phosphoprotein drug target signaling activation measurements in human lung cancer: implications for personalized medicine. Proteomics Clin Appl
59. Espina V, Edmiston KH, Heiby M, Pierobon M, Sciro M, Merritt B, Banks S, Deng J, VanMeter AJ, Geho DH, Pastore L, Sennesh J, Petricoin EF 3rd, Liotta LA (2008) A portrait of tissue phosphoprotein stability in the clinical tissue procurement process. Mol Cell Proteomics 7(10):1998–2018
60. Pinhel IF, Macneill FA, Hills MJ, Salter J, Detre S, A'hern R, Nerurkar A, Osin P, Smith IE, Dowsett M (2010) Extreme loss of immunoreactive p-Akt and p-Erk1/2 during routine fixation of primary breast cancer. Breast Cancer Res 12(5):R76
61. Mueller C, Edmiston KH, Carpenter C, Gaffney E, Ryan C, Ward R, White S, Memeo L, Colarossi C, Petricoin EF 3rd, Liotta LA, Espina V (2011) One-step preservation of phosphoproteins and tissue morphology at room temperature for diagnostic and research specimens. PLoS ONE 6(8):e23780

Precision Medicine-Enabled Cancer Immunotherapy

7

John K. Lee and Saul J. Priceman

Contents

J. K. Lee
Division of Human Biology, Fred Hutchinson Cancer Research Center,
Seattle, WA, USA
e-mail: Jklee5@fredhutch.org

S. J. Priceman (✉)
Department of Hematology and Hematopoietic Cell Transplantation,
City of Hope, Duarte, CA, USA
e-mail: spriceman@coh.org

D. D. Von Hoff and H. Han (eds.), *Precision Medicine in Cancer Therapy*,
Cancer Treatment and Research 178, https://doi.org/10.1007/978-3-030-16391-4_7

7.1 Introduction

Cancer immunotherapy is a revolutionary treatment paradigm designed to stimulate or program the immune system to target cancer. It has gained remarkable attention in recent years with multiple US Food and Drug Administration (FDA) approvals of immune checkpoint pathway inhibitors and adoptive cell therapies for the treatment of patients with hematological malignancies and solid cancers. The recent onslaught of immunotherapy approaches that are either FDA approved or actively being tested in cancer patients is rooted in early observations of interactions between the immune system and cancer more than a century ago. These first scientific reports came from Germany in the late nineteenth century when the physicians W. Busch and F. Fehleisen noted regression of cancers in patients after accidental infection with erysipelas. After the discovery of group A Streptococcus bacterium as the causative agent of erysipelas, a few years later, another German physician, P. Bruns, intentionally administered the organism to a cancer patient and observed tumor shrinkage. Thereafter, the American surgeon, William Coley, began to inject heat-inactivated bacteria ("Coley's toxins") into patients with inoperable sarcomas and identified a high rate of tumor regression in hundreds of patients [1]. Regrettably, this approach was not adopted during Coley's lifetime due to concerns about his scientific protocols and the inconsistency of his results. In the latter half of the twentieth century, Lloyd Old showed that the bacterium Bacillus Calmette-Guérin (BCG), a tuberculosis vaccine, could inhibit tumor growth in a mouse model [2]. William Coley and bacterial immunotherapy as a cancer treatment were vindicated when subsequent clinical studies stemming from Old's findings demonstrated the effectiveness of BCG in treating superficial bladder tumors [3], which was ultimately approved by the FDA for the treatment of patients with bladder cancer in 1990. By the late twentieth century, multiple parallel immune-stimulating approaches were providing fundamental evidence for utility in redirecting the immune system to target cancer. For instance, interferon alpha, a cytokine that boosts immune responses in multiple tumor types, was the first biological cancer therapy tested in humans (late 1970s), receiving FDA approval in 1986.

In the late 1990s and early 2000s, seminal studies uncovered that the immune system not only played a key role in protection against tumor formation, but was also instrumental in shaping tumor immunogenicity, and ultimately, in promoting cancer progression. The cancer immunoediting theory emerged, which summarizes the dual and opposing roles that the immune system can play in cancer patients, which is comprised of three sequential stages: "elimination," "equilibrium," and "escape." Elimination is, in principal, cancer immune surveillance, where the immune system recognizes and destroys tumors before they become clinically detectable. If elimination in incomplete, the equilibrium phase ensues, accompanied by control or inhibition of tumor outgrowth. If tumors progress through this stage, escape occurs where growing tumor populations that have reduced immunogenicity and/or establish immune-suppressive mechanisms can bypass immune recognition and tumor targeting.

In addition to BCG and cytokine therapies which have shown promise in the treatment of some cancers, more personalized immunotherapies in the form of the dendritic cell cancer vaccine, sipuleucel-T, for the treatment of patients with metastatic castration-resistant prostate cancer (mCRPC), checkpoint pathways inhibitors to bypass suppressive mechanisms in solid and hematological malignancies, and more recently, adoptive cell therapy using CD19-directed chimeric antigen receptor (CAR)-engineered T-cell therapy for the treatment of patients with relapsed/refractory B-cell malignancies, have highlighted the tremendous opportunities for immunotherapy to effectively treat patients even with advanced refractory disease. Today, several hundred immunotherapy clinical trials aimed at redirecting the host immune system to selectively target cancer cells are underway. While we have made remarkable headway in developing effective immunotherapies for certain cancers, we are still in relative infancy when it comes to understanding the complexities of the immune system in human diseases. Therefore, it is increasingly evident that precision medicine will be required in driving personalized immunotherapies forward to create safe and effective treatments for each and every patient (Table 7.1).

7.2 Immunotherapy Strategies

7.2.1 Cancer Vaccines

7.2.1.1 Autologous and Allogeneic Tumor Cell Vaccines

Cancer vaccines using patient tumor cells were first evaluated in the late 1970s [4]. Whole tumor cells are collected, often irradiated, combined with a stimulatory adjuvant, and administered back into the patient. The main potential benefit of this approach is the ability to present all tumor-associated antigens (TAAs) to the patient's immune system. However, as this strategy requires the acquisition of tumor tissue for processing, it is inherently limited by tumor type and disease bulk. Given the limitations of autologous tumor cell vaccines, allogeneic whole tumor vaccines that combine several established human tumor cell lines have been developed. In contrast to autologous tumor cell vaccines, these allogeneic tumor vaccines can be standardized and readily produced at a larger scale in a cost-effective manner.

One technology designed to enhance immune stimulation by tumor cell vaccines has been the genetic engineering of tumor cells to secrete granulocyte-macrophage colony-stimulating factor (GM-CSF) prior to irradiation. These GM-CSF-transduced autologous tumor cell vaccines (GVAX) recruit dendritic cells for tumor antigen presentation and priming of cytotoxic lymphocytes [5]. GVAX-PCa, a prostate cancer vaccine containing two irradiated prostate cancer cell lines that express GM-CSF, showed promising early results in patients with mCRPC. In a phase I/II trial, GVAX-PCa was found to be safe and appeared to extend survival

Table 7.1 Overview of the targets and current status of different immunotherapy strategies

Immunotherapy strategy	Common targets	FDA-approved therapies	Indication
Cancer vaccines —Autologous and allogeneic tumor cell vaccines	GVAX-PCa: irradiated prostate cancer cell lines expressing GM-CSF	None, terminated in phase III trials	mCRPC
—Peptide-based cancer vaccines	TERT, EGFRvIII, MUC, MAGE	None, ongoing trials	Multiple solid tumor types
—Dendritic cell vaccines	PAP-GM-CSF	Sipuleucel-T (2010)	mCRPC
—Viral vaccines	PSA (PROSTVAC)	None, ongoing combination trials	mCRPC
—DNA vaccines	CpG	None, ongoing combination trials	Melanoma and other solid tumor types
Recombinant proteins	IL-2	Proleukin (1992, 1998)	mRCC, melanoma
	IL-12	None, ongoing combination trials	Multiple solid tumor types
	IL-15	None, ongoing trials	Multiple solid tumor types
Agonistic antibodies	CD137 (4-1BB)	None, ongoing combination trials	Multiple solid tumor types
	OX40	None, ongoing combination trials	Multiple solid tumor types
	CD40	None, ongoing combination trials	Multiple solid tumor types
Checkpoint pathway inhibitors	CTLA-4	Ipilimumab (2011)	Metastatic melanoma
	PD-1/PD-L1	—Pembrolizumab and —Nivolumab (2014), —Atezolizumab (2016), —Avelumab and —Durvalumab (2017)	Refractory melanoma NSCLC MCC mUC
	LAG-3, TIM-3, TIGIT	None, ongoing trials	Multiple solid tumor types

(continued)

Table 7.1 (continued)

Immunotherapy strategy	Common targets	FDA-approved therapies	Indication
Oncolytic viruses	HSV	T-VEC (2015)	Metastatic melanoma
	Other HSV, adenoviruses, vaccinia viruses, PV, RV, NDV	None, ongoing trials	Multiple solid tumor types
Adoptive T-cell therapies —Tumor-infiltrating lymphocytes (TILs)	Specific TAAs (e.g., ERBB2IP, SLC3A2)	None, ongoing trials	Multiple solid tumor types
—TCR T-cell therapy	NYESO-1, MART-1, MAGEs, HPV, CEA	None, ongoing trials	Multiple solid tumor types
CAR T-cell therapy	Hematological malignancies (CD19, BCMA, CD123, CD33)	— Tisagenlecleucel (2017) —Axicabtagene ciloleucel (2018)	B-ALL NHL
	Solid tumors (GD2, HER2 IL13Ra2, mesothelin, PSMA, PSCA)	None, ongoing trials	Multiple solid tumor types

with a high-dose boost [6]. However, two phase III trials evaluating GVAX-PCa in combination with docetaxel in mCRPC were terminated early due to increased mortality and lack of therapeutic efficacy.

7.2.1.2 Peptide-Based Cancer Vaccines

Recombinant vaccines, based on peptides from TAAs, represent an alternative to autologous or allogeneic cancer vaccines. TAAs encompass antigens overexpressed in cancer (e.g., TERT and mesothelin), oncofetal antigens (e.g., MUC1 and CEA), cancer–testis antigens (e.g., MAGE, NY-ESO-1, and SSX-2), lineage-restricted antigens shared by both normal tissue and tumors (e.g., PSA and PAP in prostate epithelium and prostate cancer), and tumor-specific antigens such as mutated oncogenes (e.g., $BRAF^{V600E}$) or oncogenic viral antigens (e.g., E7 from HPV-16). TAAs are not highly immunogenic, and therefore, recombinant vaccines are generally co-administered with an adjuvant or an immune modulator to boost immune responses.

Most of the peptide-based vaccines that have been investigated in clinical trials have targeted oncofetal antigens, cancer–testis antigens, and lineage-restricted antigens. In phase III studies, a peptide-based vaccine targeting the lineage-specific melanocyte antigen gp100 did not show added therapeutic benefit in patients with unresectable stage III or IV melanoma when added to ipilimumab [7], but did show improved clinical responses and a longer progression-free survival when added to IL-2 [8]. Several other vaccines have demonstrated promising activities in early phase studies, but failed to demonstrate a benefit in phase III studies. One example is rindopepimut, a vaccine targeting the EGFR deletion mutation, EGFRvIII, which when combined with temozolomide did not increase survival in patients with newly diagnosed glioblastoma [9]. Similarly, tecemotide, a MUC antigen-specific vaccine, provided no survival benefit after chemoradiotherapy for unresectable stage III non-small cell lung cancer [10].

One issue facing peptide-based vaccines is that targeting either one or a few epitopes of the TAA increases the potential for immune escape of cancer. Improved efficacy has been suggested with multi-peptide vaccine cocktails than with single-peptide vaccines [11]. In a phase II study, IMA901, a renal cell carcinoma vaccine with ten tumor-associated peptides, appeared to induce immune responses and prolong overall survival in a phase II study. Disappointingly, a phase III study of IMA901 in combination with sunitinib in the first-line treatment of metastatic renal cell carcinoma did not improve overall survival [12]. Additional multi-peptide vaccine cocktails, long peptide vaccines designed to present epitopes to both cytotoxic and T helper lymphocytes, and combination vaccine strategies are currently under active clinical investigation.

7.2.1.3 Dendritic Cell Vaccines

Dendritic cells (DCs) are professional antigen-presenting cells (APCs) that are involved in the interplay between the innate and adaptive immune systems. DCs present antigenic peptides from pathogens or the host to activate or prime naïve antigen-specific T lymphocytes in lymphoid organs. Human DCs can be isolated from peripheral blood mononuclear cells or from cultures of $CD34^+$ hematologic progenitor cells. DC vaccines are generated by loading TAAs onto the DCs and stimulating with adjuvants, after which the DCs are introduced back into the patient. Sipuleucel-T, an autologous cellular vaccine in which APCs (including DCs) obtained from leukapheresis are incubated with prostatic acid phosphatase (PAP) fused to GM-CSF, was FDA approved in 2010 as the first anti-cancer vaccine for the treatment of mCRPC. Sipuleucel-T demonstrated a favorable toxicity profile and was found to provide an overall survival benefit of 4.1 months (25.8 months vs. 21.7 months) when compared to placebo [13]. While Sipuleucel-T is considered a clinical success, its anti-tumor effects are quite modest with a 4.1-month improvement in overall survival. Recent clinical studies with DC vaccines have incorporated new adjuvants and concomitant immune modulatory agents to enhance immunogenicity and T-cell stimulation with the hope of enhancing anti-tumor activity.

7.2.1.4 Viral Vaccines

Pathogens like viruses contain numerous molecules that can induce immune activation pathways. The use of a viral vector to deliver tumor antigens can therefore potentially increase immune stimulation. Viruses have been used for direct immunization, but the development of neutralizing antibodies can prevent repeated use. One strategy to circumvent this has been virus-based prime boost in which the immune system is first primed with one vaccine followed by a boost of the response with a second, different vaccine. An example of this approach is PROSTVAC, in which recombinant vaccinia encoding PSA and three immune co-stimulatory molecules (LFA-3, ICAM-1, and B7.1), collectively called TRICOM, are administered subcutaneously to prime and then followed by six boost doses of fowlpox-expressing PSA and TRICOM [14]. A phase II study showed that patients with minimally symptomatic mCRPC receiving PROSTVAC had a 9.9-month overall survival benefit compared to those receiving the control empty vector (26.2 months vs. 16.3 months) [15]. However, the phase III PROSPECT trial in minimally symptomatic mCRPC patients did not demonstrate an improvement in overall survival. Ongoing studies are exploring PROSTVAC in combination with immune checkpoint inhibitors or with chemotherapy.

7.2.1.5 DNA Vaccines

Bacterial DNA induces innate immune responses through stimulation of Toll-like receptors (TLRs) which recognize structurally conserved molecules found in microbes. For instance, unmethylated deoxycytidylate-phosphate-deoxyguanylate (CpG) dinucleotide motifs found in bacterial and viral but not mammalian DNA activate TLR9, leading to increased inflammatory cytokine production [16]. Bacterial DNA plasmids are therefore used to stimulate an immune response while enabling expression of TAAs by the host. DNA vaccines are generally introduced via intradermal or intramuscular injections to transfect cells in the skin or muscles. Current studies are aimed at improving delivery, increasing immune stimulation with molecular adjuvants, and enhancing TAA transgene expression from modified bacterial plasmids.

7.2.1.6 Personalized Vaccine Approaches

The sets of somatic mutations found in each individual tumor are very distinct. These mutations lead to the alteration of protein sequences, generating neoantigens from which neoepitopes may be processed and presented on major histocompatibility complex (MHC) molecules. Several observations point to the importance of immune recognition of neoepitopes. First, neoepitope-specific T cells appear to have significant anti-tumor activity in the context of immune checkpoint inhibition and adoptive transfer of autologous tumor-infiltrating lymphocytes (TILs) [17, 18]. Second, there is a positive correlation between the mutational frequency found in a tumor, the immune cell infiltration of a tumor, and overall survival [19]. Personalized vaccines, using any variety of the vectors described above, are designed to target neoantigens in order to stimulate the immune system against the individual's tumor. However, this approach is both costly and slow as it requires the identification of mutations by next-generation sequencing of a patient's tumor DNA, prediction of neoepitopes from the mutational data based on algorithms, and personalized design and production of the vaccine.

7.2.2 Recombinant Proteins

There is a long history of physicians and healers, including Hippocrates, documenting the shrinkage of tumors in patients with high fevers. Fevers are induced by a subset of cytokines, which are a group of proteins secreted by the immune system that modulate cell signaling. Immune-stimulating cytokines can activate innate or adaptive immune responses, and a few also demonstrate anti-tumor effects. Class I interferons are a type of cytokine, which have been shown to induce cell death and block angiogenesis in tumors [20]. Recombinant interferon-α2a (IFN-α2a) and interferon-α2b (IFN-α2b) were approved for clinical use in 1986 for the treatment of various cancers, including chronic myeloid leukemia, hairy cell leukemia, and malignant melanoma [21]. Another cytokine, recombinant interleukin-2 (IL-2), which has immunostimulatory effects on lymphocytes and natural killer (NK) cells that mediate anti-tumor activity, was first generated and characterized by Steven Rosenberg and colleagues [22]. High-dose IL-2 was clinically approved for patients with metastatic renal cell carcinoma in 1992. Multiple clinical studies of high-dose IL-2 in metastatic renal cell carcinoma showed a complete response rate of 9%, and over 80% of the patients with complete responses had durable remissions amounting to a cure [23]. High-dose IL-2 was subsequently approved for malignant melanoma in 1998, based on a series of studies showing an overall response rate of 16% with 6% of patients achieving complete responses [24]. These early findings were critical to the development of adoptive cell therapy (described below), which was also spearheaded by Rosenberg.

Similar to IL-2, IL-15 is also able to stimulate lymphocytes and NK cells to induce anti-tumor effects. IL-15 may potentially be superior to IL-2 for cancer immunotherapy because it enhances immune memory through propagation of memory T cells, prevents activation-induced T-cell death, and does not expand immunosuppressive regulatory T cells (T_{regs}) [25]. However, IL-15 is limited by a short half-life and poor bioavailability. IL-12, which has shown both immune and non-immune anti-tumor effects, is another cytokine that has been of high interest to the field. IL-12 increases interferon-gamma (IFN-γ) production, activates NK cells and T lymphocytes, and remodels the tumor microenvironment. Findings by Judah Folkman demonstrate that IL-12 also inhibits tumor-associated angiogenesis [26], which may play a significant role in its anti-tumor activity. Although recombinant IL-12 appeared promising in preclinical studies, clinical trials of IL-12 monotherapy did not show clinical efficacy. Multiple clinical trials investigating recombinant IL-15 or IL-12 therapy in cancer, including enhanced formulations and combinations with chemotherapy or other immunotherapies, are currently ongoing.

Since endogenous cytokines have valuable anti-tumor potential, several strategies are under development to enhance their efficacy. One approach has been the engineering of novel fused cytokines to deliver signals that induce immune responses in subsets of cells, such as the fusion of GM-CSF to various interleukins, each of which have unique immunomodulatory effects. These fusions not only have the potential to benefit cancer immunotherapy but can also be applied to the treatment of infections and amelioration of autoimmune diseases [27]. Another strategy is the fusion of cytokines to antibodies in order to localize cytokine effects to specific cells or tissue compartments. An early demonstration of this technology came in the form of a fusion protein encoding an anti-GD2 ganglioside binding site and recombinant IL-2, which showed enhanced lysis of neuroblastoma cells and disease control relative to systemic IL-2 administration in a preclinical xenograft model [28]. Furthermore, conjugation of cytokines with chemical moieties such as polymer polyethylene glycol (PEG) has been performed to enhance protein half-life. Successful PEGylation of IFN-α2a and granulocyte colony-stimulating factor (G-CSF) has been achieved and is clinically available.

7.2.3 Agonistic Antibodies

A number of co-stimulatory molecules are expressed on T cells that provide signals to sustain an optimal response and promote expansion. 4-1BB is a co-stimulatory molecule found on activated T cells and NK cells. Engagement of 4-1BB leads to pro-survival signaling and enhanced T-cell effector functions even in dysfunctional T cells [29]. Agonistic 4-1BB antibodies have shown anti-tumor effects in preclinical mouse models [30], and currently ongoing clinical trials show early evidence of safety and clinical benefit. OX40 is another co-stimulatory molecule expressed on $CD8^+$ T cells, NK cells, natural killer T (NKT) cells, and neutrophils. It is engaged by the OX40 ligand (OX40L), which is presented on APCs only after activation. In preclinical studies, both antibodies against OX40 and OX40L-Fc fusion proteins enhanced anti-tumor responses in mouse models [31]. OX40 agonists, either alone or in combination with other immune modulatory agents, are in clinical trials for cancer immunotherapy. For example, the combination of OX40 agonists and CpG has demonstrated exceptional preclinical anti-tumor activity against multiple tumor types and is now being investigated in early clinical trials [32]. However, a recent study indicated that the anti-tumor effects of OX40 agonistic antibody therapy can be negated by simultaneous PD-1 inhibition [33]. These findings underscore the need for preclinical validation of combination and sequential immunotherapies prior to clinical translation. Additional agonistic antibodies or recombinant ligands designed to engage CD27, CD28, CD40, ICOS, and others are in various stages of development for cancer therapy.

7.2.4 Checkpoint Pathway Inhibitors

Immune activation requires strict regulation, and several negative regulators or checkpoints of T-cell response have been identified. James Allison and Jeffrey Bluestone discovered cytotoxic T lymphocyte-associated protein 4 (CTLA-4), which was found to translocate to the cell surface in activated T cells and compete with CD28 for binding to co-stimulatory molecules [34, 35]. Blockade of CTLA-4 with an antibody was found to induce tumor regression in mouse cancer models, warranting its investigation in the clinic. Treatment of patients with metastatic melanoma with the anti-CTLA-4 antibody, ipilimumab, resulted in a 15% objective response rate with many patients experiencing durable remissions [36]. Ipilimumab was found to extend overall survival in metastatic melanoma leading to its clinical approval in 2011 [7].

The programmed cell death 1 (PD-1) receptor is an immune checkpoint that acts by inhibiting downstream signaling of the TCR [37]. PD-1 has two ligands: programmed cell death ligand 1 (PD-L1) and programmed cell death ligand 2 (PD-L2). PD-L1 is broadly expressed by cells in response to inflammatory cytokines while PD-L2 expression is restricted to APCs [38]. In contrast to CTLA-4, PD-1 appears to have a more restricted effect on regulating immune responses. Blockade of PD-1 appears to preferentially de-repress anti-tumor T cells, leading to greater activity against tumors and less autoimmune toxicity [39]. PD-1 blocking antibodies, pembrolizumab and nivolumab, were approved for the treatment of refractory melanoma in 2014 and advanced non-small cell lung cancer (NSCLC) in 2015. The PD-L1 blocking antibodies, atezolizumab and avelumab, were approved for urothelial cancer in 2016 and for Merkel cell carcinoma in 2017, respectively. Importantly, anti-PD1 antibodies were found to be effective across a number of solid tumors with microsatellite instability [40], a hypermutated phenotype associated with impaired DNA mismatch repair (MMR). High neoantigen load associated with the increased mutational burden is thought to make these tumors more susceptible to T-cell responses after checkpoint blockade.

7.2.5 Oncolytic Viruses

Oncolytic viruses (OVs) are a promising treatment modality for cancer, largely because of their tumor selectivity, desirable immunogenic properties, and ability to incorporate transgenes into their genome for targeted delivery to tumors [41]. OVs have gained significant momentum in recent years due to their immune-stimulating effects in both the local tumor microenvironment and systemically creating a more immunologically active tumor for improved immunotherapy responses. The first clinically approved OV, talimogene laherparepvec (T-VEC), is a genetically modified type I herpes simplex virus that expresses granulocyte-macrophage colony-stimulating factor (GM-CSF). T-VEC was approved by the FDA in 2015 as an intralesional virotherapy for the treatment of metastatic melanoma [42]. In addition to, and in some respects as a consequence of, the tumor cell-selective replication and direct tumor cell lysis, T-VEC is capable of producing soluble tumor antigens and inducing host anti-tumor immunity. Recent combination immunotherapy approaches have exploited OV, which is desirable for "cold" tumors that otherwise show poor immunotherapy responses. Additionally, newer OV versions have been engineered to express genes, including ones for cytokines that may further improve tumor recruitment of T cells to enhance anti-tumor immunity of other immunotherapeutic agents [43].

7.2.6 Adoptive T-Cell Therapy

7.2.6.1 Tumor-Infiltrating Lymphocytes (TILs)

In the 1960s and 1970s, T cells were becoming widely appreciated for their potential capacity to treat cancer through preclinical adoptive transfer studies [44]. However, expanding human T-cells ex vivo was only feasible following the identification and characterization of IL-2 and its use in manufacturing T cells in culture, as well as providing survival and growth signals to adoptively transferred T-cells in vivo [45]. In the early 1980s, Rosenberg's group at the NCI was the first to document the use of adoptively transferred T cells, ex vivo expanded in IL-2 as well as in vivo administered IL-2, for the effective treatment of murine lymphoma [46, 47]. In 1985, they also demonstrated a complete tumor regression in a metastatic melanoma patient and multiple objective responses in patients following adoptive transfer of tumor-infiltrating lymphocytes (TILs) with supplemental administration of IL-2 [48]. These early results of personalized medicine spawned an entire platform dedicated to isolation and expansion of autologous TILs for adoptive T-cell therapy. While advanced melanoma has become a poster child for cancer immunotherapy, TIL therapy has been effective across multiple tumor types, such as colon and cervical cancers [49, 50], and more recently demonstrated a complete and durable regression in a patient with metastatic breast cancer with TIL specificity for selected tumor-associated mutated antigens [51]. Recent advances in the field have facilitated the identification of unique and immunogenic gene mutations allowing for selective expansion of TILs. These discoveries will ultimately drive the broader utility of this approach to multiple cancer types.

7.2.6.2 TCR T-Cell Therapy

The identification of specific tumor-associated mutations recognized by TILs, as well as the difficulties associated with isolating and expanding TILs from many cancers, led to the idea that specific T-cell receptors (TCRs) could be genetically engineered into peripheral blood-derived T cells to redirect their specificity toward the tumor [52]. TCRs are responsible for recognition of TAA peptides presented by MHC class I molecules. This platform was first successfully demonstrated in 2006 when adoptively transferred T cells engineered to express a TCR specific for the TAA, MART-1, mediated cancer regression in patients with metastatic melanoma [53]. A similar approach was used generate TCR-engineered T-cell therapy specific for the NYESO-1 cancer–testis antigen [54], human papillomavirus (HPV) [55], carcinoembryonic antigen (CEA) [56], and other TAAs. However, TCR specificity must be comprehensively examined, as one clinical experience with TCR-engineered T cells specific for MAGE-A3, a cancer–testis antigen, resulted in two fatalities from unexpected targeting of a related protein expressed at low levels in normal tissue [57].

7.2.6.3 CAR T-Cell Therapy

While TCR-engineered T-cell therapy has tremendous utility in redirecting immune recognition of MHC:peptide complexes on tumor cells, one major immune escape strategy used by tumor cells is the downregulation or loss of MHC class I expression and/or dysfunctional antigen processing and presentation [58], which may limit this approach for many solid cancers. In the late 1980s, research led by Zelig Eshhar at the Weizmann Institute in Israel, attempted to redirect specificity of T cells using chimeric antigen receptors (CARs), termed immunoglobin-T-cell receptor chimeric molecules at the time [59]. CARs are modular synthetic immunoreceptors consisting of three major functional components: the antigen-binding domain for redirecting specificity of T cells, the extracellular nonsignaling spacer, and the intracellular signaling domain that initiates cytolytic activity. Together, this molecule recapitulates native T-cell effector function, including antigen-dependent cytokine production, proliferation, and serial tumor cell killing. The major advantage of this approach is its ability to target TAAs independent of MHC:peptide complex-mediated presentation to endogenous or engineered TCR on T cells.

While this CAR approach was preclinically validated with exceptional tumor killing abilities, early clinical responses were relatively unimpressive. It became evident that first-generation CARs, which lacked co-stimulation, also demonstrated limited T-cell persistence and function in vivo. So-called second-generation CARs, which incorporate intracellular co-stimulatory domains in tandem with the cytolytic domain, have been extensively evaluated over the last decade both preclinically and clinically for multiple cancer types [60, 61]. The breakthrough for CAR T-cell therapy came with the targeting of CD19 antigen for the treatment of B-cell malignancies, including acute lymphoblastic leukemia (ALL) and non-Hodgkin's lymphoma (NHL). In patients with relapsed/refractory ALL treated with CD19-specific CAR T cells, the complete response (CR) rate has typically reached over 85% as best outcome, across clinical trials using different co-stimulatory domains, antigen-binding domains, and ex vivo T-cell manufacturing practices. Similar, but lower overall response rates have been observed for NHL and for chronic lymphocytic leukemia (CLL) patients treated with CD19-CAR T cells. These impressive clinical responses have recently resulted in two landmark FDA approvals for patients with B-cell ALL (Tisagenlecleucel, Novartis) and diffuse large B-cell lymphoma (Axicabtagene Ciloleucel, Kite/Gilead). Recent trials have focused on additional targets for B-cell malignancies, including CD20 and CD22, as well as targets for other hematological malignancies, including acute myelogenous leukemia (including CD123 and CD33) and multiple myeloma (including BCMA), which have also shown impressive early clinical responses.

With successes in treating hematologic diseases with CAR T-cell therapy, broader application of this approach to solid tumors is under intense investigation. CARs targeting multiple solid tumor antigens have been evaluated to date, including GD2, ErbB2/HER2, IL13Ralpha2, CEA, and mesothelin [62]. Clinical responses have not yet reached the levels observed for hematological malignancies, due, in part, to the unique and challenging tumor microenvironment of solid tumors, which can significantly hamper anti-tumor immunity. In addition to second-generation CARs, third-generation CARs incorporating multiple co-stimulatory domains, and fourth-generation or armored CARs are also currently being investigated with the goal of improving the specificity and potency of CAR T cells. Redirecting effector function with CARs has also been extended to other immune cell types, including NK cells as well as non-conventional T cells like NKT and gamma delta (γδ) T cells, that are expanded ex vivo for adoptive transfer, or genetically engineered with CAR for enhanced tumor targeting. CAR therapy, while demonstrating striking clinical responses for patients with relapsed/refractory and often bulky disease, has been associated with a variety of toxicities that can be life-threatening [63]. In addition to the often expected cytokine release syndrome and neurotoxicities following CD19-CAR T-cell therapy, other severe complications due to off-tumor on-target effects of CAR T cells have been observed. For instance, an early trial using CAR T-cells-targeting HER2 resulted in an acute death of a patient with metastatic colorectal cancer [64]. These examples underscore the need to further improve CAR design and clinical trial design to achieve maximal therapeutic benefits for patients with hematological malignancies or solid cancers.

7.3 Big Data-Enabled Precision Medicine

The declining costs associated with next-generation sequencing (NGS) have led to the increased adoption of focused sequencing panels, whole exome sequencing, and whole genome sequencing in clinical oncology. As these platforms become widespread, the major question will be how healthcare providers and patients will use this information to guide care. For instance, the identification of microsatellite instability in a tumor by sequencing may become an indication for treatment with pembrolizumab. However, few genetic mutations found in cancer are otherwise therapeutically actionable at present. Multiple studies aimed at evaluating therapeutics that target specific cancer mutations in a tissue agnostic manner, known as basket trials, are currently underway to address this gap. Tumor mutational sequencing leading to the identification of neoantigens specific to tumors has also brought forth advances in personalized immunotherapies. As an example, personalized neoantigen vaccines are now made possible by NGS and computational prediction of antigenic epitopes. In early clinical trials, this approach has shown the ability to induce tumor immunity in patients with melanoma [65].

Big data from NGS also provide insight into biomarkers associated with response or resistance to immunotherapies. High tumor mutational burden appears to be a strong predictor of objective response, durable benefit, and survival with checkpoint inhibition therapy [66]. Recent studies have also described transcriptomic features that predict response to anti-PD1 therapy [67, 68]. Additionally, NGS of tumors has uncovered mechanisms of primary and acquired resistance to PD-1 blockade, including loss-of-function mutations in Janus kinase 1 and 2 (JAK1/2) and truncating mutations in beta-2-microglobulin (B2M) [69, 70]. Lastly, NGS may be useful in monitoring immune responses in patients undergoing cancer immunotherapy by quantifying immune repertoires. For instance, the diversification of T-cell receptor immune repertoires has been shown to serve as a biomarker of clinical response in patients with breast and pancreatic cancer receiving immunotherapy [71, 72].

Single cell technologies are also rapidly advancing and poised to provide even larger sets of tumor data. Single cell genomics, transcriptomics, and mapping technologies have the potential to uncover rich information about interactions between cell types, genetic mutations, epigenetic states, transcriptional programs, and clonal and spatial organization within a tumor, both pretreatment and in response to therapeutic perturbations. The major goal of big data-enabled precision medicine in the context of immunotherapy is to dramatically increase the 15–30% overall response rates and the safety profile observed across multiple immunotherapy approaches. These deep interrogations into responses and resistance patterns will also inform the field on future combination immunotherapy strategies utilizing multiple treatment modalities listed above to maximize therapeutic responses for patients.

References

1. Coley WB (1910) The treatment of inoperable sarcoma by bacterial toxins (the mixed toxins of the Streptococcus erysipelas and the Bacillus prodigiosus). Proc R Soc Med 3(Surg Sect):1–48
2. Old LJ, Clarke DA, Benacerraf B (1959) Effect of Bacillus Calmette-Guerin infection on transplanted tumours in the mouse. Nature 184(Suppl 5):291–292
3. Morales A, Eidinger D, Bruce AW (1976) Intracavitary Bacillus Calmette-Guerin in the treatment of superficial bladder tumors. J Urol 116(2):180–183
4. Hanna MG Jr, Peters LC (1978) Specific immunotherapy of established visceral micrometastases by BCG-tumor cell vaccine alone or as an adjunct to surgery. Cancer 42(6):2613–2625
5. Dranoff G et al (1993) Vaccination with irradiated tumor cells engineered to secrete murine granulocyte-macrophage colony-stimulating factor stimulates potent, specific, and long-lasting anti-tumor immunity. Proc Natl Acad Sci U S A 90(8):3539–3543
6. Higano CS et al (2008) Phase 1/2 dose-escalation study of a GM-CSF-secreting, allogeneic, cellular immunotherapy for metastatic hormone-refractory prostate cancer. Cancer 113 (5):975–984
7. Hodi FS et al (2010) Improved survival with ipilimumab in patients with metastatic melanoma. N Engl J Med 363(8):711–723
8. Schwartzentruber DJ et al (2011) gp100 peptide vaccine and interleukin-2 in patients with advanced melanoma. N Engl J Med 364(22):2119–2127
9. Weller M et al (2017) Rindopepimut with temozolomide for patients with newly diagnosed, EGFRvIII-expressing glioblastoma (ACT IV): a randomised, double-blind, international phase 3 trial. Lancet Oncol 18(10):1373–1385
10. Butts C et al (2014) Tecemotide (L-BLP25) versus placebo after chemoradiotherapy for stage III non-small-cell lung cancer (START): a randomised, double-blind, phase 3 trial. Lancet Oncol 15(1):59–68
11. Walter S et al (2012) Multipeptide immune response to cancer vaccine IMA901 after single-dose cyclophosphamide associates with longer patient survival. Nat Med 18(8):1254–1261

12. Rini BI et al (2016) IMA901, a multipeptide cancer vaccine, plus sunitinib versus sunitinib alone, as first-line therapy for advanced or metastatic renal cell carcinoma (IMPRINT): a multicentre, open-label, randomised, controlled, phase 3 trial. Lancet Oncol 17(11):1599–1611
13. Kantoff PW et al (2010) Sipuleucel-T immunotherapy for castration-resistant prostate cancer. N Engl J Med 363(5):411–422
14. Gulley JL et al (2014) Immune impact induced by PROSTVAC (PSA-TRICOM), a therapeutic vaccine for prostate cancer. Cancer Immunol Res 2(2):133–141
15. Kantoff PW, Gulley JL, Pico-Navarro C (2017) Revised overall survival analysis of a phase II, randomized, double-blind, controlled study of PROSTVAC in men with metastatic castration-resistant prostate cancer. J Clin Oncol 35(1):124–125
16. Ohto U et al (2015) Structural basis of CpG and inhibitory DNA recognition by Toll-like receptor 9. Nature 520(7549):702–705
17. van Rooij N et al (2013) Tumor exome analysis reveals neoantigen-specific T-cell reactivity in an ipilimumab-responsive melanoma. J Clin Oncol 31(32):e439–e442
18. Robbins PF et al (2013) Mining exomic sequencing data to identify mutated antigens recognized by adoptively transferred tumor-reactive T cells. Nat Med 19(6):747–752
19. Rizvi NA et al (2015) Cancer immunology. Mutational landscape determines sensitivity to PD-1 blockade in non-small cell lung cancer. Science 348(6230):124–128
20. Medrano RFV et al (2017) Immunomodulatory and antitumor effects of type I interferons and their application in cancer therapy. Oncotarget 8(41):71249–71284
21. Creagan ET et al (1986) Recombinant leukocyte A interferon (rIFN-alpha A) in the treatment of disseminated malignant melanoma. Analysis of complete and long-term responding patients. Cancer 58(12):2576–2578
22. Rosenberg SA et al (1984) Biological activity of recombinant human interleukin-2 produced in Escherichia coli. Science 223(4643):1412–1414
23. Fyfe GA et al (1996) Long-term response data for 255 patients with metastatic renal cell carcinoma treated with high-dose recombinant interleukin-2 therapy. J Clin Oncol 14 (8):2410–2411
24. Atkins MB et al (1999) High-dose recombinant interleukin 2 therapy for patients with metastatic melanoma: analysis of 270 patients treated between 1985 and 1993. J Clin Oncol 17(7):2105–2116
25. Marks-Konczalik J et al (2000) IL-2-induced activation-induced cell death is inhibited in IL-15 transgenic mice. Proc Natl Acad Sci U S A 97(21):11445–11450
26. Voest EE et al (1995) Inhibition of angiogenesis in vivo by interleukin 12. J Natl Cancer Inst 87(8):581–586
27. Ng S, Galipeau J (2015) Concise review: engineering the fusion of cytokines for the modulation of immune cellular responses in cancer and autoimmune disorders. Stem Cells Transl Med 4(1):66–73
28. Sabzevari H et al (1994) A recombinant antibody-interleukin 2 fusion protein suppresses growth of hepatic human neuroblastoma metastases in severe combined immunodeficiency mice. Proc Natl Acad Sci U S A 91(20):9626–9630
29. Williams JB et al (2017) The EGR2 targets LAG-3 and 4-1BB describe and regulate dysfunctional antigen-specific CD8+ T cells in the tumor microenvironment. J Exp Med 214 (2):381–400
30. Melero I et al (1997) Monoclonal antibodies against the 4-1BB T-cell activation molecule eradicate established tumors. Nat Med 3(6):682–685
31. Weinberg AD et al (2000) Engagement of the OX-40 receptor in vivo enhances antitumor immunity. J Immunol 164(4):2160–2169
32. Sagiv-Barfi I et al (2018) Eradication of spontaneous malignancy by local immunotherapy. Sci Transl Med 10(426)
33. Shrimali RK et al (2017) Concurrent PD-1 blockade negates the effects of OX40 agonist antibody in combination immunotherapy through inducing T-cell apoptosis. Cancer Immunol Res 5(9):755–766

34. Chambers CA et al (2001) CTLA-4-mediated inhibition in regulation of T cell responses: mechanisms and manipulation in tumor immunotherapy. Annu Rev Immunol 19:565–594
35. Walunas TL et al (1994) CTLA-4 can function as a negative regulator of T cell activation. Immunity 1(5):405–413
36. Schadendorf D et al (2015) Pooled analysis of long-term survival data from phase II and phase III trials of ipilimumab in unresectable or metastatic melanoma. J Clin Oncol 33 (17):1889–1894
37. Ribas A, Wolchok JD (2018) Cancer immunotherapy using checkpoint blockade. Science 359 (6382):1350–1355
38. Baumeister SH et al (2016) Coinhibitory pathways in immunotherapy for cancer. Annu Rev Immunol 34:539–573
39. Robert C et al (2015) Pembrolizumab versus ipilimumab in advanced melanoma. N Engl J Med 372(26):2521–2532
40. Le DT et al (2015) PD-1 blockade in tumors with mismatch-repair deficiency. N Engl J Med 372(26):2509–2520
41. Kaufman HL, Kohlhapp FJ, Zloza A (2015) Oncolytic viruses: a new class of immunotherapy drugs. Nat Rev Drug Discov 14(9):642–662
42. Rehman H et al (2016) Into the clinic: talimogene laherparepvec (T-VEC), a first-in-class intratumoral oncolytic viral therapy. J Immunother Cancer 4:53
43. Martin NT, Bell JC (2018) Oncolytic virus combination therapy: killing one bird with two stones. Mol Ther 26(6):1414–1422
44. Delorme EJ, Alexander P (1964) Treatment of primary fibrosarcoma in the rat with immune lymphocytes. Lancet 2(7351):117–120
45. Morgan DA, Ruscetti FW, Gallo R (1976) Selective in vitro growth of T lymphocytes from normal human bone marrows. Science 193(4257):1007–1008
46. Donohue JH et al (1984) The systemic administration of purified interleukin 2 enhances the ability of sensitized murine lymphocytes to cure a disseminated syngeneic lymphoma. J Immunol 132(4):2123–2128
47. Eberlein TJ, Rosenstein M, Rosenberg SA (1982) Regression of a disseminated syngeneic solid tumor by systemic transfer of lymphoid cells expanded in interleukin 2. J Exp Med 156 (2):385–397
48. Rosenberg SA et al (1985) Observations on the systemic administration of autologous lymphokine-activated killer cells and recombinant interleukin-2 to patients with metastatic cancer. N Engl J Med 313(23):1485–1492
49. Tran E et al (2015) Immunogenicity of somatic mutations in human gastrointestinal cancers. Science 350(6266):1387–1390
50. Tran E et al (2016) T-cell transfer therapy targeting mutant KRAS in cancer. N Engl J Med 375(23):2255–2262
51. Zacharakis N et al (2018) Immune recognition of somatic mutations leading to complete durable regression in metastatic breast cancer. Nat Med 24(6):724–730
52. Rosenberg SA, Restifo NP (2015) Adoptive cell transfer as personalized immunotherapy for human cancer. Science 348(6230):62–68
53. Morgan RA et al (2006) Cancer regression in patients after transfer of genetically engineered lymphocytes. Science 314(5796):126–129
54. Robbins PF et al (2011) Tumor regression in patients with metastatic synovial cell sarcoma and melanoma using genetically engineered lymphocytes reactive with NY-ESO-1. J Clin Oncol 29(7):917–924
55. Stevanovic S et al (2015) Complete regression of metastatic cervical cancer after treatment with human papillomavirus-targeted tumor-infiltrating T cells. J Clin Oncol 33(14):1543–1550
56. Parkhurst MR et al (2011) T cells targeting carcinoembryonic antigen can mediate regression of metastatic colorectal cancer but induce severe transient colitis. Mol Ther 19(3):620–626
57. Morgan RA et al (2013) Cancer regression and neurologic toxicity following anti-MAGE-A3 TCR gene therapy. J Immunother 36(2):133–151

58. Drake CG, Jaffee E, Pardoll DM (2006) Mechanisms of immune evasion by tumors. Adv Immunol 90:51–81
59. Gross G, Waks T, Eshhar Z (1989) Expression of immunoglobulin-T-cell receptor chimeric molecules as functional receptors with antibody-type specificity. Proc Natl Acad Sci U S A 86 (24):10024–10028
60. Priceman SJ, Forman SJ, Brown CE (2015) Smart CARs engineered for cancer immunotherapy. Curr Opin Oncol 27(6):466–474
61. Sadelain M, Brentjens R, Riviere I (2013) The basic principles of chimeric antigen receptor design. Cancer Discov 3(4):388–398
62. Hartmann J et al (2017) Clinical development of CAR T cells-challenges and opportunities in translating innovative treatment concepts. EMBO Mol Med 9(9):1183–1197
63. Neelapu SS et al (2018) Chimeric antigen receptor T-cell therapy—assessment and management of toxicities. Nat Rev Clin Oncol 15(1):47–62
64. Morgan RA et al (2010) Case report of a serious adverse event following the administration of T cells transduced with a chimeric antigen receptor recognizing ERBB2. Mol Ther 18(4):843–851
65. Ott PA et al (2017) An immunogenic personal neoantigen vaccine for patients with melanoma. Nature 547(7662):217–221
66. Goodman AM et al (2017) Tumor mutational burden as an independent predictor of response to immunotherapy in diverse cancers. Mol Cancer Ther 16(11):2598–2608
67. Hugo W et al (2015) Non-genomic and immune evolution of melanoma acquiring MAPKi resistance. Cell 162(6):1271–1285
68. Auslander N et al (2018) Robust prediction of response to immune checkpoint blockade therapy in metastatic melanoma. Nat Med
69. Zaretsky JM et al (2016) Mutations associated with acquired resistance to PD-1 blockade in melanoma. N Engl J Med 375(9):819–829
70. Shin DS et al (2017) Primary resistance to PD-1 blockade mediated by JAK1/2 mutations. Cancer Discov 7(2):188–201
71. Page DB et al (2016) Deep sequencing of T-cell receptor DNA as a biomarker of clonally expanded TILs in breast cancer after immunotherapy. Cancer Immunol Res 4(10):835–844
72. Hopkins AC et al (2018) T cell receptor repertoire features associated with survival in immunotherapy-treated pancreatic ductal adenocarcinoma. JCI Insight 3(13)

Part III
Future Precision Medicine

Use of Precision Imaging in the Evaluation of Pancreas Cancer

8

Ronald L. Korn, Syed Rahmanuddin and Erkut Borazanci

Contents

R. L. Korn (✉) · E. Borazanci
Virginia G Piper Cancer Center at HonorHealth, Scottsdale, AZ, USA
e-mail: rkorn@imagingendpoints.com

R. L. Korn · E. Borazanci
Translational Genomics Research Institute, An Affiliate of City of Hope, Phoenix, AZ, USA

S. Rahmanuddin
City of Hope, Duarte, CA, USA

R. L. Korn
Imaging Endpoints Core Lab, Scottsdale, AZ, USA

D. D. Von Hoff and H. Han (eds.), *Precision Medicine in Cancer Therapy*,
Cancer Treatment and Research 178, https://doi.org/10.1007/978-3-030-16391-4_8

8.1 Introduction

Pancreatic ductal adenocarcinoma (PDAC) is currently the third leading cause of cancer-related deaths in the USA [1] and will become related to the second leading cause of cancer deaths by the year 2030 [2]. The location of the pancreas deep in the retroperitoneum makes early detection difficult since most patients with this disease will present with non-specific symptoms such as weight loss, abdominal or epigastric pain, diarrhea, and nausea [3]. As opposed to breast cancer, melanoma, and prostate cancer, most cases of PDAC are diagnosed in the advanced disease stage [1]. The five-year survival in PDAC across all stages is 8%, although in localized disease it is 32% [1]. While there are several promising approaches to PDAC therapy that are currently under investigation [4], the overall survival beyond 3 years has not matched that of other malignancies. This is thought to be related to both the aggressive nature of the disease and its initial manifestation as metastatic disease in most patients. Therefore, two of the most critical unmet needs in PDAC are (1) to detect the cancer in its earlier stages while curative intent is still possible and (2) to be able to rapidly identify the effective therapies for the control and reversal of this aggressive disease.

The use of imaging in the care of patients with known or suspected PDAC has a pivotal role to play in this regard. It is not an overstatement to suggest that in the era of rapid biologic discovery into the hallmarks of cancer combined with the use of novel precision-based treatment regimens, the need for better non-invasive approaches to detect, stage, and monitor the disease is urgent. Early detection of pancreas cancer in high-risk families and swift detection of treatment responses to novel therapies underlie the belief that the best chance for long-term survival, if not cure, is based upon reducing tumor burden so that surgical intervention may be undertaken. While documenting the presence of disease on CT, MRI and ultrasound will remain an integral part of the care of PDAC patients and high-risk groups [5], emerging molecular imaging modalities with MRI, PET, and SPECT-based radiopharmaceutical agents will continue to grow. In order to ultimately conquer this disease, novel biomarkers that can detect PDAC at its precursor stage and/or rapidly detect effective responses to avoid ineffective therapies would be highly desirable. Recently, innovative approaches in the use of imaging fueled by advanced computer technologies and artificial intelligence (AI) are actively being pursued. This has led to the burgeoning field of radiomics whereby the high information content inherent on cross-sectional images can be extracted to provide large volume datasets for correlation with the biologic drivers of this disease ("omics") and then used to derive clinically useful surrogates via big data approaches, all elements necessary for precision imaging. This chapter will provide an overview into some of the novel approaches being considered for the early detection and treatment response assessments in PDAC using radiomic approaches. More detailed descriptions of the engines which help drive this new field of precision imaging can be found in many excellent references [6–9]. It is the authors hope that this overview will help to stimulate further interest into the development of innovative technologies and techniques that will contribute to a better understanding of PDAC and ultimately conquer this aggressive disease.

8.2 Novel Biomarkers for Evaluation of PDAC

Previous work from Yachida et al. has shown that the development of inciting mutations in the pancreas eventually leading to metastatic pancreatic disease can take up to seventeen years prior to initial clinical presentation [10]. This insight leads one to hope that more sensitive and specific testing may yield better clinical outcomes. Current biomarker testing for detecting pancreatic cancer is not perfect. The utilization of the serum marker CA 19-9, the most commonly used blood test for pancreatic cancer monitoring and detection, has a limited sensitivity, particularly with small malignancies [11]. Furthermore, 10% of the patient population do not express the Lewis body antigen needed to have an elevated CA 19-9 [12]. Another tumor marker that may be utilized to supplement CA 19-9 testing is CEA, which also carries a modest sensitivity to detecting PDAC [13]. Recently, several novel biomarkers have been examined to provide more sensitive and specific data regarding the detection and monitoring of disease activity. For example, the use of micro-RNAs (miRNA) which are short non-coding RNA that are expressed uniquely in malignancy may be captured through the use of peripheral blood tests either from cell-free miRNA or exosomal miRNA assays [14, 15]. Circulating tumor DNA has also been advocated as a means for screening and detection of PDAC along with assessment of response [16]. Other approaches have found a unique profile of branched chain amino acid combinations of isoleucine, leucine, and valine as being elevated up to 8.7 years prior to the diagnosis of recurrent pancreatic cancer metabolites in peripheral blood [17]. The ability of using minimally invasive blood tests to yield better sensitivity and specificity for malignancy is promising but has yet to be fully integrated into routine clinical care. Although the above methods have their appeal compared to more invasive procedures such as tissue biopsy, there are limitations related to the content and quantity-of-source material and uncertainty as to the location and origin of the contributing lesion(s). Because of these limitations, other methodologies are being explored. It is here that there has been a growing interest in using imaging as a noninvasive source of biomarker development owing to its widespread use in patients known or suspected of harboring cancer. This new field of investigation has been referred to as

Radiomics as it combines radiologic information with biologic ("omic") data to provide better precision in the evaluation of the cancer patient.

8.3 Radiomic Background and Significance for Precision Medicine

Radiomics allows for the identification, extraction, quantitation, and processing of the high content information contained within a radiographic image to produce imaging signatures or phenotypes. When combined with a variety of demographic, biologic ("omic") and outcomes driven information surrogate imaging biomarkers can be developed for clinical use in precision medicine. Such precise imaging biomarkers have been described in a variety of tumors and conditions including CNS [18–21], breast [22–24], lung [25–28], liver [29–31], renal [32–35], pancreas [36, 37], gastric [38, 39], colorectal [40–42], hematological [43] and prostate [44–48] cancers, and precursor tumor lesions [49–51] as well as for CNS disorders of dementia, hepatic and pulmonary fibrosis, and cardiovascular disease. Recently, we and others have found interesting radiomic signatures correlated with the hallmarks of cancer, prognosis, treatment prediction (especially with immunotherapy), and early detection of response [52–54].

The underlying mechanism and biologic underpinning which creates a radiomic signature(s) is currently being tested. Both the tumor microenvironment including the fibrotic status of the tumor milieu, its proliferative, metabolic and hypoxic status, and tissue/tumor vascularity appears to contribute to radiomic signature. Although the complexity of tumor composition and behavior along with the cellular changes visible only at the microscopic and/or molecular level makes direct correlation with imaging signals difficult, these factors likely contribute to the varied appearance of lesions on radiographic studies which in turn contribute the radiomic signature(s). Regardless of the physical, morphological, and biological nature of the tumor, radiomics can offer fundamental advantages over current techniques for assessment of malignant lesions and tissues. These advantages include (1) the availability of radiologic studies due to the necessity to use imaging on a frequent basis for diagnosis, staging, and monitoring treatment responses in people with non-superficial cancer lesions, (2) the ability to provide detailed and important information regarding both spatial and temporal evolution of tumor behavior and response, (3) the permanent nature of radiographic images compared to the consumption of tissue samples required for analysis obtained through biopsy or blood samples, (4) the large field of anatomic coverage (whole body) that can potentially interrogate each and every lesion and diseased organ compared to sampling errors from lesion heterogeneity of biopsied tissues, and (5) the relative safety profile of imaging rather than tissue biopsy. Thus, radiomics and the precision that it may offer has the potential to allow for early detection, treatment monitoring, outcome prediction, and/or biomarker discovery and shed light into some of the radiographic changes noted in the hallmarks of cancer as described by Hanahan and Weinberg

[55]. Additionally, given the heterogenous appearance of PDAC lesions on imaging, its widespread tumor burden in most patients at the time of either diagnosis and/or recurrence and the frequent use of multimodality imaging required for patient care creates an ideal testing ground for the use of radiomics in precision medicine. The essential elements required for the generation of radiomic signatures are provided in the sections below.

8.4 Essential Elements for Radiomic Signatures

Radiomics requires the extraction of both quantitative and qualitative imaging signals to generate a meaningful signature in which to correlate with outcomes, responses, and "omics." These extracted signal features can be divided into three major categories: (I) structural (syntactic), (2) statistical, and (3) textural (spectral) [7, 8, 56].

8.4.1 Structural Elements for Radiomic Signatures

Structural elements include descriptive features like lesion size, volume, and shape (e.g., spherical, asphericity, etc.), boundary morphology (spiculated, rounded, well-defined, sharp, ill-defined, amorphous, indistinct, etc.), and spatial enhancement properties (contrast enhancement properties across or within a lesion and surrounding tissues). These features typically require reader input to make assessments. As such, these features are much harder to extract automatically from the image datasets and are dependent upon reader training of exemplar cases and are susceptible to reader experience and judgment. This can lead to higher inter- and intravariability of image interpretation. In addition, the same lesion may share overlapping features depending upon whether the analysis is conducted on a single imaging slice (i.e., on either the axial, coronal or sagittal 2D planes) or whole tumor and/or organ volume (i.e., 3D reconstructions). For example, a tubular-shaped lesion may appear as a round lesion on axial images but a cylindrical lesion on coronal or sagittal views. Nevertheless, this category of elements is one of the first important steps in radiomic signature generation. An illustration of some of the structural elements on single slice image is shown in Fig. 8.1.

8.4.2 Statistical Elements for Radiomic Signatures

Statistical features are quantitative by nature and involve the determination of the grayscale signal intensity value contained within each pixel of a region of interest (ROI), volume of interest (VOI) or object. These grayscale signal intensity values can be extracted using either semi-automated or automated computer-based segmentation and automation approaches thereby reducing inter- and intrareader

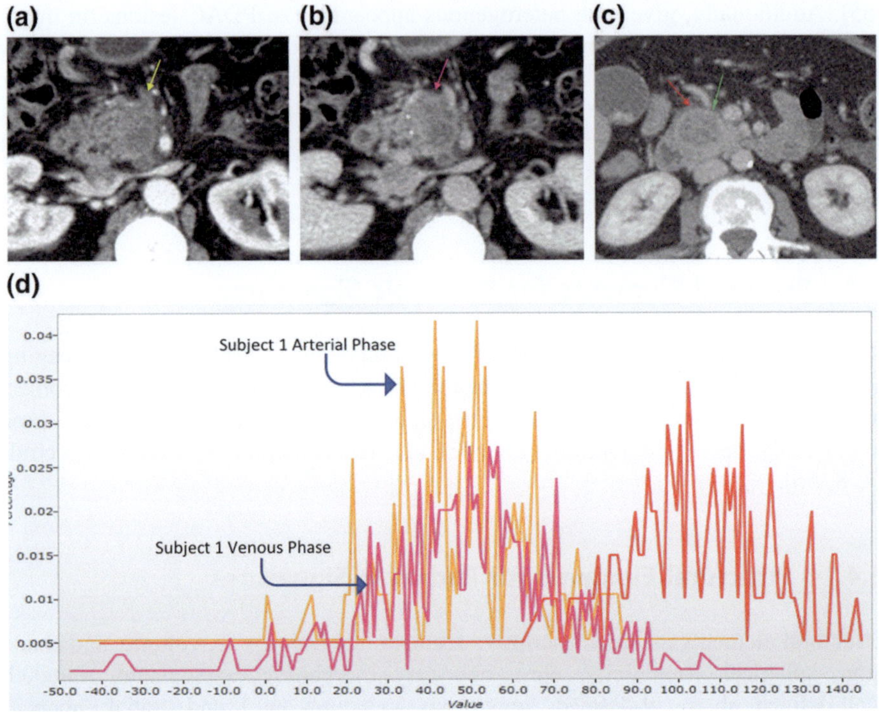

Fig. 8.1 Examples of axial contrast-enhanced CT images of PDAC. Panel **a** shows a poorly defined spherical-shaped 3.2 cm mass in the head of the pancreas (yellow arrow) on arterial phase. Panel **b** is acquired during the portal venous phase (rouge arrow). Note that the tumor is better seen on venous compared to arterial phase due to the less vascular nature of PDAC [57] compared to surrounding normal pancreatic parenchymal tissue and delayed tumor enhancement. The white asterisk highlights a penetrating vascular structure in the mass lesion which can be an important radiomic finding occasionally associated with enhanced neovascular gene expression. Panel **c** represents the axial portal venous phase from a different patient demonstrating a well-defined 2.8 cm hypodense lesion (red arrow) with a pseudocapsule (green arrow). There is internal haziness seen within the low-density portion of the tumors suggesting mixed areas of viability and necrosis. Panel **d** demonstrates histogram frequency curves (HFC) derived from the tumor in each image. The x-axis represents the density values (Hounsfield Units) of each pixel in the region of interest while the y-axis is the frequency (fraction) at which each density is observed. Note that the profile of the yellow and rouge curves overlaps each other except that the yellow HFC is more peeked (higher kurtosis) during arterial enhancement. The red curve from the second lesion is shifted to the right (higher density) but otherwise has a similar shape. These HFCs form the basis for deriving statistical elements for radiomics feature analysis

variability. Commonly used statistical elements (grayscale signal intensity values) obtained from the images are referred to as first-order statistical features. They provide measurements of the mean pixel signal value, standard deviation skewness, and kurtosis. The results of first-order statistical features are usually displayed either as single values or as histogram frequency curves (HFC). Either display method highlights the grayscale signal intensity values within a ROI. The grayscale intensities are, however, unique to the imaging modality from which they are derived. These non-deterministic values include signal intensity (SI) units or apparent diffusion constant (ADC) values from MRI, Hounsfield Units (HU) from CT and decay-corrected radioactive counts from PET. Since the signal intensity value derived from each pixel is unique to CT, MRI, US, or PET, they cannot be directly combined or compared. For example, a lesion or object with central necrosis may have high grayscale intensity values on T2W MRI but low grayscale intensity values on contrast-enhanced CT. Nonetheless, the information from each modality can be collectively integrated to provide a quantitative summary of a target region's intensity pattern. Although first-order statistical features are attractive to use in radiomic analysis because of their simplicity, there is no spatial information contained within their values.

The use of second-order statistical features can provide spatial information regarding the distribution of grayscale intensities within a lesion or object. The second-order statistical features take into account the grayscale intensities of nearest neighbor pixels in order to provide the necessary spatial information. Frequently used second-order statistical descriptors include gray level co-occurrence matrices (GLCM) [58] and gray level run length matrices (GLRLM) [59]. In GLCM, the frequencies with which the pixel of the same signal intensity are found adjacent to each other (co-occurrence) is provided as a matrix and is used to describe the coarseness of signal intensity in a particular direction. In GLRLM, the frequency that nearest neighbor pixels match each other in intensity or have "runs of same signal intensity" can be calculated to determine the heterogeneity of signal intensity within a ROI. For example, if the signal intensity of all pixels in all directions within a lesion or object is identical, then the run length would be unity (i.e., 1) and the lesion or object would be considered homogeneous. In contrast, for lesions or objects in which all pixels in all directions are different, then the run length would be 0 reflecting extreme heterogeneity. Note that with these methods, the location of the local or regional zones of uniformity and/or heterogeneity may not be delineated within the ROI, lesion, or object. In this regard, local binary patterns (LBP) and other algorithms [60] can be used because of their focus on the patterns of intensity within a subregion of a ROI which is obtained by applying a centroid mask on top of nearest neighbor pixels within lesion or object. The signal within the nearest neighbors is then converted to a binary signal intensity of either greater than or less than the center pixel within the centroid. In this way can a threshold approach of statistical analysis be used to estimate local-regional difference in signal within a lesion or object. An illustration of statistical approaches is shown in Fig. 8.2.

8.4.3 Textural (Spectral) Analysis Elements for Radiomic Signatures

Texture analysis is a quantitative approach that helps to characterize the local spatial organization of signal intensity values that are repeated within a ROI by applying and adjusting filters in multidimensional space yielding a representative

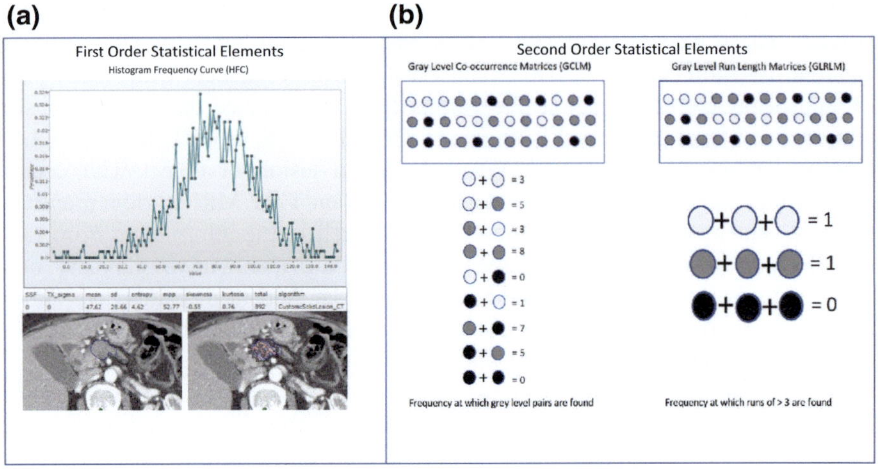

Fig. 8.2 Examples of statistical elements for radiomic signatures. Panel A shows a histogram frequency curve (HFC) from an infiltrating PDAC lesion located in the head of the pancreas as seen in the axial images below the graph. The *x*-axis represents the density values (Hounsfield Units) of each pixel in the region of interest while the *y*-axis is the frequency (fraction) at which each density is observed. First-order statistical values as displayed in the table below the HFC are derived from this curve and include mean pixel value, standard deviation (SD), mean positive pixel value (MPP which represents average value of those pixels with HU > 0), skewness, and kurtosis. Entropy is derived from the natural log of the pixel signal over the area of the ROI and represents heterogeneity of a lesion. The axial CT image at the bottom right contains a fused color overlay representing the spatial distribution of pixels containing positive pixel values (red) or negative pixel values (blue) derived from a textural analysis platform (TexRad®, Essex, UK). Panel B demonstrates the logic behind second-order statistical elements. Each circle represents the signal intensity of individual pixels. The darker the shade of gray, the higher the signal intensity. In this example, pixel elements of only three discrete intensities are represented in the boxed areas. The GCLM provides an estimate of the frequency that pixels of near identical intensities are found adjacent to one another (nearest neighbor co-occurrence) while the GLRLM estimates the frequency at which runs of neighboring pixels of near equal intensity are found. Unlike first-order statistical elements, second-order statistical elements contain information regarding the spatial relationships of pixels

mathematical model of texture. These elements are usually derived through a Fournier transformation (FT) of the grayscale values that converts spatial information to the frequency space and then a reversal of the process back to the spatial domain. Typical techniques include discrete orthonormal stockwell transform (DOST) [61], Gabor filter banks [62] Wavelet transform (WT) [63], Riesz transform [64], Stockwell transform (ST) [65], and Laplacian of the Gaussian [66]. The later technique uses a Laplacian filtering technique specified as a spatial frequency ranging from 2 to 6 pixels clustered together to obtain texture information in the form of mean, standard deviation, skewness, entropy, kurtosis displayed as histogram frequency curves (see Fig. 8.1a).

8.4.4 Radiomic Workflows

The methods of feature extraction outlined above have often been used in radiomic studies because they are intrinsically simple to calculate and can rapidly produce a large number of imaging traits in which to apply in a high-input manner for statistical correlation and model building using bioinformatic approaches and machine learning (ML). In order to apply these elements successfully for precision imaging, a radiomic workflow is needed.

The radiomic workflow is a multistep process (Fig. 8.3). These steps include (1) image acquisition with or without spatial registration, (2) lesion and/or object segmentation, (3) voxel resampling (discretization) to limit the range of intensity values, (4) feature extraction, (5) feature analysis, and (6) model building for biomarker testing, training, and validation. Ideally each step should be carefully controlled and automated, if possible, to provide the robustness needed for clinical application and to control for variations due to scanner-related differences, patient-derived factors variations of lesion, organ, and/or body function, and statistical noise due to data overfitting which has historically limited the accuracy and precision of many imaging biomarkers. The importance of variations in imaging has been tested both using phantom studies and in the clinical setting. For example, Makin et al. [67] created a texture phantom to determine the variability in radiomic features across 17 scanner sites and compared it to radiomic analysis in cases of non-small cell lung cancer (NSCLC). Their study demonstrated that variability in radiomic features extracted from phantoms was comparable to the variability observed with the same radiomic features in NSCLC tumors meaning that much of the statistical elements extracted from radiomic evaluation can be related to technical rather than biological differences. In addition, several reports have found a high degree of test–retest instability between imaging scans [68, 69]. For example, in one study of 219 radiomic features in NSCLC on CT, only 30% of them had intraclass correlation coefficient >0.9 when scans were repeated 15 min apart [69]. In order to reduce such variability in the future, the need for acquisition standardization, phantom qualification, and patient preparation harmonization will be important aspects for ensuring the robustness of radiomics in the clinical setting.

8.5 Precision Imaging with Radiomics in the Evaluation of Pancreas Cancer

8.5.1 General Comments

There are several interesting features of pancreatic cancer that make precision imaging with radiomic feasible. These includes both classical and atypical appearances of primary and metastatic lesions on CT, MRI, and PET and their changes with effective therapies (either shrinkage and/or developing necrosis on CT/MRI and with improvement in free water diffusion and hypometabolism on

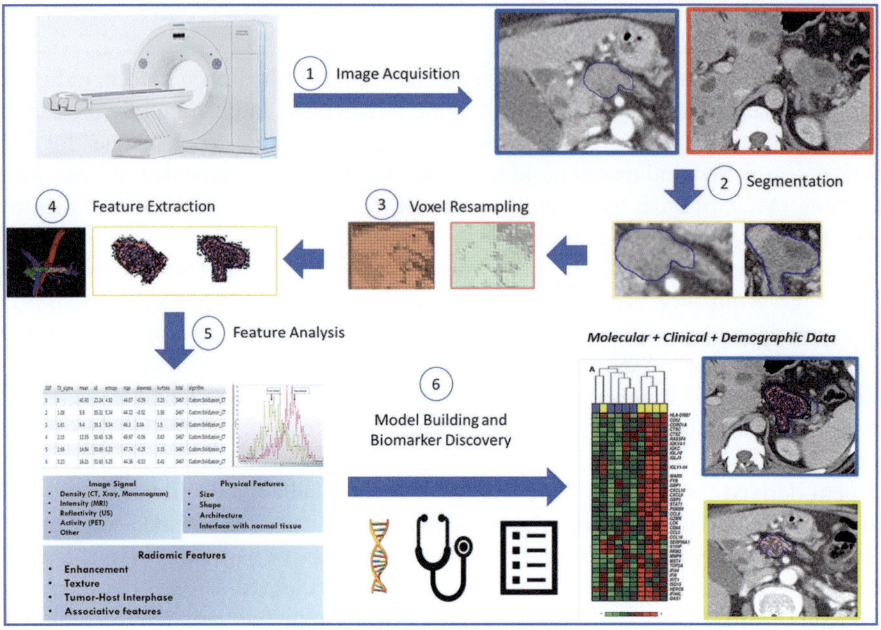

Fig. 8.3 General workflow for radiomic signature development beginning with (1) image acquisition, (2) lesion segmentation (blue outlines of PDAC from two separate subjects, (3) voxel resampling to reduce noise and normalize pixel grayscale intensities, (4) feature extraction (both 3D volumetric lesion shape determination and texture analysis profiles obtained), (5) feature analysis with the various components of first- and second-order statistical evaluation and additional ingredients integrated for imaging signature discovery and validation, and (6) final step of model building which explores the relationship between radiomic traits and clinical and molecular associations

FDG PET) versus ineffective treatments with the associated development of recurrence and/or treatment resistance (lesion growth, reduction in free water diffusion from increased cellularity on MRI and hypermetabolism on FDG PET).

Conventional imaging plays an essential role in PDAC given the reported sensitivity for detection of PDAC ranges from 76 to 96% for [70–75] depending on tumor size. Representative appearances of PDAC on multiphasic CT/MRI include a hypoattenuating (low density) mass on CT, hypo/hyperintense signal abnormalities on MRI (T1W/T2W hypointensity/hyperintensity, respectively), and hypermetabolic uptake on FDG PET. Each of these findings can be associated with pancreatic duct dilatation and upstream atrophy of the pancreas. However, up to approximately 20% of subjects do not have a distinct low-density mass on CT [75, 76]. The lack of mass detection on CT is presumably due to the well-differentiated nature of these tumors with lower tumor cellularity and less necrosis at the microscopic level [77] which provides an opportunity for using radiomic signatures to detect malignant transformation. In the liver, space occupying lesions (hypoattenuating mass lesions on CT/MRI with/without central necrosis most conspicuous on the portal venous phase and/or T1W-T2W hypo/hyperintense focus, respectively) is commonly observed. These lesions may or may not have distinct boundaries, contain pseudocapsular rinds, have penetrating vascular branches leading into the center of the lesion, and display rim-like peripheral enhancement in a corona-like pattern during both the arterial and portal venous phases. Some of these features have been shown to represent important radiomic traits for microvascular thrombosis and tumor invasion [29] in HCC and similar work is ongoing in pancreas cancer.

In addition to the lesion's statistical and textural feature elements that might be extracted for radiomic analysis, indirect structural features of pancreatic tumors including pancreatic and/or common bile duct dilatation especially in tumors within the head of the pancreas (so-called double duct sign), abrupt pancreatic duct caliber change, and atrophy may be important components for prediction/prognosis and aid in early detection especially in high-risk patients for PDAC [78–82]. In addition, many patients with PDAC have associated inflammatory changes in the pancreas due either to the obstructing nature of tumor lesion, stent reaction, and/or superimposed cholangitis. The imaging changes affiliated with inflammatory changes can be difficult to distinguish by conventional means but may be more readily delineated using a multifeatured extraction (radiomic) approach as has been demonstrated in other tumor types [83]. One additional unique feature of radiomic analysis on MRI imaging that can also be used for diagnosis and monitoring treatment response involves the detection of free water molecule movement on diffusion weighted images (DWI). This highly quantitative MRI sequence obtained during most standards of care MRI procedures allows for the calculation of apparent diffusion constant (ADC) maps. Due to the increased cellularity and/or fibrosis in many tumors, lower ADC values are noted compared to higher ADC values for normal tissue and/or necrosis [84, 85]. Since pancreas cancer can incite a fibrotic reaction, the movement of water can be restricted on ADC maps and used for radiomic trait discovery.

The following sections will illustrate some specific uses of radiomic evaluation for PDAC including examples of early detection and characterization of the tumor microenvironment and monitoring of treatment response.

8.5.2 Early Detection for PDAC

Current efforts have focused on developing screening programs for earlier detection of pancreatic cancer. The International Cancer of the Pancreas Screening (CAPS) Consortium is one such organization composed of experts from several different disciplines including epidemiology, genetics, gastroenterology, radiology, oncology, surgery, and pathology examining the literature and providing recommendations on screening individuals thought to be at risk for developing pancreatic cancer [86]. A prospective study of 51 individuals who presented to a single clinic at Columbia University Medical Center/New York Presbyterian Hospital that helped formed the basis of the recommendations of the CAPS consortium [87] was able to classify patients according to risk factors for PDAC. In this study, individuals were stratified into different risk categories by the presence of the age and number of relatives affected with pancreatic cancer along with the presence of germ line mutations associated with a risk of pancreatic cancer (i.e., *BRCA 1/2*, *CDKN2A*, those with Lynch syndrome, etc.). Individuals were offered to undergo imaging tests through MRI/MRCP, blood tests through CA 19-9 and glucose tolerance, and endoscopic ultrasound if indicated. Up to 40% of asymptomatic individuals had actionable findings including potentially malignant disease (two were found to have pancreatic cancer—one localized and one with metastatic disease along with two cases of ovarian cancer, four with intraductal papillary mucinous neoplasm, one with thyroid cancer, and one with neuroendocrine cancer [87]). A more recent study found that individuals with CDKN2A germ line mutations had an overall survival benefit with yearly EUS along with MRI/MRCP [88]. Currently, there are no guidelines for pancreatic cancer screening from the American Cancer Society, National Comprehensive Cancer Network (NCCN), or the United States Preventative Task Force (USPTSF) [89]. Therefore, further work in detecting pancreatic cancer utilizing what is available in the clinic with an eye toward promising biomarker research is needed to change the current paradigm of pancreatic cancer detection. Recent experience at the author's clinical site is currently offering a holistic approach to the care of these families at risk including the adoption of the prior guidelines from CAPS along with other published studies through the use of MRI/MRCP along with blood testing and emphasis on the tumor markers CEA and CA 19-9. Individuals are presented weekly at a tumor board composed of radiologists, gastroenterologist, surgeons, genetic counselors, oncologists, nurses, and social workers. If indicated, the individual may be recommended to undergo further evaluation with an EUS procedure or surgery. To date, over 180 individuals have been enrolled in the screening program with one case of pancreatic cancer and one case of melanoma detected.

Radiomics may offer a distinct advantage over other techniques in early detection programs. Due to the slow nature of malignant change over a 18-year period prior to the appearance of PDAC on cross-sectional imaging, a change in the texture pattern may be noted (Fig. 8.4) prior to its manifestation on imaging. Borazanci et al. [89] are currently applying both 2D and 3D radiomic techniques for detection of these changes and integrating the finding with other liquid biomarkers. Furthermore, the integration of advanced imaging tests, such as the utilization of hyperpolarized [1-^{13}C]-pyruvate magnetic resonance spectroscopy which was able to detect early changes concerning for pancreatic cancer in a preclinical model, warrants further study in individuals with pancreatic cancer [90].

A precursor lesion can be found in up to one-third patients who develop PDAC. Referred to as intraductal papillary mucinous neoplasms (IPMNs), these cystic lesions can undergo malignant transformation if left unmonitored. Detected early, however, they can be removed to prevent the development of PDAC. Not all IPMNs, though, undergo malignant transformation, and many can be followed with imaging for documentation of long-term stability. Given the cystic nature of the

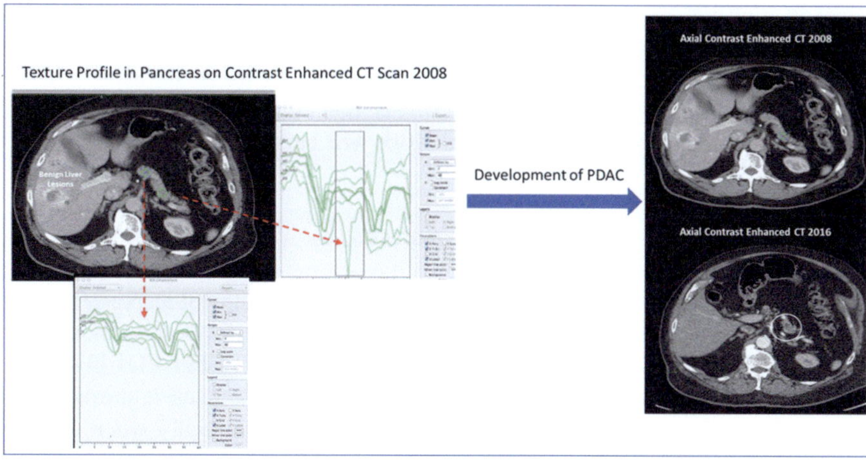

Fig. 8.4 An example of the potential use of radiomics for the early detection of pancreas cancer. Since molecular events may occur several decades before the manifestation of PDAC on conventional imaging, the evaluation of the pancreas texture may provide some evidence of transformation. In this subject, a retrospective look at the texture profile in pancreas tissue in 2008 (green circles) noted a difference in the histogram frequency curve in the body of the pancreas (downward peaks) compared to the pancreatic neck tissue. A 2.1-cm PDAC subsequently developed in the body of the pancreas 8 years later (white circle)

lesion, MRI is the more superior modality for the detection and longitudinal assessment in patients harboring these lesions.

The use of radiomics to characterize IPMN lesions has yielded interesting results compared to established Fukuoka guidelines for determining the malignant potential of IPMNs [91]. Fukuoka guidelines define high-risk stigmata and worrisome features to assess malignant potential and need for surgical intervention. These features include obstructive jaundice, enhancing mural nodules, pancreatic duct dilatation > 10 mm, cysts > 3 cm, thickened enhancing walls, abrupt changes in PD caliber, distal pancreatic atrophy, pancreatitis, and lymphadenopathy [91]. Since surgical resection of IPMNs is not a gentle procedure with its attendant complications of infection/abscess, bowel obstruction, pancreatic duct leakage and pancreatic insufficiency, any biomarker(s) that can accurately distinguish high-risk from low-risk lesions would be attractive. Recently, Hanania et al. correlated radiomics signatures of IPMN to pathology. They found that GLCM statistical features within the wall of the cystic lesions differentiated low-grade and high-grade lesions better than the Fukuoka criteria with an AUC of 0.82 at a sensitivity of 85% and specificity of 68% suggesting the advantage of radiomics compared to more conventional grading systems [92]. However, additional work including the integration of molecular tests on the fluid and cellular contents found within these cystic lesions (e.g., CA19-9, miRNA, Kras, etc.) with the radiomic signature is needed to better define the high-risk features for PDAC development. Although MRI/MRCP with the use of low molecular weight gadolinium (LMWG) contrast agents in high-risk patients is the most appropriate manner to screen these individuals, theoretical concerns have been raised regarding the long-term effects of LMWG agents potentially causing neurotoxicity due to its accumulation in the dentate nucleus and globus pallidus [93]. As the clinical significance of brain accumulation remains unclear, additional work will be needed.

8.5.3 Monitoring Treatment Responses

The only truly objective biomarker for the assessment of treatment response in solid tumors is tumor shrinkage on imaging and/or clinical examination. Although the Response Evaluation Criteria in Solid Tumor Guidelines (RECIST v1.1 [94]) have been applied in almost all pivotal trials since its publication as a surrogate for anti-tumor activity, it suffers from the lack of sensitivity especially when targeted and novel therapies are used. Indeed, many treatment regimens can lead to tumor death without tumor shrinkage, and when shrinkage does occur, it can be slow to develop. Therefore, better methods are required to demonstrate effective therapies and more rapid monitoring of results. This is particularly true in PDAC in which the median progression-free survival in frontline therapy is approximately 8–11 months [95, 96]. Thus, a rapid detection and assessment of response (RaDAR) system is needed. In PDAC, Korn et al. have shown that the use of FDG PET can be an effective means of assessing early response to gemcitabine and nab-paclitaxel [97]. Indeed, patients with an early metabolic response in patients with metastatic PDAC (mPDAC) on FDG PET at 8 weeks have significantly better progression-free survival and overall survivals than patients without an early metabolic response. Furthermore, Hindorani et al. demonstrated [98] that early improvements can be noted (sometimes within days of administration therapy) in FDG PET metabolism within weeks of receiving gemcitabine-based therapy in combination with drugs that alter the tumor microenvironment. Although compelling, not all patients with mPDAC can obtain an early FDG PET scan due to local insurance carrier policies. Therefore, other means of developing a RaDAR system seem warranted.

The exploration of radiomic signatures in this environment seems ideal for detection of early changes in tumor texture. Several investigators have focused efforts on ADC maps and histogram analysis to show treatment responses in head and neck and CNS tumors [99, 100] using first-order statistical radiomic traits of kurtosis and skewness, as well as perfusion metrics (K-trans skewness) as predictors of PFS and OS. Furthermore, Zhang et al. [101] evaluated 20 subjects with esophageal cancer to predict pathologic response to neoadjuvant therapy using several multivariates and found that radiomic models contributed to pathologic prediction compared tumor size and straightforward SUV assessments on FDG PET. Current efforts are being focused on using a similar approach in PDAC.

Like these other tumor types, radiomic response assessments have shown early changes in the textural pattern in treatment response in mPDAC within 4–8 weeks of onset of chemotherapy in front-line subjects on CT (Fig. 8.5), in the neoadjuvant setting and in therapies that can alter the tumor microenvironment (Fig. 8.6). In addition, distinctive patterns of favorable healing have recently been described by Amer et al. [102] who demonstrated that patients in whom their pancreatic lesions develop more distinct borders after treatment have better outcomes (PFS and event-free survival) than those lesions with ill-defined margins [102]. Despite these encouraging examples of radiomics, several key areas need to be addressed prior to adoption of this form of precision imaging into the clinical environment beyond testing for sensitivity, specificity, and accuracy including (1) earliest time that a significant radiomic change can be seen, (2) the best modality or combination of modalities to use for identifying a radiomic response signature, (3) the best bioinformatic model(s) to provide the most accurate prediction of response either alone or in combination with other biomarkers, (4) the universal applicability of the radiomic response signature in frontline versus recurrent/resistant line therapy and whether the signature is tumor specific and/or treatment specific, and (5) issues regarding the impact of quality-of-life impacts and economic benefits of applying the signature to the general or selected PDAC population. Certainly, a well-planned, well-executed, prospective trial(s) will be required to address almost all these issues.

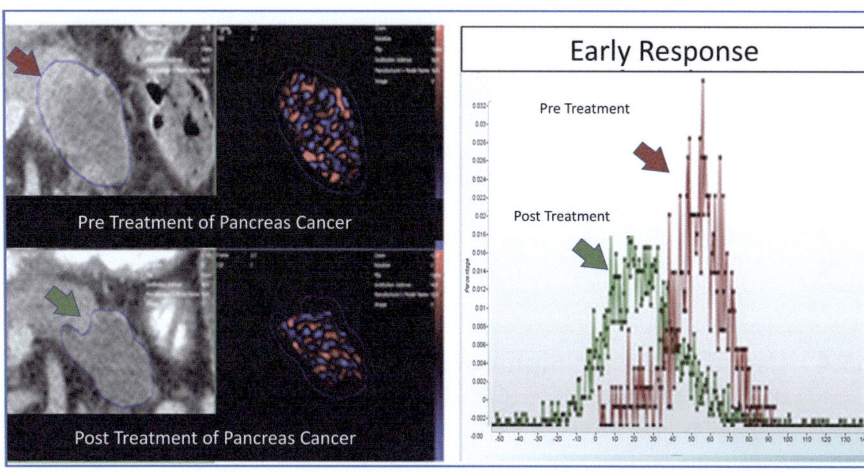

Fig. 8.5 Early response to therapy using radiomic quantitative textural analysis. Radiomic changes within 4 weeks of start of combination therapy (gemcitabine, nab-paclitaxel, and cisplatin) in a patient with metastatic pancreas cancer are depicted. A 7.2-cm hypodense lesion in the body of the pancreas was noted prior to therapy. The lesion remained stable to slightly smaller over time, but the texture profile changed substantially within 4 weeks of starting treatment. There was a clear shift in the HFC toward necrosis

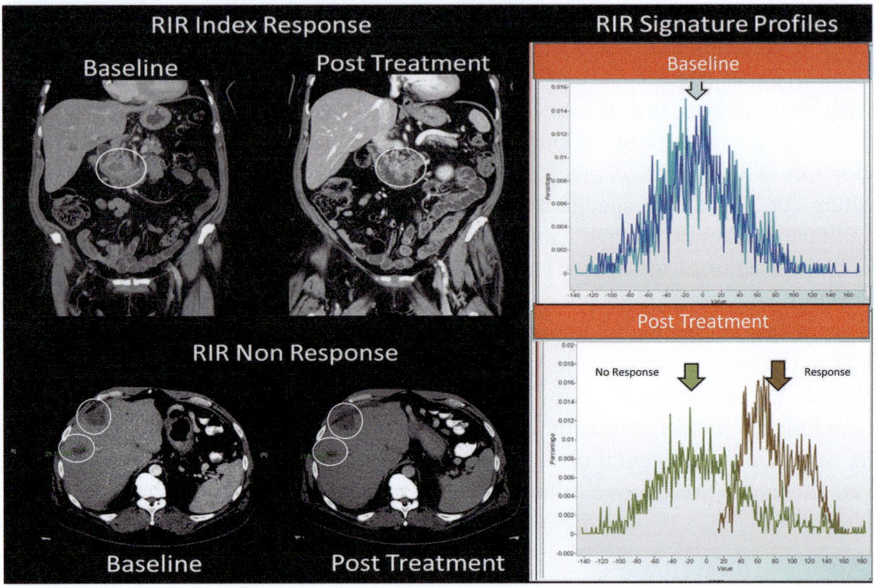

Fig. 8.6 Evaluation of tumor texture to determine context of vulnerability to treatments that can alter the tumor microenvironment. Two subjects were treated with chemotherapy + TME disrupting agents. The subject on top had a ~4 cm PDAC in the head of the pancreas (white circle and brown arrow) that resolved within 6 months of treatment as did their hepatic metastasis. The subject on the bottom had both pancreatic (not shown) and hepatic metastasis but did not see any benefit from therapy (white circles and green arrow). Texture analysis on the baseline scan showed highly similar HFCs between responders and non-responders. However, first follow-up scan (8 weeks after therapy) demonstrated differences in tumor profiles (note the shape and shift of the HFC and highlighted pixel elements (color images). Such information could be used to help rapidly detect responses when conventional imaging remains stable. RIR = regional index of response

8.5.4 Use of Radiomic Signatures for the Prediction and Prognosis

Many publications on radiomics have focused upon the prognostic and predictive value as a biomarker. A prognostic biomarker provides information about the patient's overall cancer outcome, regardless of therapy, while a predictive biomarker provides information on the effect of a therapeutic intervention. Both prognostic and predictive radiomic biomarkers have been described in a variety of settings in solid tumor and lymphoma [43, 103–106]. Recently, the ability to predict response to immunotherapy using a radiomic approach has been reported. This type of imaging biomarker may be useful in the future as work focused on converting immune isolated tumors such as PDAC into inflamed lesion that would respond to immune therapies is an area of great interest. An example of using quantitative textural analysis (QTA) to predict response to PDL-1 inhibitors from our own radiomics laboratory is shown in Fig. 8.7.

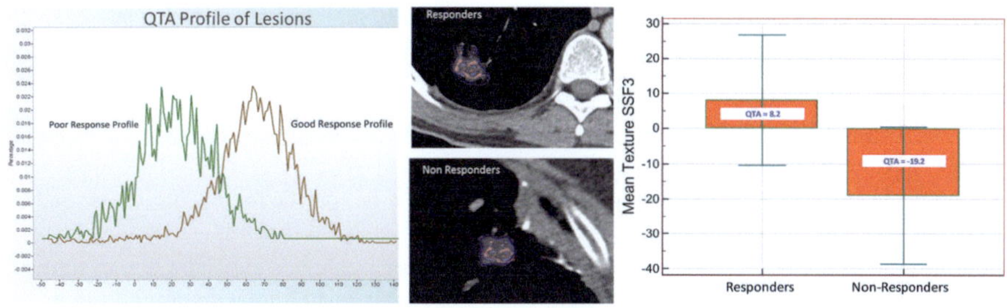

Fig. 8.7 The feasibility of using of quantitative texture analysis to evaluate baseline scans for sensitivity to immune check point inhibitor therapy. Radiomic was used to predict which subjects may respond to immunotherapy with PD-L1 agents. Baseline CT scans from 28 subjects with solid tumors amenable to check point inhibition were evaluated retrospectively using quantitative textural analysis to determine if there were potential imaging biomarkers that would predict response. The HFC shows different texture profiles between responders and non-responders with the texture trait of MPP being the most sensitive to distinguishing between the two groups ($p = 0.41$). Prospective clinical trials will be needed to translate this signature for clinical use. Such imaging biomarkers may be of great utility in exploration of therapeutic strategies of converting immune isolated tumors such as PDAC into inflamed lesions

In regard to the radiomics of PDAC, Sandrassegaran et al. applied quantitative textural analysis to provide a prognostic signature for overall survival in subjects with mPDAC and found that lesion with high kurtosis and mean positive pixel values had poor outcomes [107]. Borazanci et al. have demonstrated that radiomic signatures using texture analysis can predict response to PARP inhibitors [108]. Furthermore, preliminary work has shown that texture features of entropy and kurtosis in the primary tumor in mPDAC are associated with interchromosomal heterogeneity and that the textural features of the adjacent pancreas provide prognostic information regarding overall survival [36].

8.5.5 Limitations of Radiomics in Precision Imaging

Despite the promise of radiomics in a variety of settings in PDAC, there are significant limitations and challenges that must be addressed before radiomics can be fully implemented clinically. The degree of radiomic signature stability which can occur even within single institutional reporting can be problematic as can overfitting the data. For example, Chalkidou et al. [109] recreated a dataset from 100 features obtained in 21 esophageal cancer patients and found that about half of the recreated features had reasonable accuracy for predicting OS (AUC 0.68–0.80). Such high degree of false discovery rate can be overcome either using statistical corrections or larger number of patients. The lack of standards and harmonization across tumor types, patient preparation, image acquisition, data sampling, feature extraction, feature analysis, clinical and pathologic gold standards, and model building also can contribute to the limitation of using radiomics for precision imaging. Table 8.1 provides a more comprehensive list of the current issues facing radiomics.

Table 8.1 An overview of limitations of each component of radiomic analysis and strategies for overcoming them

Radiomic properties [relevant references]	Limiting factor
Tumor-specific factors	
Tumor type	• Radiomic signature may only be specific for the tumor type under consideration and not applicable to other tumor types
Lesion location [110]	• Lesion location may influence radiomic signature due to tumor motion (e.g., lung or upper abdomen), imaging artifacts (e.g., metal or air or improper attention correction) and partial volume effects from surrounding tissues
Lesion size and morphology [111–113]	• Small lesions may have poor signal and count statistics (especially with PET radiomic analysis). Minimum tumor size (volume) suitable for radiomics has been reported in ranges from >3 to 10 cm^3 • Image shape, boundaries, and borders can influence the placement of region and volumes of interest and affect segmentation programs. Standardization of common lexicon and definition of tumor margins are needed
Organ involvement	• Background organ (liver, lung, bone, brain) may affect the lesion texture measurement creating different radiomic signatures based upon tissue background
Pathology and molecular tests as truth standards [16]	• Significant variability can be seen during pathologic review of tissue data (local site vs central review) as well as during molecular analysis which can influence surrogate imaging biomarker performance
Image acquisition parameters	
Scanner configurations [8]	• Radiomic feature quantification is sensitive to acquisition modes, reconstruction parameters, smoothing, and segmentation • Scanner performance reporting is lacking in most studies to assess the influence of equipment differences on radiomic signatures
Modality and acquisition parameters [8]	• Radiomic signatures across different modalities cannot be directly compared • Phantom standardization and performance characteristics have not been used or not reported in most studies to help standardized image signal intensities across subjects and centers
Lesion analysis	
ROI placement and lesion definition [114, 115]	• ROI placement upon a lesion or object of interest can influence radiomic signatures. These factors include ROI size, shape, and boundaries • ROI placement by manual versus semiautomatic region growing and tumor contouring approaches can each introduce bias based upon reader preference versus segmentation algorithms
Single lesion versus multiple lesions combination [8]	• The influence of using single lesion versus multiple lesion inputs into a radiomic analysis is unknown

(continued)

Table 8.1 (continued)

Radiomic properties [relevant references]	Limiting factor
Feature analysis [112]	• Multiple radiomic features can be extracted from an image ranging from tumor size to higher order textural (spectral) features, and many of the methodologies used to capture this information have not been standardized • The same radiomic features may be implemented differently based upon the use of different platforms
Radiomic platforms [67]	• Variability across platforms based upon open source code, commercial products, and in-house systems without clear understanding of the advantages and biases of one platform over another • Different platforms can lead to different feature extraction outputs even when the same lesion is tested
Data resampling [106, 113, 116]	• Data resampling of image signal intensities to reduce the possible number of grayscale values is needed for data extraction and noise reduction but can potentially average out important and subtle radiomic signals
Statistical model considerations	
False detection rate [109, 117]	• Selection bias from the use of more radiomic features than the number of patients potentially can lead to increased false detection rates. In general, for each significant radiomic trait, a minimum of 10 patients is needed to avoid false detection report • Adjustment for multiple hypothesis testing is not always performed but is recommended to reduce false detection rate
Test-retest variability [68, 69, 118, 119]	• Significant variation in pixel intensity values can be seen with all modalities based upon slice thickness, scanner settings, contrast phase of enhancement, and reconstruction algorithms. • Up to 40% variability in signal intensities can be encountered between scan session even within 15 min of each other
Protocol-related issues	
Protocol design	• Most publications have been from single-center retrospective studies. Large prospective multi-institutional studies are needed to validate radiomic signatures for translation into the clinic • Well-documented image protocol acquisition parameters are lacking in most studies
Reader reproducibility [105]	• No rigorously tested multireader paradigm has been conducted to date to assess the influence of reader bias. This may be less of an issue with the use of automated segmentation algorithms
Other	• Lack of cost-effectiveness analysis • Open source data to facilitate comparison across platforms, large-scale discovery, and deep learning analysis are limited • Impact of radiomics on reader Workflow and efficiency is lacking • Lack of standardized lexicons and reporting

8.6 Future Directions

The use of radiomics illustrates the power of quantitative imaging, data extraction, and model building to provide potentially predictive, prognostic, biologic, and rapid response imaging biomarkers in the care of patients at risk or harboring PDAC. Platforms that can drive this technology are leading the way in precision imaging. The use of artificial intelligence (AI) to be feed big datasets will be needed to establish robust imaging biomarkers in the next generation of discovery using machine learning technologies. Machine Learning (ML) is a branch of AI which provides for meaningful mining of patterns that is invisible to routine human endeavors. As ML moves from simple principles of learning, training, and validation to deep learning techniques using neuro network approaches, a wave of new biomarkers and decision-making tools will be forthcoming. Diagnostic imaging has always been on the forefront of these advances. For example, several computer-assisted devices (CAD) are available for clinical use today for detection of breast cancer, colonic polyps on CT colonography, and quantitative dementia analysis. Others have begun to use ML to automatically detect and segment organ systems on cross-sectional images. Current efforts are underway to apply these technologies for the detection of pancreatic tumors [120].

Finally, two additional areas of future efforts in precision imaging of PDAC include (1) 3D virtual reconstruction of cross-sectional images to provide a detailed and comprehensive look at the relationship of tumor lesions to surrounding structures for precise surgical planning and radiation therapy (especially in the era of robotic surgeries and high-precision radiation therapy treatment planning systems) and (2) molecular imaging with radiopharmaceuticals that specifically target PDAC tumor or their host-dependent cells. These radiolabeled agents are directed against such targets as CA19-9, PAM-4, EGFR2, and others. Of course the newly approved ^{68}Ga-Labeled Octreotide agents for the detection of NET tumors and its companion theragnostic agents (177Lu-DotaTate: Netspot) are making a large impact in cancer care. The development of these agents will no doubt continue to grow over the next decade.

Acknowledgements The authors would like to acknowledge the generous support of the following Foundations and Granting Agencies: Marley Foundation and NCI U01 grant for early detection of pancreas program at the participating institutions; Virginia G Piper Foundation at HonorHealth for RaDAR program; Senna Magovitz Foundation; SU2C. We would also like to acknowledge Drs. Daniel D. von Hoff M.D. and Haiyang Han Ph.D. for their careful reading of the chapter and to all of the patients and families who have been true warriors in the march toward conquering this disease.

References

1. Siegel RL, Miller KD, Jemal A (2018) Cancer statistics, 2018. CA Cancer J Clin 68(1):7–30
2. Rahib L, Smith BD, Aizenberg R, Rosenzweig AB, Fleshman JM, Matrisian LM (2014) Projecting cancer incidence and deaths to 2030: the unexpected burden of thyroid, liver, and pancreas cancers in the United States. Cancer Res 74(11):2913–2921
3. Porta M, Fabregat X, Malats N, Guarner L, Carrato A, de Miguel A, Ruiz L, Jariod M, Costafreda S, Coll S, Alguacil J, Corominas JM, Solà R, Salas A, Real FX (2005) Exocrine pancreatic cancer: symptoms at presentation and their relation to tumour site and stage. Clin Transl Oncol 7(5):189–197
4. Manji GA, Olive KP, Saenger YM, Oberstein P (2017) Current and emerging therapies in metastatic pancreatic cancer. Clin Cancer Res 23(7):1670–1678
5. Chu LC, Goggins MG, Fishman EK (2017) Diagnosis and detection of pancreas cancer. Cancer J 23(6):333–342
6. Sanduleanu S, Woodruff H, de Jong EEC, van Timmeren, Jochems A, Dubois, Lambin E (2018) Tracking tumor biology with radiomics: a systematic review utilizing a radiomics quality score. Radiother Oncol 127:349–360
7. Lubner MG, Smith AD, Sandraesgran K, Sahani DV, Pickhardt PJ (2017) CT texture analysis: applications, biologic correlates, and challenges. RadioGraphics 37:1483–1503
8. Yip S, Aerts HJWL (2016) Applications and limitations of radiomics. Phys Med Biol 61 (13):R150–R166
9. Kuo MD, Jamshidi N (2014) Behind the numbers: decoding molecular phenotypes with radiogenomic—guiding principles and technical considerations. Radiology 270(2):320–325
10. Yachida S, Jones S, Bozic I, Antal T, Leary R, Fu B, Kamiyama M, Hruban RH, Eshleman JR, Nowak MA, Velculescu VE, Kinzler KW, Vogelstein B, Iacobuzio-Donahue CA (2010) Distant metastasis occurs late during the genetic evolution of pancreatic cancer. Nature 467(7319):1114–1117
11. Goggins M (2005) Molecular markers of early pancreatic cancer. J Clin Oncol 23(20):4524–4531
12. Tempero MA, Uchida E, Takasaki H, Burnett DA, Steplewski Z, Pour PM (1987) Relationship of carbohydrate antigen 19-9 and Lewis antigens in pancreatic cancer. Cancer Res 47(20):5501–5503
13. Zhang Y, Yang J, Li H, Wu Y, Zhang H, Chen W (2015) Tumor markers CA19-9, CA242 and CEA in the diagnosis of pancreatic cancer: a meta-analysis. Int J Clin Exp Med 15;8 (7):11683–11691
14. Tovar-Camargo OA, Toden S, Goel A (2016) Exosomal microRNA biomarkers: emerging frontiers in colorectal and other human cancers. Expert Rev Mol Diagn 16(5):553–567
15. Goel A (2015) MicroRNAs as therapeutic targets in colitis and colitis-associated cancer: tiny players with a giant impact. Gastroenterology 149(4):859–861
16. Alizadeh AA, Aranda V, Bardelli A, Blanpain C, Bock C, Borowski C, Caldas C, Califano A, Doherty M, Elsner M, Esteller M, Fitzgerald R, Korbel JO, Lichter P, Mason CE, Navin N, Pe'er D, Polyak K, Roberts CW, Siu L, Snyder A, Stower H, Swanton C, Verhaak RG, Zenklusen JC, Zuber J, Zucman-Rossi J (2015) Toward understanding and exploiting tumor heterogeneity. Nat Med 21:846–853
17. Mayers JR, Wu C, Clish CB, Kraft P, Torrence ME, Fiske BP, Yuan C, Bao Y, Townsend MK, Tworoger SS, Davidson SM, Papagiannakopoulos T, Yang A, Dayton TL, Ogino S, Stampfer MJ, Giovannucci EL, Qian ZR, Rubinson DA, Ma J, Sesso HD, Gaziano JM, Cochrane BB, Liu S, Wactawski-Wende J, Manson JE, Pollak MN, Kimmelman AC, Souza A, Pierce K, Wang TJ, Gerszten RE, Fuchs CS, Vander Heiden MG, Wolpin BM (2014) Elevation of circulating branched-chain amino acids is an early event in human pancreatic adenocarcinoma development. Nat Med 20(10):1193–1198

18. Herlidou-Même S, Constans JM, Carsin B, Olivie D, Eliat PA, Nadal-Desbarats L, Gondry C, Le Rumeur E, Idy-Peretti I, De Certaines JD (2003) MRI texture analysis on texture test objects, normal brain and intracranial tumors. Magn Reson Imaging 21:989–993
19. Colen RR, Hassan I, Elshafeey N, Zinn PO (2016) Shedding light on the 2016 World Health Organization classification of tumors of the central nervous system in the era of radiomics and radiogenomics. Magn Reson Imaging Clin N Am 24(4):741–749
20. Jamshidi N, Diehn M, Bredel M, Kuo MD (2014) Illuminating radiogenomic characteristics of glioblastoma multiforme through integration of MR imaging, messenger RNA expression, and DNA copy number variation. Radiology 270(1):1–2
21. Pope WB (2015 Feb) Genomics of brain tumor imaging. Neuroimaging Clin 25(1):105–119
22. Yamamoto S, Maki DD, Korn RL, Kuo MD (2012) Radiogenomic analysis of breast cancer using MRI: a preliminary study to define the landscape. Am J Roentgenol 199(3):654–663
23. Yamamoto S, Han W, Kim Y, Du L, Jamshidi N, Huang D, Kim JH, Kuo MD (2015) Breast cancer: radiogenomic biomarker reveals associations among dynamic contrast-enhanced MR imaging, long noncoding RNA, and metastasis. Radiology 275(2):384–392
24. Zhu Y, Li H, Guo W, Drukker K, Lan L, Giger ML, Ji Y (2015) Deciphering genomic underpinnings of quantitative MRI-based radiomic phenotypes of invasive breast carcinoma. Sci Rep. 5:17787
25. Weiss GJ, Ganeshan B, Miles KA, Campbell DH, Cheung PY, Frank S, Korn RL (2014) Noninvasive image texture analysis differentiates K-ras mutation from pan-wildtype NSCLC and is prognostic. PLoS ONE 9(7):e100244
26. Yamamoto S, Korn RL, Oklu R, Migdal C, Gotway MB, Weiss GJ, Iafrate AJ, Kim DW, Kuo MD (2014) ALK molecular phenotype in non-small cell lung cancer: CT radiogenomic characterization Radiology. 272(2):568–576
27. Hayano K, Kulkarni NM, Duda DG, Heist RS (2016) Sahani DV exploration of imaging biomarkers for predicting survival of patients with advanced non-small cell lung cancer treated with antiangiogenic chemotherapy. Am J Roentgenol 206(5):987–993
28. Ganeshan B, Panayiotou E, Burnand K, Dizdarevic S, Miles K (2012) Tumour heterogeneity in non-small cell lung carcinoma assessed by CT texture analysis: a potential marker of survival. Eur Radiol 22(4):796–802
29. Banerjee S, Wang DS, Kim HJ, Sirlin CB, Chan MG, Korn RL, Rutman AM, Siripongsakun S, Lu D, Imanbayev G, Kuo MD (2015) A computed tomography radiogenomic biomarker predicts microvascular invasion and clinical outcomes in hepatocellular carcinoma. Hepatology 62(3):792–800
30. Jiang Han-Yu, Chen Jie, Xia Chun-Chao, Cao Li-Kun, Duan Ting, Song Bin (2018) Noninvasive imaging of hepatocellular carcinoma: from diagnosis to prognosis. World J Gastroenterol 24(22):2348–2362
31. Jansen RW, van Amstel P, Martens RM, Kooi IE, Wesseling P, de Langen AJ, Menke-Van der Houven van Oordt CW, Jansen BHE, Moll AC, Dorsman JC, Castelijns JA, de Graaf P, de Jong MC (2018) Non-invasive tumor genotyping using radiogenomic biomarkers, a systematic review and oncology-wide pathway analysis. Oncotarget 9(28):20134–20155
32. Jamshidi N, Jonasch E, Zapala M, Korn RL, Aganovic L, Zhao H, Tumkur Sitaram R, Tibshirani RJ, Banerjee S, Brooks JD, Ljungberg B, Kuo MD (2015) The radiogenomic risk score: construction of a prognostic quantitative, noninvasive image-based molecular assay for renal cell carcinoma. Radiology 277(1):114–123
33. Jamshidi N, Jonasch E, Zapala M, Korn RL, Brooks JD, Ljungberg B, Kuo MD (2016) The radiogenomic risk score stratifies outcomes in a renal cell cancer phase 2 clinical trial. Eur Radiol 26(8):2798–2807
34. Matoori S, Thian Y, Koh D, Sohaib A, Larkin J, Pickering L, Gutzeit A (2017) Contrast-enhanced CT density predicts response to sunitinib therapy in metastatic renal cell carcinoma patients. Transl Oncol. 10(4):679–685

35. Sala E, Mema SE, Himoto Y, Veeraraghavan H, Brenton JD, Snyder A, Weigelt B, Vargas HA (2017) Unravelling tumour heterogeneity using next-generation imaging: radiomics, radiogenomics, and habitat imaging. Clin Radiol 72(1):3–10
36. Campbell DH, Barrett M, Ramanathan RK, Von Hoff DD, Korn RL (2014) Quantitative Textural Analysis (QTA) in CT imaging: identifying markers for genetic instability and overall survival in cohort of previously treated metastatic pancreatic cancer (mPC). Cancer Res 74(19 Supplement):1885
37. Jamshidi N, Korn R, Wu H, Donahue T, Dawson D, Bilow M, Kuo M (2011) Elucidating the radiogenomic landscape of pancreatic adenocarcinoma. In: Radiological Society of North America 2011 Scientific Assembly and Annual Meeting, Nov 26–Dec 2, 2011, Chicago IL
38. Woolsey JG, Cardenas-Rodriguez JC, Lee JY, Burkett A, Korn RL (2018) Prediction of clinical outcomes for early gastric cancer using radiomic signatures derived from the quantitative texture analysis of conventional CT scans and machine learning. J Clin Oncol 36 (suppl; abstr e16091)
39. Yoon SH, Kim YH, Lee YJ, Park J, Kim JW, Lee HS, Kim B (2016) Tumor heterogeneity in human epidermal growth factor receptor 2 (HER2)-positive advanced gastric cancer assessed by CT texture analysis: association with survival after trastuzumab treatment. PLoS ONE 11 (8):e0161278
40. Ng F, Ganeshan B, Kozarski R, Miles KA, Goh V (2013) Assessment of primary colorectal cancer heterogeneity by using whole-tumor texture analysis: contrast-enhanced CT texture as a biomarker of 5-year survival. Radiology 266(1):177–184
41. Lubner MG, Stabo N, Lubner SJ, del Rio AM, Song C, Halberg RB, Pickhardt PJ (2015) CT textural analysis of hepatic metastatic colorectal cancer: pre-treatment tumor heterogeneity correlates with pathology and clinical outcomes. Abdom Imaging 40(7):2331–2337
42. Wagner F, Hakami YA, Warnock G, Fischer G, Huellner MW, Veit-Haibach P (2017) Comparison of contrast-enhanced CT and [18F] FDG PET/CT analysis using kurtosis and skewness in patients with primary colorectal cancer. Mol Imaging Biol 19(5):795–803
43. Ganeshan B, Miles KA, Babikir S, Shortman R, Afaq A, Ardeshna KM, Groves AM, Kayani I (2017) CT-based texture analysis potentially provides prognostic information complementary to interim FDG-PET for patients with Hodgkin's and aggressive non-Hodgkin's lymphomas. Eur Radiol 27(3):1012–1020
44. Penzias G, Singanamalli A, Elliott R, Gollamudi J, Shih N, Feldman M, Stricker PD, Delprado W, Tiwari S, Böhm M, Haynes AM, Ponsky L, Fu P, Tiwari P, Viswanath S, Madabhushi A (2018) Identifying the morphologic basis for radiomic features in distinguishing different Gleason grades of prostate cancer on MRI: preliminary findings. PLoS ONE 13(8):e0200730
45. Algohary A, Viswanath S, Shiradkar R, Ghose S, Pahwa S, Moses D, Jambor I, Shnier R, Böhm M, Haynes AM, Brenner P, Delprado W, Thompson J, Pulbrock M, Purysko AS, Verma S, Ponsky L, Stricker P, Madabhushi A (2018) Radiomic features on MRI enable risk categorization of prostate cancer patients on active surveillance: preliminary findings. J Magn Reson Imaging (Epub ahead of print)
46. Shiradkar R, Ghose S, Jambor I, Taimen P, Ettala O, Purysko AS, Madabhushi A (2018 May 7) Radiomic features from pretreatment biparametric MRI predict prostate cancer biochemical recurrence: preliminary findings. J Magn Reson Imaging (Epub ahead of print)
47. Singanamalli A, Rusu M, Sparks RE, Shih NN, Ziober A, Wang LP, Tomaszewski J, Rosen M, Feldman M, Madabhushi A (2016) Identifying in vivo DCE MRI markers associated with microvessel architecture and gleason grades of prostate cancer. J Magn Reson Imaging 43(1):149–158
48. Chaddad A, Kucharczyk MJ, Niazi T (2018) Multimodal radiomic features for the predicting gleason score of prostate cancer. Cancers. 10(8):249–254
49. Hanania AN, Bantis LE, Feng ZD et al (2016) Quantitative imaging to evaluate malignant potential of IPMNs. Oncotarget 7:85776–85784

50. Song B, Zhang G, Lu H, Wang H, Zhu W, J Pickhardt P, Liang Z (2014) Volumetric texture features from higher-order images for diagnosis of colon lesions via CT colonography. Int J Comput Assist Radiol Surg 9(6):1021–1031
51. Hu Y, Liang Z, Song B, Han H, Pickhardt PJ, Zhu W, Duan C, Zhang H, Barish MA, Lascarides CE (2016) Texture feature extraction and analysis for polyp differentiation via computed tomography colonography. IEEE Trans Med Imaging 35(6):1522–1531
52. Aerts HJ (2016) The potential of radiomic-based phenotyping in precision medicine: a review. JAMA Oncol. 2(12):1636–1642
53. Lee JW, Lee SM (2018) Radiomics in oncological PET/CT: clinical applications. Nucl Med Mol Imaging 52(3):170–189
54. Sun R, Limkin EJ, Dercle L, Reuzé S, Zacharaki EI, Chargari C, Schernberg A, Dirand AS, Alexis A, Paragios N, Deutsch É, Ferté C, Robert C (2017) Computational medical imaging (radiomics) and potential for immuno-oncology. Cancer Radiother 21(6–7):648–654
55. Hanahan D, Weinberg RA (2011) Hallmarks of cancer: the next generation. Cell 144 (5):646–674
56. Srinivasan V, Shobha G (2008) Statistical texture analysis. PWASET 36:1264–1269
57. Von Hoff DD, Korn RL, Mousses S (2009) Pancreatic cancer—could it be that simple? A different context of vulnerability. Cancer Cell 16:7–8
58. Haralick RM (1979) Statistical and structural approaches to texture. Proc IEEE 67:786–804
59. Galloway M (1975) Texture analysis using gray level run lengths. Comput Graph Image Process 4(2):172–179
60. Timo O, Pietikainen M, Maenpaa T (2002) Multiresolution gray-scale and rotation invariant texture classification with local binary patterns. IEEE Trans Pattern Anal Mach Intell 24 (7):971–987
61. Drabycz S, Stockwell RG, Mitchell JR (2009) Image texture characterization using the discrete orthonormal S-transform. J digital Imaging 22(6):696–712
62. Jain AK, Farrokhnia F (1991) Unsupervised texture segmentation using Gabor filters. Pattern Recogn 24(12):1167–1186
63. Mallat SG (1989) A theory for multiresolution signal decomposition: the wavelet representation. IEEE Trans Pattern Anal Mach Intell 11(7):674–693
64. Adrien Depeursinge A, Foncubierta-Rodriguez A, Van de Ville D, Müller H (2011) Lung texture classification using locally–oriented Riesz components. In: International conference on medical image computing and computer-assisted intervention. Springer, Berlin, pp 231–238
65. Stockwell RG, Mansinha L, Lowe RP (1996) Localization of the complex spectrum: the S transform. IEEE Trans Signal Process 44(4):998–1001
66. Davnall F, Yip CSP, Ljungqvist G, Ng MSF, Sanghera B, Ganeshan B, Miles KA, Cook GJ, Goh V (2012) Assessment of tumor heterogeneity: an emerging imaging tool for clinical practice? Insights Imaging 3(6):573–589
67. Mackin D, Fave X, Zhang L, Fried D, Yang J, Taylor B, Rodriguez-Rivera E, Dodge KC, Jones AK, Court L (2015) Measuring computed tomography scanner variability of radiomics features. Invest Radiol 50:757–765
68. Balagurunathan Y, Gu Y, Wang H, Kumar V, Grove O, Hawkins S, Kim J, Goldgof DB, Hall LO, Gatenby RA, Gillies RJ (2014) Reproducibility and prognosis of quantitative features extracted from CT images. Transl Oncol 7:72–87
69. Balagurunathan Y, Kumar V, Gu Y, Kim J, Wang H, Liu Y, Goldgof D, Hall L, Korn R, Zhao B, Schwartz L, Basu S, Eschrich S, Gatenby R, Gillies R (2014) Test-retest reproducibility analysis of lung CT image features. J Digit Imaging 27:805–823
70. Bluemke DA, Cameron JL, Hruban RH, Pitt HA, Siegelman SS, Soyer P, Fishman EK (1995 Nov) Potentially resectable pancreatic adenocarcinoma: spiral CT assessment with surgical and pathologic correlation. Radiology 197(2):381–385; Ichikawa T, Haradome H, Hachiya J, Nitatori T, Ohtomo K, Kinoshita T, Araki T (1997) Pancreatic ductal

adenocarcinoma: preoperative assessment with helical CT versus dynamic MR imaging. Radiology 202:655–662
71. Sheridan MB, Ward J, Guthrie JA, Spencer JA, Craven CM, Wilson D, Guillou PJ, Robinson PJ (1999) Dynamic contrast-enhanced MR imaging and dual-phase helical CT in the preoperative assessment of suspected pancreatic cancer: a comparative study with receiver operating characteristic analysis. AJR 173:583–590
72. Fletcher JG, Wiersema MJ, Farrell MA, Fidler JL, Burgart LJ, Koyama T, Johnson CD, Stephens DH, Ward EM, Harmsen WS (2003) Pancreatic malignancy: value of arterial, pancreatic, and hepatic phase imaging with multi-detector row CT. Radiology 229:81–90
73. Bronstein YL, Loyer EM, Kaur H, Choi H, David C, DuBrow RA, Broemeling LD, Cleary KR, Charnsangavej C (2004) Detection of small pancreatic tumors with multiphasic helical CT. Am J Roentgenol 182(3):619–623
74. Tamm EP, Loyer EM, Faria SC, Evans DB, Wolff RA, Charnsangavej C (2007) Retrospective analysis of dual-phase MDCT and follow-up EUS/EUS-FNA in the diagnosis of pancreatic cancer. Abdom Imaging 32:660–667
75. Chen FM, Ni JM, Zhang ZY, Zhang L, Li B, Jiang CJ (2016) Presurgical evaluation of pancreatic cancer: a comprehensive imaging comparison of CT versus MRI. Am J Roentgenol 206:526–535
76. Ishigami K, Yoshimitsu K, Irie H, Tajima T, Asayama Y, Nishie A, Hirakawa M, Ushijima Y, Okamoto D, Nagata S, Nishihara Y, Yamaguchi K, Taketomi A, Honda H (2009) Diagnostic value of the delayed phase image for iso-attenuating pancreatic carcinomas in the pancreatic parenchymal phase on multidetector computed tomography. Eur J Radiol 69:139–146
77. Tamada T, Ito K, N Kanomata, N Sone T, Kanki A, Higaki A, Hayashida M, Yamamoto A (2016) Pancreatic adenocarcinomas without secondary signs on multiphasic multidetector CT: association with clinical and histopathologic features. Eur Radiol 26:646–655
78. Gangi S, Fletcher JG, Nathan MA, Christensen JA (2004) Time interval between abnormalities seen on CT and The clinical diagnosis of pancreatic cancer: retrospective review of CT scans obtained before diagnosis. Am J Roentgenol 182:897–903
79. Pelaez-Luna M, Takahashi N, Fletcher JG, Chari St. (2007) Resectability of presymptomatic pancreatic cancer and its relationship to onset of diabetes: a retrospective review of CT scans and fasting glucose values prior to diagnosis. Am J Gastroenterol 102:2157–2163
80. Ahn SS, Kim MJ, Choi JY, Hong HS, Yong EC, Seok JL (2009) Indicative findings of pancreatic cancer in prediagnostic CT. Eur Radiol 19:2448–2455
81. Tamada T, Ito K, Kanomata N, Sone T, Kani A, Higaki A, Hayashida M, Yamamoto A (2016) Pancreatic adenocarcinomas without secondary signs on multiphasic multidetector CT: association with clinical and histopathologic features. Eur Radiol 26:646–655
82. Gonoi W, Hayashi TY, Okuma H, Akahane M, Naki Y, Mizuno S, Tateishi R, Isayama H, Koike K, Ohtomoet K (2017) Development of pancreatic cancer is predictable well in advance using contrast enhanced CT: a case-cohort study. Eur Radiol 27(12):4941–4950
83. Bogowicz M, Riesterer O, Sabrina Stark L, Studer G, Unkelbach J, Guckenberger M, Tandini-Lang S (2017) Comparison of PET and CT radiomics for local tumor control in head and neck squanous cell carcinoma. Acta Oncol 56(11):1531–1536
84. Muraoka N, Uematsu H, Kimura H, Imamura Y, Fujiwara Y, Murakami M, Yamaguchi A, Itoh H (2008) Apparent diffusion coefficient in pancreatic cancer: characterization and histopathological correlations. J Magn Reson Imaging 27:1302–1308
85. Park MJ, Kim YK, Choi SY, Rhim H, Lee WJ, Choi D (2014) Preoperative detection of small pancreatic carcinoma: value of adding diffusion-weighted imaging to conventional MR imaging for improving confidence level. Radiology 273:433–443
86. Canto MI, Harinck F, Hruban RH, Offerhaus GJ, Poley JW, Kamel I, Nio Y, Schulick RS, Bassi C, Kluijt I, Levy MJ, Chak A, Fockens P, Goggins M, Bruno M (2013) International Cancer of Pancreas Screening (CAPS) Consortium. International Cancer of the Pancreas

Screening (CAPS) Consortium summit on the management of patients with increased risk for familial pancreatic cancer. Gut. 62(3):339–347
87. Verna EC, Hwang C, Stevens PD, Rotterdam H, Stavropoulos SN, Sy CD, Prince MA, Chung WK, Fine RL, Chabot JA, Frucht H (2010) Pancreatic cancer screening in a prospective cohort of high-risk patients: a comprehensive strategy of imaging and genetics. Clin Cancer Res 16(20):15–25
88. Vasen H, Ibrahim I, Ponce CG, Slater EP, Matthäi E, Carrato A, Earl J, Robbers K, van Mil AM, Potjer T, Bonsing BA, de Vos Tot Nederveen Cappel WH, Bergman W, Wasser M, Morreau H, Klöppel G, Schicker C, Steinkamp M, Figiel J, Esposito I, Mocci E, Vazquez-Sequeiros E, Sanjuanbenito A, Muñoz-Beltran M, Montans J, Langer P, Fendrich V, Bartsch DK (2016 June 10) Benefit of surveillance for pancreatic cancer in high-risk individuals: outcome of long-term prospective follow-up studies from three European expert centers. J Clin Oncol 34(17):2010–2019
89. Borazanci E, Haag S (2017) Chapter 6: Hereditary pancreatic cancer. In: Challenges in pancreatic pathology. ISBN 978-953-51-3116-8. Published April 26, 2017. https://www.intechopen.com/books/challenges-in-pancreatic-pathology
90. Penheiter AR, Deelchand DK, Kittelson E, Damgard SE, Murphy SJ, O'Brien DR, Bamlet WR, Passow MR, Smyrk TC, Couch FJ, Vasmatzis G, Port JD, Marjańska M, Carlson SK (2018) Identification of a pyruvate-to-lactate signature in pancreatic intraductal papillary mucinous neoplasms. Pancreatology 18(1):46–53
91. Fonseca AL, Kirkwood K, Kim MP, Mairta A, Koyay EJ (2018) Intraductal papillary mucinous neoplasms of the pancreas. Current understanding and future directions for stratification of malignancy risk. Pancreas 47:272–279
92. Hanania AN, Bantis LE, Feng ZD, Wang H, Tamm Ep, Katz MH, Maitra A, Koay KJ (2016) Quantitative imaging to evaluate malignant potential of IPMNs. Oncotarget 7:85776–85784
93. Olchowy C, Cebulski K, Tasecki M, Chaber R, Olchowy A, Kałwak K, Zaleska-Dorobisz U (2017) The presence of the gadolinium-based contrast agent depositions in the brain and symptoms of gadolinium neurotoxicity—a systematic review. PLoS ONE 12(2):e0171704
94. Eisenhauer EA, Therasse P, Bogaerts J, Schwartz LH, Sargente D, Ford R, Dancey J, Arbuckh S, Gwyther S, Mooney M, Rubinstein L, Shankar L, Dodd L, Kaplan R, Lacombe D, Verweij J (2009) New response evaluation criteria in solid tumours: revised RECIST guideline (version 1.1). Eur J Can 45:228–247
95. Von Hoff DD, Ramanathan RK, Borad MJ, Latheru DA, Smith LS, Wood TE, Korn RL, Desai N, Trieu V, Iglesias JL, Zang H, Soon-Shiong P, Shi T, Rajeshkumar NV, Maitra A, Hildalgo M (2011) Gemcitabine plus nab-paclitaxel is an active regimen in patients with advanced pancreatic cancer: a phase I/II trial. J Clin Oncol 29(34):4548–4554
96. Conroy T, Desseigne F, Ychou M, Bouche O, Adenis A, Raoul JL, Gourgou-Bourgade S, de la Fouchardiere C, Bennouna J, Bachet JB, Khemissa-Akouz F, Pere-Verge D, Delbaldo C, Assenat E, Bhauffert B, Michel P, Montoto-Grillot C, Ducreux M (2011) FOLFIRINOX versus gemcitabine for metastatic pancreas cancer. N Engl J Med 364:1817–1825
97. Korn RL, Von Hoff DD, Borad MJ, Renschler MF, McGovern D, Bay RC, Ramanathan RK (2017) 18F-FDG PET/CT response in a phase 1/2 trial of nab-paclitaxel plus gemcitabine for advanced pancreatic cancer. Cancer Imaging 17:23–33
98. Hingorani SR, Harris WP, Beck JT, Berdov BA, Wagner SA, Pshevlotsky EM, Tjulandin SA, Gladkov OA, Holcombe RF, Korn R, Natarajan R, Dycter S, Ping J, Shepard M, Devoe CE (2016) Phase Ib study of PEGylated recombinant human hyaluronidase and gemcitabine in patients with advanced pancreatic cancer. Clin Canc Res 22(12):2848–2854
99. Shukla-Dave A, Lee NY, Jansen JFA, Thaler HT, Stambuk HE, Fury MG, Patel SG, Moreira AL, Sherman E, Karimi S, Wang Y, Kraus D, Shah JP, Pfister DG, Koutcher JA (2012) Dynamic contrast-enhanced magnetic resonance imaging as a predictor of outcome in head-and-neck squamous cell carcinoma patients with nodal metastases. Int J Radiat Oncol Biol Phys 82:1837–1844

100. Baek HJ, Kim HS, Kim N, Choi YJ, Kim YJ (2012) Percent change of perfusion skewness and kurtosis: a potential imaging biomarker for early treatment response in patients with newly diagnosed glioblastomas. Radiology 264:834–843
101. Zhang H, Tan S, Chen W, Kligerman S, Kim G, D'Souza WD, Suntharalingam M, Lu W (2014) Modeling pathologic response of esophageal cancer to chemoradiation therapy using spatial-temporal 18F-FDG PET features, clinical parameters, and demographics. Int J Radiat Oncol *Biol* Phys 88:195–203
102. Amer AM, Zaid M, Chaudhury B, Elganainy D, Lee Y, Wilke CT, Cloyd J, Wang H, Maitra A, Wolff RA, Varadhachary G, Overman MJ, Lee JE, Fleming JB, Tzeng CW, Katz MH, Holliday EB, Krishnan S, Minsky BDE, Herman JM, Tanguchi CM, Das P, Crane CH, Le O, Bhosale P, Tamm EP, Koay EJ (2018) Imaging-based biomarkers: changes in the tumor interface of pancreatic ductal adenocarcinoma on computed tomography scans indicate response to cytotoxic therapy. Cancer 124(8):1701–1709
103. Johansen R, Jensen LR, Rydland J, Goa PE, Kvistad KA, Bathen TF, Axelson DE, Lundgren S, Gribbestad IS (2009) Predicting survival and early clinical response to primary chemotherapy for patients with locally advanced breast cancer using DCE-MRI. J Magn Reson Imaging 29:1300–1307
104. Yip C, Landau D, Kozarski R, Ganeshan B, Thomas R, Michaaelidou A, Goh V (2014) Primary esophageal cancer: heterogeneity as potential prognostic biomarker in patients treated with definitive chemotherapy and radiation therapy. Radiol 270(1):141–148
105. Smith AD, Gray MR, del Campo SM et al (2015) Predicting overall survival in patients with metastatic melanoma on antiangiogenic therapy and RECIST stable disease on initial posttherapy images using CT texture analysis. AJR Am J Roentgenol 205(3):W283–W293
106. Doumou G, Siddique M, Tsoumpas C, Goh V, Cook G (2015) The precision of textural analysis in 18F-FDG-PET scans of oesophageal cancer. Eur Radiol 25:2805–2812
107. Sandrasegaran K, Lin Y, Asare-Sawiri M, Taiyini T and Tann, M (2018 Aug 16) CT texture analysis of pancreatic cancer. Eur Radiol. https://doi.org/10.1007/s00330-018-5662-1 (Epub ahead of print)
108. Boranzanci EH, Guarnieri C, Haag S, Korn RL, Snyder CE, Hendrickson K, Caldwell D, Von Hoff DD (2018) Retrospective analysis of patients using olaparib (O) in pancreatic cancer (PC). J Clin Oncol 36(4) suppl:389
109. Chalkidou A, O'Doherty MJ, Marsden PK (2015) False discovery rates in PET and CT studies with texture features: a systematic review. PLoS ONE 10:e0124165
110. Bashir U, Siddique MM, Mclean E, Goh V, Cook GJ (2016) Imaging heterogeneity in lung cancer: techniques, applications, and challenges. Am J Roentgenol 207(3):534–543
111. Hatt M, Cheze-le Rest C, van Baardwijk A, Lambin P, Pradier O, Visvikis D (2011) Impact of tumor size and tracer uptake heterogeneity in 18F-FDG PET and CT non-small cell lung cancer tumor delineation. J Nucl Med 52:1690–1697
112. Hatt M, Majdoub M, Vallières M, Tixier F, Le Rest CC, Groheux D, Hindié E, Martineau A, Pradier O, Hustinx R, Perdrisot R, Guillevin R, El Naqa I, Visvikis D (2015) 18F-FDG PET uptake characterization through texture analysis: investigating the complementary nature of heterogeneity and functional tumor volume in a multi-cancer site patient cohort. J Nucl Med 56:38–44
113. Orlhac F, Soussan M, Maisonobe J-A, Garcia CA, Vanderlinden B, Buvat I (2014) Tumor texture analysis in 18F-FDG PET: relationships between texture parameters, histogram indices, standardized uptake values, metabolic volumes, and total lesion glycolysis. J Nucl Med 55:414–422
114. Velazquez ER, Parmar C, Jermoumi M, Mak RH, van Baardwijk A, Fennessy FM, Lewis JH, De Ruysscher D, Kikinis R, Lambin P, Aerts HJWL (2013) Volumetric CT-based segmentation of NSCLC using 3D-Slicer. Sci Rep. 3:3529
115. Parmar C, Rios Velazquez E, Leijenaar R, Jermoumi M, Carvalho S, Mak RH, Mitra S, Shankar BU, Kikinis R, Haibe-Kains B, Lambin P, Aerts HJWL (2014) Robust radiomics feature quantification using semiautomatic volumetric segmentation. PLoS ONE 9:e102107

116. Cheng N-M, Fang Y-H, Yen T-C (2013) The promise and limits of PET texture analysis. Ann Nucl Med 27:867–869
117. Alic L, Niessen WJ, Veenland JF (2014) Quantification of heterogeneity as a biomarker in tumor imaging: a systematic review. PLoS ONE 9:e110300
118. Tixier F, Hatt M, Le Rest CC, Le Pogam A, Corcos L, Visvikis D (2012) Reproducibility of Tumor uptake heterogeneity characterization through textural feature analysis in 18F-FDG PET. J Nucl Med 53:693–700
119. Leijenaar RTH, Carvalho S, Velazquez ER, van Elmpt WJC, Parmar C, Hoekstra OS, Hoekstra CJ, Boellaard R, Dekker ALAJ, Gillies RJ, Aerts HJWL, Lambin P (2013) Stability of FDG-PET radiomics features: an integrated analysis of test-retest and inter-observer variability. Acta Oncol 52:1391–1397
120. Zhou Y, Xie L, Fishman EK (2017) Deep supervision for pancreatic cyst segmentation in abdominal CT scans. arXiv:1706.073462017. Available at: https://arxiv.org/abs/1706.07346. Accessed Sept 29, 2017

Single-Cell Sequencing in Precision Medicine

9

Julia E. Wiedmeier, Pawan Noel, Wei Lin, Daniel D. Von Hoff and Haiyong Han

Contents

J. E. Wiedmeier · D. D. Von Hoff
Mayo Clinic, Scottsdale, AZ, USA

P. Noel · W. Lin · D. D. Von Hoff · H. Han (✉)
Molecular Medicine Division, Translational Genomics Research Institute, Phoenix, AZ, USA
e-mail: hhan@tgen.org

D. D. Von Hoff and H. Han (eds.), *Precision Medicine in Cancer Therapy*,
Cancer Treatment and Research 178, https://doi.org/10.1007/978-3-030-16391-4_9

9.1 Background

The advent of next-generation sequencing (NGS) platforms made it possible to sequence DNA more efficiently and economically than Sanger sequencing. In addition, the application of NGS in cancer genomics allowed for a deeper understanding of the underlying genetics and pathogenesis of cancer. The human body is composed of trillions of cells that belong to approximately 200 different cell types; however, individual cells from defined cell types are diverse with unique expression profiles [1]. Many cell types/subtypes have few reliable markers that can be used for purification which is in part due to the fact that even cell types with well-established markers contain diversity [1]. Standard techniques for cancer analysis involve averaging signals from mixed populations of cells, which may mask or hide rare/small tumor clones and subclones that contribute to cell diversity [2]. However, with the use of single-cell genomics, the underlying genetics, expression levels, and epigenetics of every gene in the genome can now be analyzed across thousands of individual cells.

The first report of RNA transcriptome sequencing of single-cell mammalian cells occurred in 2009, and the first report of single human cancer cell DNA genome sequencing occurred in 2011 [2, 3]. Since that time, studies on single-cell exome and whole genome sequencing in varying types of cancers including renal, myeloproliferative, colon, lung, glioblastoma, breast, and prostate have been conducted [4–11]. The original single-cell sequencing method combined flow sorting, whole genome amplification, and NGS to generate genomewide datasets from single cancer cells; however, it had only $\sim 10\%$ physical coverage of a single cell's genome, sufficient for measuring large-scale copy number changes, but insufficient for resolving mutations at base-pair resolution [2]. Since that time, several other methods have been developed that can achieve high coverage (>90%) from single mammalian cells.

The data now available by single-cell sequencing has revolutionized cancer cell biology. The underlying mechanisms of how tumor and clonal diversity contribute to cancer biological processes remain largely unknown. Intratumor heterogeneity, clonal evolution, underlying mechanisms of tissue invasion, metastasis, and response to cancer-related therapies can potentially be elucidated by investigating molecular signatures at the single-cell level (Fig. 9.1). Tumor diversity is impacted by selection pressures, which can impact the underlying genetics of a cancer cell population. Examples of selection pressures include effects of the immune system, hypoxia, nutrient deprivation, geographical barriers, pH changes, and chemotherapy [2]. Understanding the underlying genetics of intratumor heterogeneity at the single-cell level has the potential to reveal cancer therapy resistance mechanisms that are lost at the bulk level. Single-cell tumor phylogenic evolutionary trees have the potential to reveal driver mutations which can be used for targeted cancer therapies for those small populations of cells that harbor resistant mutations after treatment [12].

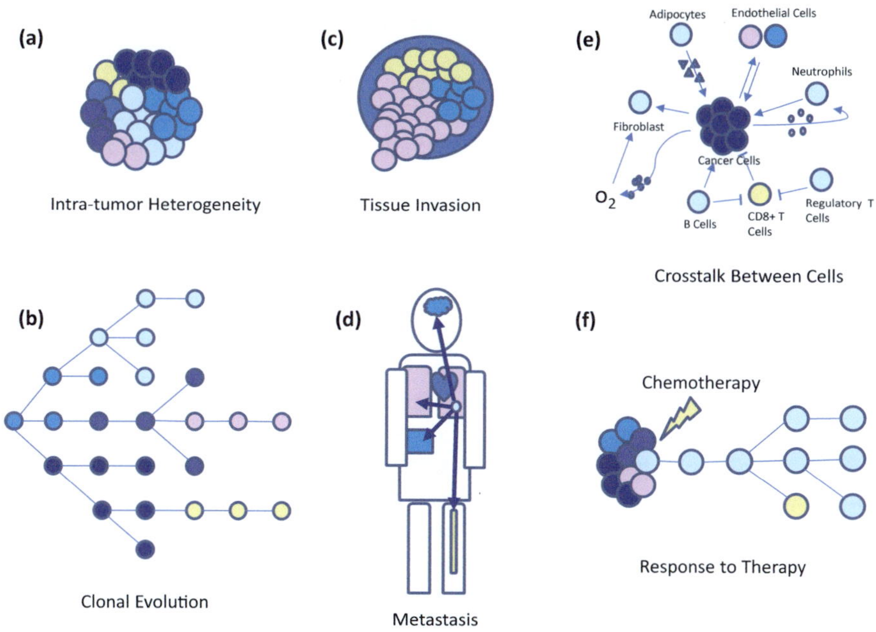

Fig. 9.1 Applications of single-cell sequencing. Mechanisms behind **a** Intratumor heterogeneity, where different tumor cells show distinct genotypic and phenotypic variability (represented by different colored cells), **b** clonal evolution, or genetic diversification and clonal selection where different colored cells represent genetic changes, **c** tissue invasion, where mutant cells invade adjacent tissues (pink cells) with the potential to **d** travel to different sites, or metastasis, **e** crosstalk between cells with newer technologies, and **f** response to cancer-related therapies and subsequent clonal evolution can be elucidated by investigating the molecular signature at the single-cell level

Identification of cancer therapy resistance mechanisms at the single-cell level may also reveal novel mutations after induction of therapeutic agents (which generate clonal and subclonal populations of cells). In fact, NGS studies on single-cell mutations that drive tumorigenesis have revealed that resistance mutations vary from tumor to tumor [13]. Single-cell sequencing also has the potential to illuminate the mechanisms behind metastatic dissemination. For instance, several groups have used circulating tumor cells (CTCs) to study genomic and transcriptomic data from metastatic colon cancer, lung adenocarcinoma, and melanoma [2].

Bulk tumor gene expression studies are composites of transcriptional changes of heterogeneous cell populations; however, analysis of tumor cell expression at the single-cell level expands *average* tumor expression profiles of specific cell types, including non-malignant stromal, immune, and tissue-specific cells. In addition, single-cell transcriptomics aids in the detection of novel variants after treatments that may potentially drive drug resistance or serve as biomarkers of therapeutic success [14]. Furthermore, single-cell sequencing can detect low abundance of expression and/or novel RNA variants that are not detectable in bulk cell populations.

9.2 Single-Cell Sequencing Modalities

9.2.1 Sample Type and Preparation

Current single-cell technologies assay a single cell's gene expression, DNA variation, epigenetic state, and nuclear structure (see Table 9.1). In order to analyze genomics at the single-cell level, cells need to be isolated from extracellular matrix and cell–cell adhesion for downstream processes. One of the major limitations of single-cell sequencing from solid tissues includes unbiased disaggregating of the tissue into a suspension of single cells [15]. This is important as preferential processing or lysis of one cell type over another may skew data generation and thus analysis of results.

Single cells can be obtained from virtually any tissue, and current research focuses on circulating blood cancer cells, solid tumors, or circulating tumor cells (CTCs). Single cells from solid tumors can be obtained either following surgical removal, sampling/biopsy of the primary tumor or other organs with overt metastasis, or bone marrow aspiration. Solid tumors, especially in the invasive metastatic stages, are also known to shed cells into systemic circulation. These cells in the patient's blood stream are known as circulating tumor cells (CTCs), and those that disseminate to distant organs are termed disseminated tumor cells (DTCs).

Different methods for isolating single cells of interest from a suspension have been developed. Early studies used manual methods of cell isolation, using specialized pipettes or micromanipulation devices to isolate single cells [17]. This method of single-cell isolation has low throughput but can be used when a small number of cells are to be analyzed [22]. Other methods include fluorescence-activated cell sorting (FACS), magnetic-activated cell sorting (MACS), laser capture microdissection (LCM), and microfluidics, all of which can generally be used for larger numbers of cells. Microfluidics is a common method of single-cell isolation and allows for high throughput investigation of complex cellular systems using nanoliters of material. Microfluidics technologies isolate and encapsulate single cells in reaction chambers or droplets followed by standardized and automated nanoliter reactions, including barcoded sequence library prep for RNA and DNA sequencing. Commercially available microfluidic devices include Fluidigm C1 system, the 10× Genomics Chromium, and Illumina Biorad SureCell system [23].

9.2.2 Single-Cell DNA Sequencing

Whole genome amplification (WGA) followed by DNA sequencing identifies the underlying genetics and mutation frequencies of a single cell. Various methods for DNA whole genome amplification (WGA) at the single-cell level are available (multiple displacement amplification (MDA), PCR, or combination of both, see Table 9.1). These methods can now achieve >90% coverage of a single-cell

Table 9.1 Comparison of single-cell sequencing modalities

Single-cell sequencing modality	Technique	Description	Strengths	Weaknesses	Reference
DNA	Nuc-Seq Single nucleus exome sequencing (SNES)	Combines flow sorting of single nuclei)	High coverage data High detection efficiencies for single-nucleotide variants and indels Suitable for analyzing highly proliferative cells Reduced cost	Not suitable for analyzing normal or slow cell division Less genomic coverage than whole genome sequencing Time limited	Leung et al. [16]
	DNA seq Whole genome amplification approaches	Multiple genome amplification (MDA) Multiple-annealing, looping-based amplification-based cycle method (MALBAC)	High coverage Can generate genomic changes based on copy number alterations, structural variants, or single-nucleotide mutations	Artifacts Poor physical coverage High error rates	Van Loo and Voet [17] Trapnell [15] Navin [2]
RNA	RNA seq	MDA based or in vitro transcription based amplification of reverse transcribed single-cell mRNA (see above)	Most widely used and therefore many single-cell genomic assays available Inter- and intra-subclonal differences in expressed genes and expression level	Non-reliable amplification and deletion of transcripts expressed <10 copies/cell Only selectively amplify the polyA RNAs of a cell—bias in transcript coverage (3′ UTR)	Van Loo and Voet [17] Trapnell [15] Navin [2]

(continued)

Table 9.1 (continued)

Single-cell sequencing modality	Technique	Description	Strengths	Weaknesses	Reference
DNA/ RNA	Microfluidics: DropSeq (RNA) Compartmented droplet multiple displacement amplification (cd-MDA) (16)	Droplets containing individual cells with a barcoded RNA capture bead Bead contains cell identification and unique molecular identifier (UMI) Reverse transcription the bead oligonucleotides as templates Pool cDNA for library construction and subsequent sequencing	Can integrate labor-intensive experimental WGA processes in a single, closed device Improved reaction efficiency and detection sensitivity at the single-molecule level	Doublets can increasing sequencing depth leads to plateau Expensive	Hosokawa et al. [18] Islam et al. [19]
Epigenetic	ATAC-seq	Uses engineered transposase to construct sequencing library from accessible DNA elements	Can take place within intact nuclei	Integration w/mutational and transcriptome analysis is challenging	Cusanovic et al. [20]
	Single-cell Hi-C	Active chromatin domains in cell nuclei localize to the surface of spatial chromosome territories Measures physical proximity between sites in the genome in three dimensions	Can take place within intact nuclei	Integration with mutational and transcriptome analysis is challenging	Cusanovic et al. [20] Buenrostro et al. [21]

genome, and mutations can be detected at a single base-pair resolution [17, 2]. Technical challenges remain, however, including effective isolation and lysis of single cells, uniform amplification of whole genome, quality assessment of single-cell amplified genomes, sequencing library preparation, and data analysis [18].

Detection of point mutations or base substitutions in single cells has to be discriminated from polymerase base infidelities and sequencing errors. Such errors can occur during the WGA process, including allelic dropout (one allele is not amplified), transcripts can be over or under amplified, false-positive errors due to the infidelity of the DNA polymerase, and uneven amplification [2, 12]. By nature of the amplification process using DNA polymerases, errors that occur in the initial rounds of amplification are then inherited by all subsequent molecules [17]. Single-cell genomewide DNA sequencing is more challenging than single-cell transcriptomics due to the fact that there is simply less template available for single-cell genomics with DNA sequencing. Whereas single cells contain thousands of copies of each mRNA molecule, there are only two copies of each chromosome (or gene for that matter), and therefore only two template DNA molecules for WGA reactions.

9.2.3 Single-Cell RNA Sequencing

Single-cell RNA sequencing essentially reveals the transcriptional status at the single-cell level. Whole transcriptome sequencing, or RNA seq, where exclusively messenger RNA is assayed from single cells, is the most widely used method of single-cell analysis [24, 17, 25, 26]. It measures global gene expression by reverse transcription of mRNA into cDNA, and downstream sequencing libraries are made of hundreds to thousands of individual cells (Fig. 9.2). Gene expression is measured directly by counting the number of reads or the unique molecular index (UMI) that originate from each gene in a single cell. RNA seq of single cells achieves greater sequencing resolution than cell populations at the cost of less coverage [14]. The challenge with single-cell transcriptomics, as with most of the sequencing methods, is the "noise" generated from such experiments [27, 28, 12]. For example, biological variation is derived from genetic, epigenetic, environmental, and cellular factors. Technical noise can be introduced in the course of processing from sample handling, cell isolation, reverse transcription, cDNA amplification, sequencing, and analysis.

New techniques and methods are continuously been developed and reformed to limit the aforementioned challenges [29]. A crucial step of single-cell RNA seq is the unbiased amplification of cDNA before sequencing [27, 30, 28]. The use of unique molecular identifiers (UMIs), which bar codes each molecule, allows a robust quantification by intercepting amplification. Cell throughput is high, and the use of unique molecular identifiers to barcode individual transcripts also helps distinguish heterogeneous gene expression differences [19]. Microfluidics uses a process of capturing cells within nanofluidic chambers and has considerably

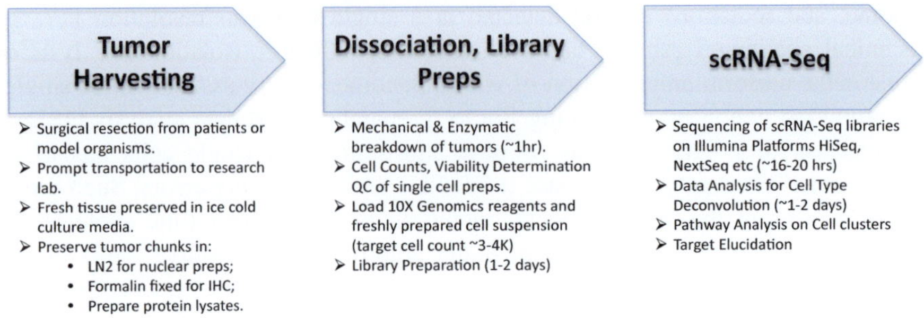

Fig. 9.2 Workflow of the single-cell RNA sequencing process. Starting from harvesting tumors from patients or model organisms, fresh tissues are rapidly broken down into single cells, which are the input material for the 10× Genomics pipeline to generate sequencing libraries from single cells. Finally, the libraries are sequenced and data is analyzed to elucidate the cellular heterogeneity and biology of individual tumors

improved sensitivity for mutation detection by minimizing allelic dropouts [19, 12]. Drawbacks include reduced sensitivity such that only the 10–20% of the most abundant transcripts can be quantitated. In addition, reliable amplification and deletion of transcripts expressed at less than 10 copies per cell is a challenge and can lead to inaccurate quantification of low abundancy transcripts [27, 28, 2]. Doublets, or cells that share the same UMI and bar codes, can also occur during sample processing; therefore, it is important to validate true single-cell capture before subsequent analysis.

9.2.4 Single-Cell Epigenetic Analysis

Whereas transcriptomics can be described as tracking "output" signals of a given genetic locus, such as a protein encoding gene, the analysis of chromatin, and epigenetic changes may be thought of as tracking the "input" signals of the locus in question (Wills 2015). With advances in technology, it is now easier to probe epigenetic phenomenon at the single-cell level including single-cell analysis of DNA accessibility, methylation status, histone modifications, and chromosome conformation by bisulfite sequencing, DNAase I hypersensitivity sequencing, ATAC-seq, and single-cell Hi-C, with the latter methods being the most developed for single-cell sequencing approaches [21, 31, 32, 33, 34, 35]. Challenges associated with these techniques are very similar to those of single-cell DNA sequencing.

Whole genome bisulfite sequencing assays identify DNA methylation (CpG islands). Chromatin immunoprecipitation sequencing (ChIP-seq) has yet to be adapted for single-cell sequencing; however, a method termed single-cell Hi-C analyzes active chromatin domains in cell nuclei [35]. This method measures proximity between sites in the genome in three dimensions, producing a "contact map" that can be used to identify looping interactions between regulatory elements and gene loci [33, 35, 15]. Single cell assays for transposase-accessible chromatin with sequencing (ATAC-seq) is another method used to identify open chromatin regions which, in cancer cells, are often associated with oncogene expression and represent sites with increased vulnerability to mutagenic assault [20].

9.2.5 Other Single-Cell Analysis Techniques

One weakness of current single-cell techniques is that it requires analysis of single cells in suspension, which does not capture information pertaining to cell-to-cell interactions [2, 12]. Moreover, tumor clones evolve dynamically in space and time, and single-cell samples from an individual tumor may reveal mutations that are clonally dominant but may not be apparent in other regions of the tumor [2]. This has been partially overcome by spatiotemporal dynamics (discussed further below) which can be obtained by serial sampling of the same patient and provides information about evolution of a tumor through time (this is easier for liquid vs. solid tumors), multiple anatomically distinct biopsies for intratumor heterogeneity, in situ sequencing and imaging techniques for spatial resolution, or laser capture microdissection, which aids with information lost with cell-to-cell interactions [12].

Finally, new methods that integrate different single-cell genomic approaches and functional assays have recently been developed and include simultaneously measuring two or more modalities, whether it be genome and transcriptome, transcriptome and methylome, or RNA and protein [36, 17]. The ultimate goal of linking phenotypes of cells and their genotypes includes validation of gene expression and further development of precision medicine [36]. There are many different approaches available, some of which include gDNA-mRNA sequencing (DR-seq), genome and transcriptome sequencing (G&T-seq), single-cell DNA methylation analysis through bisulfite sequencing (scBS-seq) and reduced representation bisulfite sequencing (scRRBS-seq), as well as single-cell methylome and transcriptome sequencing (scTrio-seq) [37]. When extracting multiple "omic" datasets from individual cells, there are similar quality compromises as discussed previously [12].

9.3 Data Analysis

Single-cell measurements preserve crucial information that is lost in bulk assays. Statistical and computational methods are critical to extract meaningful information from the data [36]. Single-cell analysis is based on the analysis of a cell modality (genetic variations, cell expression profile, changes in chromatin conformation, etc.), compared with some critical threshold. This threshold depends on the variability that exists in the assay as well as biological variability [15]. Statistical models can account for this variability.

Whole genome and whole transcriptome amplification as well as sequencing data are more difficult to analyze at the single-cell level than in bulk experiments [38, 39, 40, 1]. Bulk experiments have dozens of samples, and genome measurements cannot distinguish between fluctuations due to changes in gene regulation versus shifts in the ratio of different cell types. For single-cell genome amplification experiments, DNA is extracted from millions of cells, with intermixed sequences from different tumor clones, as well as normal cells [17]. Single-cell expression measurements can be variable; therefore, separating technical variability from biological variability is essential. Computational methods can help determine which mutations are clonal (present in all tumor cells) and which are subclonal. Point mutations and copy number data can be further analyzed with bioinformatics algorithms, and phylogenetic trees of different tumor subclones can be inferred. Analyzing expression levels in properly grouped subpopulations of cells allows a more accurate measurement of expression among different cell subpopulations [41, 15].

One of the major tasks of single-cell RNA seq data analysis is the resolution of cellular heterogeneity (Fig. 9.3). Most pathological samples such as tumor tissues consist of multiple cell types. Tumor tissues usually contain primary tumor cells, stromal cells, endothelial cells, and immune cells recruited from the peripheral blood and lymphatic organs. They are derived from different cellular lineages and play different roles in the tumor initiation, progression, and metastasis, which makes a tumor sample very complex and difficult to investigate. Before looking deeper into the tumor clonal variation, the tumor and its microenvironment should be resolved first. By identifying signature genes expressed in each cell type, one can further delineate the states of different cell types.

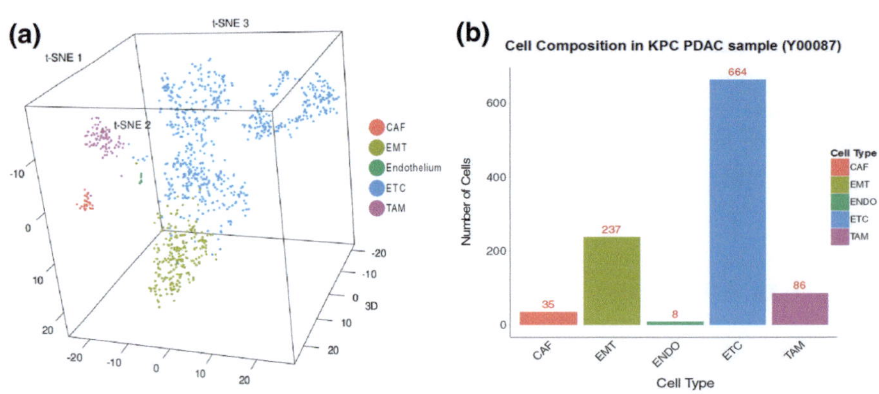

Fig. 9.3 Single-cell RNA sequencing data analysis. **a** A representative example of a three-dimensional tSNE rendering of scRNA seq data for a mouse pancreatic tumor is shown. Each dot depicts a single cell, and colored clusters represent distinct cell types identified in the tumor. **b** Quantification of each individual cell type is shown with five different most commonly observed cell types identified in this tumor. CAF: cancer-associated fibroblasts; EMT: tumor cells undergoing epithelial to mesenchymal transition; ENDO: endothelial cells; ETC: epithelial tumor cells; TAM: tumor-associated macrophages

Understanding the cellular composition and tumor evolution can facilitate the evaluation of the tumor state and aid treatment decisions. Given the assumption that biological variability is larger than the technical variability, it is generally believed that similar cell types will cluster together by the cell type-specific feature expressions. The dynamic change of a specific cell type from one state to another sometimes could also be captured by such metric, though it is very challenging.

The calculation of the similarity between cells is usually based on multiple gene expression features. The relative position of these cells in a high-dimensional space is not easy to comprehend. Principal components analysis (PCA) is one of the most commonly used algorithms for reducing the dimensionality of data. Nonetheless, for single-cell RNA seq data, the first two to three components of PCA analysis cover a very small proportion of variance and therefore make the clustering effect less representative than for those other gene expression datasets [42]. A more advanced, nonlinear dimensionality reduction algorithm called t-Distributed Stochastic Neighbor Embedding, or t-SNE [42], has been proposed to explore high-dimensional single-cell RNA seq data. t-SNE itself does not necessarily define the similarity metric between cells but makes it visualizable in low-dimensional space. This algorithm is being widely used in part because it can be adapted to many visualization tools that are easily understood and interpreted by non-computational biologists (Fig. 9.3). The relationships across cell types can be inferred by the high-dimensional calculation and explored by the low-dimensional visualization.

The single-cell clustering and trajectory method of analysis can be used to define cell types and stable cell states. For example, clustering of three different cell types from one tumor by gene expression can group single cells into those of invasive tumor cells, noninvasive tumor cells, and stromal cells. When clustering, or grouping cells by gene expression, each cell represents a point in space based on expression of genes (approximately 30,000 genes). Clustering is based on the measured distances between points, and cells are grouped based on mutual proximity.

Besides resolving the cellular composition of heterogeneous tissues, single-cell studies also aim to characterize genes in such a way so that presumptions can be made of where a cell is in time and what drives a cell to transition from one state to another [15]. Using current methods, cells are analyzed at a particular state and time. The intact sample is destroyed by, for example, cell lysis (in the case of RNA seq and qRT-PCR) or cell fixation (in the case of FISH). Time series experiments extrapolate cell transition states through time; however, they misconstrue results by averaging cell expression as they proceed through a biological process in unsynchronized manner [43, 15]. Any particular sample at a given time-point contains cells of varying stages of cell growth and transition, reflecting the underlying dynamics of transitional state relevant genes. Single-cell analysis can define genes that are differentially expressed during these transitional states. In order to recover true signal of relevant expression, cells are re-ordered in something called "pseudotime" according to biological progress (for example, percent cells differentiated instead of time). Two algorithms are currently available based on pseudotime,

Wanderlust and Monocele, both of which attempt to define those genes responsible for cell transition [43, 15].

9.4 Application of Single-Cell Analysis in Precision Cancer Therapy

The translational application of single-cell sequencing in precision cancer therapy has the potential to improve cancer diagnostics, prognostics, targeted therapy, early detection, and noninvasive monitoring [2]. It is now technically and economically feasible to sequence single-cell DNA and RNA. Single-cell sequencing allows highly sensitive detection of rare mutations and cell-specific gene expression profiles. This method can identify rare tumor tissue variants that have the potential to drive drug resistance or serve as biomarkers of therapeutic success and ultimately advancing cancer genomics [14].

The importance of single-cell techniques in the clinical setting can be illustrated in tumor sampling. A single sample from a tumor does not represent the tumor as a whole. Spatially separate samples from a single tumor (or elsewhere in the body from metastasis) is composed of varying proportions of cell types and/or diverse underlying genetic and epigenetic makeup, otherwise known as tumor heterogeneity. Greater tumor heterogeneity may predict poorer response to therapy, higher probability of metastasis, or poor overall survival [2]. Identification of founder mutations, constructed from tumor phylogenetic trees, may aid in prediction of response to treatment.

Sequencing at the single-cell level can detect low abundance mutations, facilitating the identification of drivers of drug resistance. Drug resistance dynamics have been previously modeled in metastatic breast cancer cell line using RNA seq technology [14]. When metastatic breast cancer cells were treated with paclitaxel, stressed cells arrest and die, whereas those rare drug-tolerant cells resume proliferation and their clones expand. The ability to profile both the genome and transcriptome of the same cells has potential to elucidate heterogeneity at the genome, epigenome, transcriptome level.

Drug development is a lengthy and expensive endeavor with a high failure rate [10]. Drug development includes many steps: identification of drug targets, candidates, assessing drug resistance, drug toxicity, and pharmacokinetics. Many drugs emerge from preclinical studies only to fail in clinical trials. NGS has identified new target candidates for drug development. Single-cell sequencing in drug development expands on bulk genomic data by offering a more thorough and comprehensive picture on the underlying genetics, epigenetics, and transcriptomics of responders versus non-responders at an individual cell level. This ultimately allows for improved efficiency, accuracy, and identification. Applications of single-cell sequencing in drug development include identification of drug candidates and drug targets, drug resistance, and drug responses and toxicities [10].

Single-cell sequencing has shown potential to advance early detection and noninvasive monitoring. This concept is being elucidated by studies on circulating tumor cells (CTC), ultimately providing insight on metastatic dissemination (Navin 2015). CTC studies also aid in understanding evolution of the genome in early stages of cancer by identifying clones (and their underlying genetics, transcriptomics, etc.) that invade surrounding tissue.

Algorithms like Wanderlust and Monocle allows one to reconstruct transcriptional dynamics of development, differentiation, and/or clonal evolution from single-cell transcriptome data. Given such insight, we look forward to single-cell sequencing's ability to identify signature transcriptions of tumor states, which will strongly facilitate treatment decisions and healthcare strategies for patients.

9.5 Perspectives

Single-cell sequencing will transform cancer research over the coming years as even initial experiments have revolutionized our current understanding of gene regulation and disease. Indeed, the data available with single-cell techniques has never been possible before. Since the initial single-cell sequencing experiments, there have been many technical and experimental advances and the field continues to advance at a remarkable speed.

Drawbacks to single-cell sequencing include loss of tumor characteristics including spatial information, intratumor heterogeneity, and important cell-to-cell interactions. This issue stems from the fact that single-cell preparation and isolation capture techniques require intact single cells to be dissociated from fresh tissues. Most single cells are derived from a biopsy or small piece of tissue; therefore, single-cell sequencing may not accurately represent the underlying genome/transcriptome of the original tumor. Even the process of dissociating single cells from tissues may alter the cells and their underlying gene expression. In addition, microfluidic devices lose entire cell populations and may have bias for certain cells sizes, which, along with inherent weaknesses of selective amplification, can skew results.

With increasing amounts of complex data generated by single-cell sequencing techniques, there exists the dilemma of accurate interpretation and what to do with the sheer quantity of data generated. While many tools for analysis have been developed, there is a need for further analytic improvement in filtering noise and scalability [43]. Some of the above issues, particularly spatial information, can be overcome by single-cell analysis techniques, but this highlights the need for skilled bioinformaticians to accurately analyze the data. In addition, there is currently no universal analysis technique available, allowing for potentially more bias. Another challenge that limits the wide application of whole genome single-cell sequencing in the research and clinical settings is its relatively high cost compared to other bulk sequencing techniques. For example, a single-cell RNA seq experiment using the Chromium System from 10× Genomics currently costs at least 10 times higher than a typical bulk whole genome RNA seq experiment. However, new and cheaper techniques are being developed which will greatly improve the accessibility of the technology so as time goes on.

Emerging new technologies that combine single-cell sequencing with other techniques acquire even deeper and richer genomic/biological information of cells and tissues. Spatial transcriptomics, which integrates single-cell RNA seq with the in situ hybridization (ISH), is one of such new technologies. It analyzes intact tissue sections on slides and does not require the need for cell isolation from tissue. The process involves the placement of histological sections on slides that contain reverse transcription primers with unique positional bar codes and subsequent placement of millions of oligonucleotides in micrometer subsections. This is followed by reverse transcription [23]. This method has the potential to overcome the loss of spatial information, intratumor heterogeneity, and the potential alteration of cells during the process of dissociation. Application of such technologies in clinical samples could potentially revolutionize patient care.

Acknowledgements We would like to thank the members of the Pancreatic Cancer Research Laboratory at the Translational Genomics Research Institute for their technical support and insightful discussions during the preparation of this manuscript. The work was supported in part by the Stand Up to Cancer—Cancer Research UK—Lustgarten Foundation (SU2C-CRUK-Lustgarten) Dream Team Translational Research Grant, a Program of the Entertainment Industry Foundation, and the National Foundation for Cancer Research (NFCR).

References

1. Trapnell C, Cacchiarelli D, Grimsby J et al (2014) The dynamics and regulators of cell fate decisions are revealed by pseudotemporal ordering of single cells. Nat Biotechnol 32:381. https://doi.org/10.1038/nbt.2859
2. Navin NE (2015) The first five years of single-cell cancer genomics and beyond. Genome Res 25(10):1499–507. https://doi.org/10.1101/gr.191098.115. PubMed MID: 26430160
3. Tang F, Barbacioru C, Wang Y et al (2009) mRNA-Seq whole-transcriptome analysis of a single cell. Nat Methods 6:377. https://doi.org/10.1038/nmeth.1315
4. Aceto N, Bardia A, Miyamoto DT et al (2014) Circulating tumor cell clusters are oligoclonal precursors of breast cancer metastasis. Cell 158(5):1110–1122. https://doi.org/10.1016/j.cell.2014.07.01
5. Heitzer E, Auer M, Gasch C et al (2013) Complex tumor genomes inferred from single circulating tumor cells by array-CGH and next-generation sequencing. Cancer Res 73 (10):2965 LP–2975. http://cancerres.aacrjournals.org/content/73/10/2965.abstract
6. Lohr JG, Adalsteinsson VA, Cibulskis K et al (2014) Whole-exome sequencing of circulating tumor cells provides a window into metastatic prostate cancer. Nat Biotechnol 32:479. https://doi.org/10.1038/nbt.2892
7. Ni X, Zhuo M, Su Z et al (2013) Reproducible copy number variation patterns among single circulating tumor cells of lung cancer patients. Proc Natl Acad Sci 110(52):21083 LP–21088. http://www.pnas.org/content/110/52/21083.abstract
8. Patel AP, Tirosh I, Trombetta JJ et al (2014) Single-cell RNA-seq highlights intratumoral heterogeneity in primary glioblastoma. Science (80-), 344(6190):1396–1401
9. Wang Y, Waters J, Leung ML et al (2014) Clonal evolution in breast cancer revealed by single nucleus genome sequencing. Nature 512:155. https://doi.org/10.1038/nature13600

10. Xu X, Hou Y, Yin X et al (2012) Single-cell exome sequencing reveals single-nucleotide mutation characteristics of a kidney tumor. Cell 148(5):886–895. https://doi.org/10.1016/j.cell.2012.02.025
11. Zong C, Lu S, Chapman AR, Xie XS (2012) Genome-wide detection of single-nucleotide and copy-number variations of a single human cell. Science (80-), 338(6114):1622 LP–1626. http://science.sciencemag.org/content/338/6114/1622.abstract
12. Wills QF, Mead AJ (2015) Application of single-cell genomics in cancer: promise and challenges. Hum Mol Genet 15:24(R1):R74–84. https://doi.org/10.1093/hmg/ddv235. PubMed PMID: 26113645
13. Kan Z, Jaiswal BS, Stinson J et al (2010) Diverse somatic mutation patterns and pathway alterations in human cancers. Nature 466:869. https://doi.org/10.1038/nature09208
14. Lee M-CW, Lopez-Diaz FJ, Khan SY et al (2014) Single-cell analyses of transcriptional heterogeneity during drug tolerance transition in cancer cells by RNA sequencing. Proc Natl Acad Sci 111(44):E4726–E4735. https://doi.org/10.1073/pnas.1404656111
15. Trapnell C (2015) Defining cell types and states with single-cell genomics. Genome Res 25 (10):1491–1498. https://doi.org/10.1101/gr.190595.115
16. Leung ML, Wang Y, Waters J, Navin NE (2015) SNES: single nucleus exome sequencing. Genome Biol 16(1):55. https://doi.org/10.1186/s13059-015-0616-2
17. Van Loo P, Voet T (2014) Single cell analysis of cancer genomes. Curr Opin Genet Dev 24:82–91. https://doi.org/10.1016/j.gde.2013.12.004
18. Hosokawa M, Nishikawa Y, Kogawa M, Takeyama H (2017) Massively parallel whole genome amplification for single-cell sequencing using droplet microfluidics. Sci Rep 7(1):1–12. https://doi.org/10.1038/s41598-017-05436-4
19. Islam S, Zeisel A, Joost S et al (2013) Quantitative single-cell RNA-seq with unique molecular identifiers. Nat Methods 11:163. https://doi.org/10.1038/nmeth.2772
20. Cusanovich DA, Daza R, Adey A et al (2015) Multiplex single-cell profiling of chromatin accessibility by combinatorial cellular indexing. Science (80-), 348(6237):910 LP–914. http://science.sciencemag.org/content/348/6237/910.abstract
21. Buenrostro JD, Giresi PG, Zaba LC, Chang HY, Greenleaf WJ (2013) Transposition of native chromatin for fast and sensitive epigenomic profiling of open chromatin, DNA-binding proteins and nucleosome position. Nat Methods 10:1213. https://doi.org/10.1038/nmeth.2688
22. Hu P, Zhang W, Xin H, Deng G (2016) Single cell isolation and analysis. Front Cell Dev Biol 4(116). https://doi.org/10.3389/fcell.2016.00116
23. Hedlund E, Deng Q (2018) Single-cell RNA sequencing: technical advancements and biological applications. Mol Aspects Med 59:36–46
24. Cloonan N, Forrest ARR, Kolle G et al (2008) Stem cell transcriptome profiling via massive-scale mRNA sequencing. Nat Methods 5:613. https://doi.org/10.1038/nmeth.1223
25. Mortazavi A, Williams BA, McCue K, Schaeffer L, Wold B (2008) Mapping and quantifying mammalian transcriptomes by RNA-Seq. Nat Methods 5:621. https://doi.org/10.1038/nmeth.1226
26. Nagalakshmi U, Wang Z, Waern K et al (2008) The transcriptional landscape of the yeast genome defined by RNA sequencing. Science (80-). 320(5881):1344 LP–1349. http://science.sciencemag.org/content/320/5881/1344.abstract
27. Kolodziejczyk AA, Kim JK, Svensson V, Marioni JC, Teichmann SA (2015) The technology and biology of single-cell RNA sequencing. Mol Cell 58(4):610–620. https://doi.org/10.1016/j.molcel.2015.04.005
28. Stegle O, Teichmann SA, Marioni JC (2015) Computational and analytical challenges in single-cell transcriptomics. Nat Rev Genet 16:133. https://doi.org/10.1038/nrg3833
29. Saliba AE, Westermann AJ, Gorski SA, Vogel J (2014) Single-cell RNA-seq: advances and future challenges. Nucleic Acids Res 42(14):8845–8860. https://doi.org/10.1093/nar/gku555
30. Marr C, Zhou JX, Huang S (2016) Single-cell gene expression profiling and cell state dynamics: collecting data, correlating data points and connecting the dots. bioRxi, 44743. https://doi.org/10.1101/044743

31. Buenrostro JD, Wu B, Litzenburger UM et al (2015) Single-cell chromatin accessibility reveals principles of regulatory variation. Nature 523:486. https://doi.org/10.1038/nature14590
32. Guo H, Zhu P, Wu X, Li X, Wen L, Tang F (2013) Single-cell methylome landscapes of mouse embryonic stem cells and early embryos analyzed using reduced representation bisulfite sequencing. Genome Res 23:2126–2135. https://doi.org/10.1101/gr.161679.113
33. Lieberman-Aiden E, van Berkum NL, Williams L et al (2009) Comprehensive mapping of long-range interactions reveals folding principles of the human genome. Science (80-), 326 (5950):289 LP–293. http://science.sciencemag.org/content/326/5950/289.abstract
34. Lister R, O'Malley RC, Tonti-Filippini J et al (2008) Highly integrated single-base resolution maps of the epigenome in <em>Arabidopsis</em>. Cell 133(3):523–536. https://doi.org/10.1016/j.cell.2008.03.029
35. Nagano T, Lubling Y, Stevens TJ et al (2013) Single-cell Hi-C reveals cell-to-cell variability in chromosome structure. Nature 502:59. https://doi.org/10.1038/nature12593
36. Linnarsson S, Teichmann SA (2016) Single-cell genomics: coming of age. Genome Biol 17 (1):16–18. https://doi.org/10.1186/s13059-016-0960-x
37. Macaulay IC, Ponting CP, Voet T (2017) Single-cell multiomics: multiple measurements from single cells. Trends Genet 33(2):155–168
38. Klein AM, Mazutis L, Akartuna I et al (2015) Droplet barcoding for single-cell transcriptomics applied to embryonic stem cells. Cell 161(5):1187–1201. https://doi.org/10.1016/j.cell.2015.04.044
39. Macosko EZ, Basu A, Satija R et al (2015) Highly parallel genome-wide expression profiling of individual cells using nanoliter droplets. Cell 161(5):1202–1214. https://doi.org/10.1016/j.cell.2015.05.002
40. Shalek AK, Satija R, Shuga J et al (2014) Single-cell RNA-seq reveals dynamic paracrine control of cellular variation. Nature 510:363. https://doi.org/10.1038/nature13437
41. Simpson EH (1951) The interpretation of interaction I contingency tables. J R Stat Soc Series B Stat Methodol 13:238–241
42. Hinton G (2008) Visualizing data using t-SNE visualizing data using t-SNE. J Mach Learn Res 9(2579–2605):85. https://doi.org/10.1007/s10479-011-0841-3
43. Svensson RR, Teichmann SA, Kar G (2017) Computational approaches for interpreting scRNA-seq data. FEBS Let 591(15):2213–2225. https://doi.org/10.1002/1873-3468.12684

Human Microbiota and Personalized Cancer Treatments: Role of Commensal Microbes in Treatment Outcomes for Cancer Patients

10

Stephen Gately

Contents

S. Gately (✉)
Translational Drug Development (TD2), Scottsdale, AZ, USA
e-mail: sgately@td2inc.com

D. D. Von Hoff and H. Han (eds.), *Precision Medicine in Cancer Therapy*,
Cancer Treatment and Research 178, https://doi.org/10.1007/978-3-030-16391-4_10

10.1 The Gut Microbiota

Precision oncology considers the molecular characteristics of a patient's tumor to determine an ideal approved or investigational therapy that could provide clinical benefit [1]. While prospective profiling of patient's tumors has resulted in improved selection and response to therapies [2–4], this "tumorcentric" approach can fail to account for impact of the complex microenvironment that influences tumor growth and response to therapy. The gut microbiota is a complex ecosystem of microorganisms where the total number of bacteria in the average 70 kg person is estimated to be 3.8×10^{13} [5]. The number of bacteria in the body is of the same order of magnitude as the number of human cells and has a total mass of about 0.2 kg [6]. These microbes play fundamental roles in health and survival and have been found to play a significant role in the response to cancer therapy and susceptibility to toxic side effects of those drugs.

10.2 Gut Microbiota Generate Short-Chain Fatty Acids (SCFA)

The gut microbiota produces SCFA mainly through the fermentation of carbohydrates that escape digestion and absorption in the small intestine [7]. The major SCFA products produced are formate, acetate, propionate, and butyrate and these products are detectable in the circulation [7]. SCFAs are reported to directly activate G-coupled receptors, inhibit histone deacetylases (HDACs), serve as energy substrates, and promote T-cell differentiation into both effector and regulatory T cells to promote either immunity or immune tolerance [8–10]. The SCFA's butyrate and propionate directly modulate the gene expression of CD8+ cytotoxic T lymphocytes and Tc17 cells [11]. The SCFAs appear not only optimize the function of Tregs and CD4+ T cells, but also modulate the function of CD8+ T cells to enhance anti-tumor and anti-viral activity [11, 12].

10.3 SCFAs as Regulators of Histone Post-translational Modifications (HPTM)

Human gut microbes regulate gene transcription using a variety of epigenetic marks (see Table 10.1, adapted from [13]). At least eleven types of HPTMs have been reported on over 60 different amino acid residues on histones, including methylation, acetylation, propionylation, butyrylation, formylation, phosphorylation, ubiquitylation, sumoylation, citrullination, proline isomerization, and ADP ribosylation [14], and the gut microbiota-generated SCFAs are involved in many of these modifications. While most consider lysine acetylation to be a predominant epigenetic event, a new histone modification, lysine crotonylation (Kcr) was found to be surprisingly abundant in the small intestine crypt and colon [15]. Crotonyl-CoA, the precursor of Kcr, is generated by Acidaminococcus fermentans

Table 10.1 HDACs used by human gut microbes to regulate gene transcription

HDAC	Acetyl-lysine	Propionyl-lysine	Butyryl-lysine	Crotonyl-lysine
Class I	HDAC1, HDAC2, HDAC3, HDAC8	NA	NA	HDAC1, HDAC2, HDAC3
Class IIa	HDAC4, HDAC5, HDAC7, HDAC9	NA	NA	NA
Class IIb	HDAC6, HDAC10	NA	NA	NA
Class III	SIRT1, SIRT2, SIRT3, SIRT4, SIRT6, SIRT7	SIRT1, SIRT2, SIRT3	SIRT1, SIRT2, SIRT3	SIRT1, SIRT2, SIRT3
Class IV	HDAC11	NA	NA	NA

NA, not available

[16], and depletion of gut microbiota leads to decreased histone crotonylation in the colon [15]. Class I HDAC enzymes, HDAC1, HDAC2, and HDAC3, are reported to efficiently remove the crotonyl moiety; microbiota-derived SCFAs are class I selective HDAC inhibitors and are therefore also histone decrotonylation inhibitors [15, 17]. The impact of Kcr on protein function remains to be fully elucidated; however, a variety of cancer proteins are crotonylated [18]. The gut microbiota is therefore responsible for histone post-translational modifications and alterations to the gut microbiota composition will have significant effects on transcriptional regulation and sensitivity and/or resistance to cancer therapeutics.

10.4 SCFAs and Response to Cancer Chemotherapy

10.4.1 Drug Metabolism

More than 40 drugs are reported to be directly metabolized by the gut microbiota including the anticancer drugs methotrexate and irinotecan [19]. The gut microbiota also directly or indirectly increases the metabolism of orally and systemically delivered drugs through SCFA modulation of cytochrome P450 (Cyp450) gene family members [20–22]. Germ-free mice demonstrate faster metabolism of many drugs suggesting the microbiota and SCFAs exert regulatory control over the rate of drug metabolism and detoxification [20]. The heterogeneity of clinical response to drug therapy and/or variable emergence of toxicities may be due in part to differences in gut microbiota composition and differential drug metabolism [23].

10.4.2 Response to Cancer Chemotherapy

Depletion of mouse microbiota with antibiotics results in dysbiosis that causes a drop in luminal and serum SCFAs, and increased expression of HDAC2 that has been linked to colon tumorigenesis [15, 24, 25]. Elevated HDAC2 reduces the sensitivity of non-small cell lung cancer (NSCLC) cells to cisplatin [26], melanoma cells to the alkylating drugs temozolomide, dacarbazine, and fotemustine [27], colorectal cancer cells to doxorubicin [28] and glioblastoma multiforme cells to temozolomide [29]. In breast cancer, HDAC2 overexpression is correlated with metastasis, increased Ki67, and increased multidrug resistance protein expression. HDAC2-positive breast cancer is also associated with shorter survival in patients who received chemotherapy containing anthracyclines [30]. The microbiota exerts suppressive activity on HDAC2 activity via SCFA production, suggesting the potential value of class I selective HDAC inhibitors in patients with compromised gut microbiota. Isoform-selective HDAC inhibitors could serve as SCFA-replacement therapies to support local and systemic gene regulation by acting as lysine deacetylation and decrotonylation inhibitors. The SCFA-replacement theraputics could also potentially improve clinical response to a variety of chemotherapeutic agents through the inhibition of elevated HDAC2 activity found in many cancers.

Cyclophosphamide therapeutic efficacy is due in part to the stimulation of an anti-tumor immune response. Cyclophosphamide alters the microbiota in the small intestine and causes the translocation of select Gram-positive bacteria to secondary lymphoid organs [31]. There, these bacteria stimulate the generation of pathogenic T helper 17 (pTh17) cells and memory Th1 immune responses [31]. Germ-free mice or mice treated with antibiotics showed a reduction in pTh17 cells, and tumors became resistant to cyclophosphamide [31] confirming the role of the microbiota in the anticancer mechanism for cyclophosphamide. Also, antibiotic treatment suppressed the response of subcutaneous tumors to a CpG-oligonucleotide immunotherapy and platinum chemotherapy [32]. The antibiotic treated or germ-free mice had tumor-infiltrating myeloid-derived cells that produced lower levels of cytokines after CpG-oligonucleotide treatment and produced lower amounts of reactive oxygen species (ROS) following oxaliplatin or cisplatin therapy [32]. These data demonstrate that the microbiota contributes to the modification of genotoxicity for platinum compounds independent of immunogenic cell death. Anthracyclines, alkylating agents, and camptothecins also induce ROS as part of their anticancer activity, so it is likely that the gut microbiota may influence the effectiveness of these drugs as well [32]. The role of the microbiota in modulating the response to radiation therapy needs to be characterized, but tumors in germ-free mice are less responsive to the beneficial effects of radiation when compared to normal mice with an intact microbiota; evidence in humans and experimental animals suggests that the composition of the intestinal microbiota may affect the severity of radiation-induced mucosal toxicity.

The gut microbiota also has a role in the response to tyrosine kinase inhibitors [33]. Patients with metastatic renal-cell carcinoma were treated with first-line VEGF-tyrosine kinase inhibitors and were also receiving antibiotics with either Bacteroides coverage or not. When compared to patients not receiving antibiotics, a significant improvement in PFS was observed in patients taking antibiotics that covered *Bacteroides* spp [33]. These data confirm a role for the gut microbiota in the clinical response to tyrosine kinase inhibitors.

10.5 The Gut Microbiota and the Immune System

Gut bacterial SCFAs have profound effects on the adaptive immune system, with high expression of SCFA receptors being reported on immune cells [10]. The generation of effector and regulatory T cells is influenced by the gut microbiota and is dependent on the variety of cytokines found in the microenvironment [34]. SCFAs enhance T-cell differentiation into effector T cells, such as Th1 and Th17 cells, and also anti-inflammatory IL-10þ regulatory T cells [34]. Recently, it was shown that Prevotella heparinolytica promotes the differentiation of Th17 cells colonizing the gut that migrates to the bone marrow in a transgenic mouse model of multiple myeloma [35]. In this experimental model, the commensal bacteria increase IL-17 signaling that accelerates progression of smoldering myeloma to myeloma [35].

10.6 Immunotherapy and the Microbiota

Approaches that modulate the patient immune system have demonstrated significant clinical activity in hematological and solid cancers. One of the first reports on the contribution of the gut microbiota on immune therapy was the reported diminished tumor response in mice receiving antibiotics, total body irradiation, and tumor-specific cytotoxic T cells [36]. In this study, the authors report that total body irradiation caused the translocation of the gut microbiota to mesenteric lymph nodes, and increased proliferation of the injected T cells in the tumor [36]. Similarly, when mice were treated with an intratumoral TLR9 agonist CpG-oligodeoxynucleotide, anticancer activity was observed; however, the anti-tumor effect in germ-free mice or mice treated with antibiotics was diminished demonstrating that an intact microbiota was required for optimal anticancer effects [32].

The role of the gut microbiota on clinical activity or resistance of immune checkpoint modulators has been reported [37–42]. In addition to the gut microbiota, there have been reports on the contribution of an intratumoral microbiome that could play a role in chemotherapy and immunotherapy resistance [43–46].

Anti-tumor immunity in patients can be reactivated by the immune checkpoint inhibitors (antibodies against cytotoxic T lymphocyte-associated antigen 4 CTLA4) and programmed cell death protein 1 (PD1) or its ligand PD1 ligand 1 (PDL1) [47]. Antibodies targeting these immune checkpoints have demonstrated significant clinical activity in patients with a variety of cancers; however, variability and duration of patient response remain an area of active investigation [48]. The gut microbiota regulates the anticancer activity of anti-CTLA4 and anti-PDL1 cancer therapies [41, 42]. Oral supplementation of either *B. thetaiotaomicron* or *B. fragilis* in microbiota-depleted mice restores the anti-tumor response to anti-CTLA4 antibodies [42]. Vancomycin enhances the efficacy of CTLA4 blockade in mice by decreasing the abundance of Gram-positive bacteria while preserving Gram-negative Bacteroidales and Burkholderiales [42]. Analysis of the fecal microbiota from patients with melanoma before and after treatment with anti CTLA4 showed a change in the relative proportions of three dominant enterotypes; enterotype A was dominated by Prevotella, enterotypes B and C were dominated by different Bacteroides [41, 42]. When fecal microbiota from patients with each of the three human enterotypes was transferred into tumor-bearing, germ-free mice only the enterotype C resulted in enhanced response to anti CTLA4 [42].

The response to anti-PDL1 was also found to be significantly associated with the gut microbiota of the *Bifidobacterium* genus, including *Bifidobacterium breve*, *Bifidobacterium longum,* and *Bifidobacterium adolescentis* [41]. Oral administration of a probiotic cocktail of *Bifidobacterium* including *B. breve* and *B. longum*, alone or with anti-PDL1, enhanced CD8 + T-cell-induced anti-tumor activity [41]. The effect of *Bifidobacterium* was abolished in CD8+ T-cell-depleted mice, indicating that *Bifidobacterium* action is dependent on cytotoxic T-cell activity [41]. The therapeutic effectiveness of anti-PDL1 treatment can be seen when *Bifidobacterium* are in higher numbers in the gut microbiota.

The anti-tumor activity of anti-PD-1 alone or when combined with anti-CTLA4 was significantly decreased when mice were treated with a broad-spectrum antibiotic combination (ampicillin + colistin + streptomycin) [38]. This experimental data were then confirmed and extended to patients with advanced NSCLC, RCC, or urothelial carcinoma ($n = 42$) who received PD-1/PD-L1 monoclonal antibodies. Broad-spectrum antibiotic treatment in these patients resulted in resistance to PD-1 blockade [38]. Metagenomic analysis of patient stool samples revealed correlations between clinical response to checkpoint inhibitors and the relative abundance of *Akkermansia muciniphila*, and in preclinical studies supplementation with *A. muciniphila* restored the efficacy of PD-1 blockade [38]. Other studies have reported bacterial species *B. longum*, *Collinsella aerofaciens*, and *Enterococcus faecium* [40] and relative abundance of the Ruminococcaceae family [49] in PD-1 blockade responding patients. Patients with a high abundance of Clostridiales, Ruminococcaceae, or Faecalibacterium in the gut had higher frequencies of effector CD4+ and CD8+ T cells in the systemic circulation and a preserved cytokine response to anti–PD-1 therapy, whereas patients with a higher abundance of Bacteroidales in the gut microbiome had higher frequencies of Tregs and myeloid-derived suppressor cells (MDSCs) in the systemic circulation, with a blunted cytokine response [49]. These findings highlight the therapeutic potential of modulating the gut microbiome in patients receiving checkpoint blockade immunotherapy, and warrant monitoring the gut microbiota in cancer clinical trials [49].

10.7 The Intratumoral Microbiome

The microbiota has also emerged as a contributor to cancer development in intestinal tract malignancies, including laryngeal, esophageal, gastric, and colorectal cancers, as well as in primary liver cancer [50]. A recent report described that pancreatic cancers harbor a distinct intrapancreatic microbiome that is responsible for immune suppression and failure of immune checkpoint-targeted therapeutics [51]. When the intrapancreatic microbiome was ablated in experimental animals, immunogenic reprogramming of the tumor microenvironment occurred, including a reduction in MDSCs and an increase in M1 macrophage differentiation, promoting TH1 differentiation of CD4+ T cells and CD8+ T-cell activation [51]. There was an abundance of *B. pseudolongum* in gut and tumor microbiota in pancreas cancer that was associated with enhanced oncogenesis that could be reversed by ablating the microbiome [51]. The intrapancreatic microbiome has also been shown to inactivate the chemotherapeutic drug gemcitabine by Gammaproteobacteria-generated cytidine deaminase [46]. Upon examination, 113 human pancreas cancers, 86 (76%) were positive for bacteria, primarily Gammaproteobacteria, suggesting the intrapancreatic microbiome can also negatively diminish chemotherapeutic activity [46].

Recent pathological analyses have revealed a distinct microbiota that is present in breast cancer tissue that differs from normal breast tissue with a relative decreased in the genus Methylobacterium [52]. These authors also report significantly different microbiomes compared to non-cancer patients in the urinary tract characterized by increased numbers of Gram-positive bacteria [52]. The exact role of intratumoral bacteria in carcinogenesis and response to treatment in breast and urinary tract cancers is an area of active investigation.

The liver is exposed to the gut microbiota through the portal vein and recently the role of gut bacteria in anti-tumor surveillance in the liver was reported [53]. The microbiota metabolizes bile acids that recirculate back into the liver through the enterohepatic circulation [52, 53]. Antibiotic treatment of mice with vancomycin removed Gram-positive bacteria responsible for primary to-secondary bile acid metabolism causing the expression of CXCL16 and selective increase in hepatic CXCR6 positive natural killer T (NKT) cells [53]. This chemokine-dependent accumulation of hepatic NKT cells provides anti-tumor immunity in the liver, against primary and metastatic liver disease [53]. The gut microbiota increases liver anti-tumor immunosurveillance through bile acid metabolism and recruitment of immune effector cells.

In colorectal cancer, the gut microbiota translocate across compromised epithelial layers and stimulate immune cell infiltration and proinflammatory cytokine production [54]. Tumor infiltrating lymphocytes (TILs) are reported to improve survival for patients with colorectal cancer [55]. Human colorectal cancer cells from both primary tumors and established cell lines express toll-like receptors and produce significant chemokine expression when exposed to various bacterial species [55]. Antibiotic treatment of mice bearing orthotopic colorectal cancer xenografts demonstrated significantly lower levels of tumor-derived chemokines supporting the important role of the gut microbiota in tumor cell chemokine expression [55]. The extent of T-cell infiltration in primary human colorectal cancers is associated with the presence of specific bacterial families; these specific bacterial families were also associated with induction of specific immune cell attracting chemokines, suggesting the gut microbiota is directly involved in tumor cell immune cell recruitment and potentially colorectal cancer survival [55]. Some bacterial families like Fusobacteria were reported to be associated with worse clinical outcome and were found at higher levels in poorly immune cell infiltrated cancers [56]. Other bacterial families, like *F. nucleatum*, have been shown to inhibit natural killer and T-cell functions [57]. Taken together, these data demonstrate that the specific composition of the gut and tumor microbiota could play a key role in the attraction and/or suppression of immune effector cells in the tumor microenvironment, impacting patient outcomes.

10.8 Summary

It is unclear which bacterial families are required for an improved clinical response to cancer therapies, but there is no question that the variability in gut microbiota found in patients results in heterogeneous response to therapeutic interventions. Cancer patients are taking a variety of prescription and over-the-counter concomitant medications, all of which can alter the composition of the gut microbiota. For example, the COX-2 inhibitor celecoxib alters select bacterial populations in experimental animals including decreased Lactobacillaceae and Bifidobacteriaceae and increased Coriobacteriaceae [58]. Proton-pump inhibitors have been reported to significantly increase *Lactobacillus* spp., *L. gasseri*, *L. fermentum*, *L. reuteri*, and *L. ruminis* as well Streptococcus species [59]. Even nutraceuticals influence the gut microbiota composition, and many patients are taking a large variety of over-the-counter vitamins to supplement their prescription medications. For example, curcumin alters the gut microbiota resulting in increases in most *Clostridium* spp., *Bacteroides* spp., *Citrobacter* spp., *Cronobacter* spp., *Enterobacter* spp., *Enterococcus* spp., *Klebsiella* spp., *Parabacteroides* spp., and *Pseudomonas* spp. and reduced relative abundance of several Blautia spp. and most *Ruminococcus* spp. strains [60]. As a result, a new branch of pharmacogenomics, called pharmacomicrobiomics, has emerged to study drug–microbiome interactions [61]. One interesting question is the potential role of the regulatory authorities in requiring an assessment of new medicines effects on the microbiota during required GLP safety studies. Knowledge of the potential microbiota changes by these new medicines could have utility in identifying whether new drugs could negatively or positively impact the clinical activity of approved cancer medicines.

Studies to restore and/or enhance the gut microbiome by dietary modification, probiotics, prebiotics, post-biotics, autologous fecal microbiota transplant, and antibiotics could have therapeutic benefit for cancer patients to improve efficacy and reduce the toxicity of chemotherapy [62–65]. Dietary factors play a key role in the number and kind of bacterial taxa, and the production of a variety of epigenetic factors that regulate gene expression [66, 67], so close monitoring of the diets and supplements that cancer patients consume may be required to better understand and control for treatment outcomes.

To date, the majority of analyses of the gut and tumor microbiota have been through next-generation sequencing. However, gene/transcript presence does not necessarily indicate protein expression; therefore, directly measuring expressed proteins by metaproteomics will provide precise functional information on the microbiota [68, 69]. A thorough examination of the gut and intratumoral microbiota in cancer patients should include metaproteomic analysis which can reveal both human and microbial functional changes indicative of the host–microbiome interactions [70, 71].

Because cancer patients are already closely monitored when participating in clinical trials it will be important to add comprehensive microbiome assessments, including metaproteomic assessments to treatment protocols to fully understand baseline microbiota in cancer patients and to study the impact of therapies on specific bacterial families and their contribution to therapeutic outcomes.

References

1. Kurnit KC et al (2018) Precision oncology decision support: current approaches and strategies for the future. Clin Cancer Res 24(12):2719–2731
2. Jameson GS et al (2014) A pilot study utilizing multi-omic molecular profiling to find potential targets and select individualized treatments for patients with previously treated metastatic breast cancer. Breast Cancer Res Treat 147(3):579–588
3. Von Hoff DD et al (2010) Pilot study using molecular profiling of patients' tumors to find potential targets and select treatments for their refractory cancers. J Clin Oncol 28(33):4877–4883
4. Weiss GJ et al (2013) A pilot study using next-generation sequencing in advanced cancers: feasibility and challenges. PLoS ONE 8(10):e76438
5. Sender R, Fuchs S, Milo R (2016) Revised estimates for the number of human and bacteria cells in the body. PLoS Biol 14(8):e1002533
6. Sender R, Fuchs S, Milo R (2016) Are we really vastly outnumbered? Revisiting the ratio of bacterial to host cells in humans. Cell 164(3):337–340
7. Morrison DJ, Preston T (2016) Formation of short chain fatty acids by the gut microbiota and their impact on human metabolism. Gut Microbes 7(3):189–200
8. Krautkramer KA et al (2017) Metabolic programming of the epigenome: host and gut microbial metabolite interactions with host chromatin. Transl Res 189:30–50
9. Krautkramer KA et al (2016) Diet-microbiota interactions mediate global epigenetic programming in multiple host tissues. Mol Cell 64(5):982–992
10. Koh A et al (2016) From dietary fiber to host physiology: short-chain fatty acids as key bacterial metabolites. Cell 165(6):1332–1345
11. Luu M et al (2018) Regulation of the effector function of CD8(+) T cells by gut microbiota-derived metabolite butyrate. Sci Rep 8(1):14430
12. Luu M, Steinhoff U, Visekruna A (2017) Functional heterogeneity of gut-resident regulatory T cells. Clin Transl Immunology 6(9):e156
13. Ellmeier W, Seiser C (2018) Histone deacetylase function in CD4(+) T cells. Nat Rev Immunol 18(10):617–634

14. Tan M et al (2011) Identification of 67 histone marks and histone lysine crotonylation as a new type of histone modification. Cell 146(6):1016–1028
15. Fellows R et al (2018) Microbiota derived short chain fatty acids promote histone crotonylation in the colon through histone deacetylases. Nat Commun 9(1):105
16. Cook GM et al (1994) Emendation of the description of acidaminococcus fermentans, a trans-aconitate- and citrate-oxidizing bacterium. Int J Syst Bacteriol 44(3):576–578
17. Wei W et al (2017) Class I histone deacetylases are major histone decrotonylases: evidence for critical and broad function of histone crotonylation in transcription. Cell Res 27:898–915
18. Huang H, Wang DL, Zhao Y (2018) Quantitative crotonylome analysis expands the roles of p300 in the regulation of lysine crotonylation pathway. Proteomics, e1700230
19. Haiser HJ, Turnbaugh PJ (2013) Developing a metagenomic view of xenobiotic metabolism. Pharmacol Res 69(1):21–31
20. Bjorkholm B et al (2009) Intestinal microbiota regulate xenobiotic metabolism in the liver. PLoS ONE 4(9):e6958
21. Selwyn FP et al (2016) Regulation of hepatic drug-metabolizing enzymes in germ-free mice by conventionalization and probiotics. Drug Metab Dispos 44(2):262–274
22. Selwyn FP, Cui JY, Klaassen CD (2015) RNA-seq quantification of hepatic drug processing genes in germ-free mice. Drug Metab Dispos 43(10):1572–1580
23. Roy S, Trinchieri G (2017) Microbiota: a key orchestrator of cancer therapy. Nat Rev Cancer 17(5):271–285
24. Zhu P et al (2004) Induction of HDAC2 expression upon loss of APC in colorectal tumorigenesis. Cancer Cell 5(5):455–463
25. Ashktorab H et al (2009) Global histone H4 acetylation and HDAC2 expression in colon adenoma and carcinoma. Dig Dis Sci 54(10):2109–2117
26. Chen JH et al (2017) Valproic acid (VPA) enhances cisplatin sensitivity of non-small cell lung cancer cells via HDAC2 mediated down regulation of ABCA1. Biol Chem 398(7): 785–792
27. Krumm A et al (2016) Enhanced histone deacetylase activity in malignant melanoma provokes RAD51 and FANCD2-triggered drug resistance. Cancer Res 76(10):3067–3077
28. Ye P et al (2016) Histone deacetylase 2 regulates doxorubicin (Dox) sensitivity of colorectal cancer cells by targeting ABCB1 transcription. Cancer Chemother Pharmacol 77(3):613–621
29. Zhang Z et al (2016) Silencing of histone deacetylase 2 suppresses malignancy for proliferation, migration, and invasion of glioblastoma cells and enhances temozolomide sensitivity. Cancer Chemother Pharmacol 78(6):1289–1296
30. Zhao H et al (2016) HDAC2 overexpression is a poor prognostic factor of breast cancer patients with increased multidrug resistance-associated protein expression who received anthracyclines therapy. Jpn J Clin Oncol 46(10):893–902
31. Viaud S et al (2013) The intestinal microbiota modulates the anticancer immune effects of cyclophosphamide. Science 342(6161):971–976
32. Iida N et al (2013) Commensal bacteria control cancer response to therapy by modulating the tumor microenvironment. Science 342(6161):967–970
33. Hahn AW et al (2018) Targeting bacteroides in stool microbiome and response to treatment with first-line VEGF tyrosine kinase inhibitors in metastatic renal-cell carcinoma. Clin Genitourin Cancer 16(5):365–368
34. Park J et al (2015) Short-chain fatty acids induce both effector and regulatory T cells by suppression of histone deacetylases and regulation of the mTOR-S6 K pathway. Mucosal Immunol 8(1):80–93
35. Calcinotto A et al (2018) Microbiota-driven interleukin-17-producing cells and eosinophils synergize to accelerate multiple myeloma progression. Nat Commun 9(1):4832
36. Paulos CM et al (2007) Microbial translocation augments the function of adoptively transferred self/tumor-specific CD8+ T cells via TLR4 signaling. J Clin Invest 117(8): 2197–2204

37. Derosa L et al (2018) The intestinal microbiota determines the clinical efficacy of immune checkpoint blockers targeting PD-1/PD-L1. Oncoimmunology 7(6):e1434468
38. Routy B et al (2018) Gut microbiome influences efficacy of PD-1-based immunotherapy against epithelial tumors. Science 359(6371):91–97
39. Zitvogel L et al (2018) The microbiome in cancer immunotherapy: diagnostic tools and therapeutic strategies. Science 359(6382):1366–1370
40. Matson V et al (2018) The commensal microbiome is associated with anti-PD-1 efficacy in metastatic melanoma patients. Science 359(6371):104–108
41. Sivan A et al (2015) Commensal bifidobacterium promotes antitumor immunity and facilitates anti-PD-L1 efficacy. Science 350(6264):1084–1089
42. Vetizou M et al (2015) Anticancer immunotherapy by CTLA-4 blockade relies on the gut microbiota. Science 350(6264):1079–1084
43. Urbaniak C et al (2014) Microbiota of human breast tissue. Appl Environ Microbiol 80 (10):3007–3014
44. McCoy AN et al (2013) Fusobacterium is associated with colorectal adenomas. PLoS ONE 8 (1):e53653
45. Geller LT, Straussman R (2018) Intratumoral bacteria may elicit chemoresistance by metabolizing anticancer agents. Mol Cell Oncol 5(1):e1405139
46. Geller LT et al (2017) Potential role of intratumor bacteria in mediating tumor resistance to the chemotherapeutic drug gemcitabine. Science 357(6356):1156–1160
47. Ribas A, Wolchok JD (2018) Cancer immunotherapy using checkpoint blockade. Science 359 (6382):1350–1355
48. Rodig SJ et al (2018) MHC proteins confer differential sensitivity to CTLA-4 and PD-1 blockade in untreated metastatic melanoma. Sci Transl Med 10(450)
49. Gopalakrishnan V et al (2018) Gut microbiome modulates response to anti-PD-1 immunotherapy in melanoma patients. Science 359(6371):97–103
50. Plottel CS, Blaser MJ (2011) Microbiome and malignancy. Cell Host Microbe 10(4):324–335
51. Pushalkar S et al (2018) The pancreatic cancer microbiome promotes oncogenesis by induction of innate and adaptive immune suppression. Cancer Discov 8(4):403–416
52. Wang H et al (2017) Breast tissue, oral and urinary microbiomes in breast cancer. Oncotarget 8(50):88122–88138
53. Ma C et al (2018) Gut microbiome-mediated bile acid metabolism regulates liver cancer via NKT cells. Science 360(6391)
54. Grivennikov SI et al (2012) Adenoma-linked barrier defects and microbial products drive IL-23/IL-17-mediated tumour growth. Nature 491(7423):254–258
55. Cremonesi E et al (2018) Gut microbiota modulate T cell trafficking into human colorectal cancer. Gut 67(11):1984–1994
56. Mima K et al (2016) Fusobacterium nucleatum in colorectal carcinoma tissue according to tumor location. Clin Transl Gastroenterol 7(11):e200
57. Gur C et al (2015) Binding of the fap2 protein of fusobacterium nucleatum to human inhibitory receptor TIGIT protects tumors from immune cell attack. Immunity 42(2):344–355
58. Montrose DC et al (2016) Celecoxib alters the intestinal microbiota and metabolome in association with reducing polyp burden. Cancer Prev Res (Phila) 9(9):721–731
59. Hojo M et al (2018) Gut microbiota composition before and after use of proton pump inhibitors. Dig Dis Sci 63(11):2940–2949
60. Peterson CT et al (2018) Effects of turmeric and curcumin dietary supplementation on human gut microbiota: a double-blind, randomized, placebo-controlled pilot study. J Evid Based Integr Med 23:2515690X18790725
61. ElRakaiby M et al (2014) Pharmacomicrobiomics: the impact of human microbiome variations on systems pharmacology and personalized therapeutics. OMICS 18(7):402–414
62. Alexander JL et al (2017) Gut microbiota modulation of chemotherapy efficacy and toxicity. Nat Rev Gastroenterol Hepatol 14(6):356–365

63. Panebianco C, Andriulli A, Pazienza V (2018) Pharmacomicrobiomics: exploiting the drug-microbiota interactions in anticancer therapies. Microbiome 6(1):92
64. Redman MG, Ward EJ, Phillips RS (2014) The efficacy and safety of probiotics in people with cancer: a systematic review. Ann Oncol 25(10):1919–1929
65. Taur Y et al (2018) Reconstitution of the gut microbiota of antibiotic-treated patients by autologous fecal microbiota transplant. Sci Transl Med 10(460)
66. Riscuta G et al (2018) Diet, microbiome, and epigenetics in the era of precision medicine. Methods Mol Biol 1856:141–156
67. Paul B et al (2015) Influences of diet and the gut microbiome on epigenetic modulation in cancer and other diseases. Clin Epigenet 7:112
68. Erickson AR et al (2012) Integrated metagenomics/metaproteomics reveals human host-microbiota signatures of Crohn's disease. PLoS ONE 7(11):e49138
69. Verberkmoes NC et al (2009) Shotgun metaproteomics of the human distal gut microbiota. ISME J 3(2):179–189
70. Zhang X et al (2017) Deep metaproteomics approach for the study of human microbiomes. Anal Chem 89(17):9407–9415
71. Lai LA et al (2019) Metaproteomics study of the gut microbiome. Methods Mol Biol 1871:123–132

Artificial Intelligence and Personalized Medicine 11

Nicholas J. Schork

Contents

N. J. Schork (✉)
Department of Quantitative Medicine, The Translational Genomics Research Institute (TGen), Phoenix, AZ, USA
e-mail: nschork@tgen.org

The City of Hope/TGen IMPACT Center, Duarte, CA, USA

The University of California San Diego, La Jolla, CA, USA

D. D. Von Hoff and H. Han (eds.), *Precision Medicine in Cancer Therapy*, Cancer Treatment and Research 178, https://doi.org/10.1007/978-3-030-16391-4_11

11.1 Introduction: Emerging Themes in Biomedical Science

Modern biomedical science is guided, if not dominated, by many interrelated themes. Four of the most prominent and important of these themes are (see Fig. 11.1): 1. personalized medicine, or the belief that health interventions need to be tailored to the nuanced and often unique genetic, biochemical, physiological, exposure, and behavioral features individuals possess; 2. the exploitation of emerging data-intensive assays, such as DNA sequencing, proteomics, imaging protocols, and wireless health monitoring devices; 3. 'big data' research paradigms in which massive amounts of data, say of the type generated from emerging data-intensive biomedical assays, are aggregated from different sources, harmonized, and made available for analysis in order to identify patterns that would normally not be identified if the different data points were analyzed independently; and 4. artificial intelligence (AI; which we consider here to include machine learning, deep learning, neural network constructs, and a wide variety of related techniques [1]), which can be used to find relevant patterns in massive data sets.

These four themes are highly interrelated in that, e.g., personalizing a medicine or tailoring an intervention to a patient requires a very deep understanding of that patient's condition and circumstances, and this requires the extensive use of sophisticated assays that generate massive amounts of data, such as DNA sequencing or an imaging protocol. Essentially, the data produced by these assays needs to be organized so that analyses can be pursued to identify features that the patient possesses that may indicate the optimal intervention. In addition, research associated with each of these themes is often pursued independently of the others because of the very specialized expertise required. For example, there are scientific journals devoted to personal medicine (e.g., 'Personalized Medicine,' 'Journal of Personalized Medicine'), emerging assays (e.g., 'Nature Biotechnology,' 'Nature

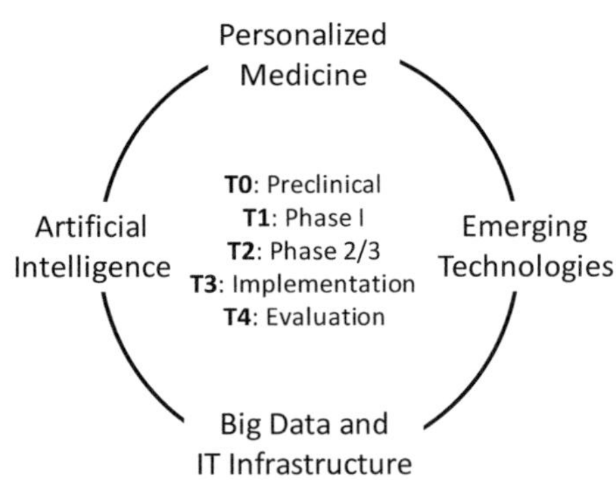

Fig. 11.1 Four emerging complementary themes in biomedical science: personalized medicine, emerging data-intensive technologies, big data and information technologies (IT) infrastructure, and artificial intelligence (AI). These technologies can be fuel, and be fueled by, AI in all phases of the development (T0–T4) of personalized medicines (see Fig. 11.2)

Digital Medicine'), big data (e.g., 'Big Data,' 'Journal of Big Data,' 'Gigascience'), and artificial intelligence (e.g., 'IEEE Transactions on Neural Networks and Learning Systems,' 'IEEE Transactions on Pattern Analysis and Machine Intelligence') that publish very focused studies. However, the integrated use of the insights, information, and strategies obtained from research associated with each of these themes is necessary for creating personalized health products, such as drugs and prognostic tools.

Bringing together research activities associated with these four emerging themes is not trivial, as it will require communication and participation from researchers and practitioners with a wide variety of skills and expertise, including molecular biology, genetics, pathology, informatics, computer science, statistics, clinical science, and medicine. AI will have a special role to play in this integration process if the goal is to advance personalized medicine, since it is unclear how relevant clinically-meaningful insights can be drawn from big data-generating assays that would complement or build off the insights from experts in different domains. In this light, there are a number of phases in the development of medicines, general interventions, and other products, such as diagnostics, prognostics, decision support tools, etc., where AI could have a significant impact. These different phases are emphasized in the various subsections of this chapter that describe and comment on recent studies leveraging AI. This chapter does not provide an exhaustive literature review of AI in medicine, however, as there are some excellent reviews for this [2–4], but rather considers the *potential* that AI has in developing new medicines, health devices, and products. In particular, a focus on the need for greater *integration* across the various phases of the development of health interventions and products could result in very radical yet positive changes in the way medicine is practiced. In this sense, this chapter is as much a summary of the ways in which AI can be exploited in modern medicine as it is a vision of the future.

11.2 The Translational Workflow

As noted, the development of interventions and health products, as with the diagnosis and treatment of a patient, proceeds in different phases. There are various ways of defining and referring to these phases; however, all of them point to opportunities for AI to have a substantial impact if leveraged appropriately. For example, in the context of clinical trials to vet a new drug or intervention for treating a disease like cancer, a common progression or workflow runs from phase I trials, which involve characterizing the pharmacokinetic properties of a drug using what may turn out to be non-physiologic (i.e., does not have an appreciable effect on the body) and physiologic (i.e., does have an appreciable effect on the body) doses of a drug in a very small number of individuals, to phase I trials, which involve establishing safe and effective doses of a drug in small number of individuals, to phase II trials, which seek to establish whether a drug is likely to be efficacious in a moderately sized group of individuals, to phase III trials, which attempt to establish the utility of a drug in the population at large by studying a very large number of individuals, to phase IV trials, which evaluate the adoption, uptake, and acceptance, as well as any evidence for adverse consequences, associated with the use of the drug in the population at large.

We take a broader view of the workflows behind developing new products than that reflected in the traditional clinical trial progression. This broader view is consistent with the scheme used by, for example, the National Institutes of Health (NIH)'s Clinical and Translational Science Award (CTSA) program [5]. The CTSA program focuses on all aspects of biomedical science associated with attempts to translate very basic biomedical insights concerning, e.g., pathogenic processes contributing to diseases, into clinically useful products like drugs or interventions for those diseases. The CTSA scheme does, however, incorporate elements of the phase 0–phase IV clinical trials workflow or transition scheme for developing drugs or health products to treat or manage diseases in the population at large. Thus, in accordance with the CTSA scheme (left panel of Fig. 11.2), T0 science involves very basic research focusing on that could lead to the identification of a drug or intervention target and then crafting an appropriate drug or intervention that modulates that target; T1 science focuses on testing an intervention or health device in a small clinical studies to determine if it is safe and at what dosages it should be used; T2 science involves vetting the drug or device in a large number of individuals in a well-designed study to assess its efficacy in the population at large; T3 science focuses on the implementation of the drug or device for use in the population, including adapting existing workflows (e.g., custody chains for tests or physician–patient interaction points); and T4 science involves a re-evaluation or assessment of the utility of the drug or device post deployment and implementation. Each of these phases can leverage AI techniques if the right data and motivation is present.

The actual practice of personalized medicine can be seen as involving an analogous process to the development of drugs and health devices (right panel of Fig. 11.2; see also Schork and Nazor [6]). Thus, P0 activity involves making a diagnosis or determining an individual's risk of developing a disease; P1 activity involves identifying the key pathophysiologic processes, if not known, that are causing (or likely to cause) a disease that might be amenable to modulation and improvement by an appropriate intervention; P2 considers the identification of an appropriate intervention given what was identified in the P0 and P1 stages; P3 involves testing the intervention on the relevant individual undergoing the diagnosis and pathobiology assessment; and P4 involves warehousing the result in appropriate databases so that the insights and information obtained on a patient can be exploited in assessments involving other patients or used in broader aggregated data mining initiatives to find clinically meaningful patterns.

A couple of items about these workflows are worth noting. First, as noted, although the science associated with each component involves unique insight and expertise and provides a fertile ground for collaborations with AI tools and scientists independently of the other components, the *transmission* of information from one component to another—or the transitions from one component to another—is of crucial importance (e.g., consider that a diagnostic would not be particularly useful if

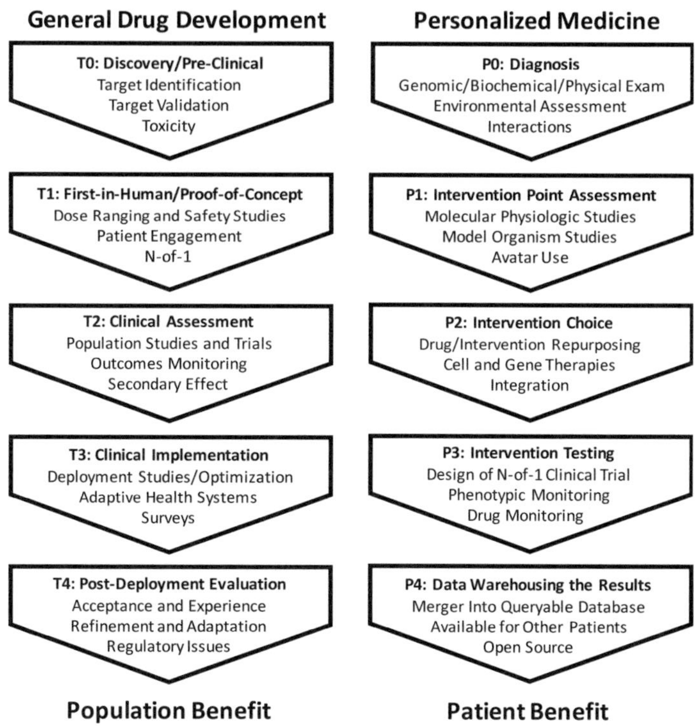

Fig. 11.2 A representation of the stages in the 'translation' of basic insights into clinical useful products considered in initiatives such as the Clinical and Translational Science Award (CTSA) initiative overseen by the National Center on Advancing Translational Science of the United States National Institutes of Health (NCATS; left panel; [5]). An analogous representation of the stages in the diagnosis and treatment of an individual patient are provided in the right-hand panel

it did not help a physician choose an appropriate course of action). Second, a goal of personalized medicine, and the improvement of health care generally, is to make workflows like those in Fig. 11.2 more efficient and reliable, and AI can have a substantial role to play in this broader goal. These two items are emphasized in Sect. 11.8 below.

11.3 Preclinical (T0) and Diagnostic (P0) Research

The identification of targets for therapies (T0 research from the left-hand side of Fig. 11.2) can be greatly aided by AI in quite a few contexts. For example, many assays used to uncover potential therapeutic targets generate massive amounts of data and as such often require sophisticated statistical methods to identify meaningful patterns. AI has been used to identify such patterns from, e.g., DNA sequence data and molecular pathology imaging protocols [7–10]. For individual patients whose comprehensive diagnosis may lay the foundation for crafting a personalized treatment or intervention plan and exploit data-intensive assays (i.e., P0 in the right-hand figure of Fig. 11.2), many AI-based tools can be leveraged. For example, mining DNA sequence information obtained from an individual in order to make a genetic diagnosis of a disease can be greatly aided by AI-based analyses [7]. In addition, facilitating, e.g., cancer diagnoses with AI-based analyses of blood analytes has been shown to have great potential [11].

If a particular therapeutic target has been identified that is likely to cause the molecular pathology underlying an individual patient's disease, then AI-based strategies can be used to identify potential compounds and drugs that modulate that target via high-throughput screening assays. Thus, AI techniques can be used to analyze drug screening data collected to determine if any of a large number of extant drugs and compounds have activity against a target and have, in fact, been shown to be very reliable [12]. In addition, AI-based studies have revealed many insights into how drugs and compounds may impact various structural and functional features of a cell [13]. Finally, web sites with large databases like DeepChem (https://deepchem.io/about.html), which leverage AI in the analysis of chemical structures of pharmacologic compounds and drugs, can be used to identify relevant properties of drugs and compounds for a given target.

An interesting research area of relevance to the identification of pathologies underlying diseases that might be amenable to pharmacological modulation involves the design of appropriate studies to tease out those pathologies. For example, if the relationships between different potential drug targets and their effect on a molecular system or pathway are not known, researchers may have to systematically perturb each element in such a system and examine the effect on the system each of these perturbations [14]. As one can imagine, such studies can be tedious and laborious. However, recent research suggest that one can use robotics and AI to conduct such experiments and, in fact, anticipate further experiments that might be called for based on the results of initial experiments [15]. The actual deployable experimental infrastructure for pursuing AI-based experiments in this manner has also been developed, but only for a few select settings [16, 17].

If an extant drug or compound is not found that could appropriately modulate a relevant target, then creating a novel pharmacotherapeutic (i.e., drug) is necessary and this often requires insights obtained from materials science in order to make sure the molecular structure of the drug produced has favorable properties inside the body. Very recent work suggests that AI can be leveraged to identify materials that may not be easily identified with traditional brute-force approaches [18, 19]. In addition, AI has been used to design new chemical and material structures, which may be relevant to crafting better interventions, whether a drug or mechanical device, and has also been used to aid in the selection of appropriate chemical syntheses [20–22]. In fact, AI has been used in studies of very basic phenomena, such as particle physics, to probe how materials interact [23]. The refinment of the design of new drugs, for example involving the refinement of the structure of a therapeutic protein or molecule, could also be greatly facilitated by AI. It has been shown that in many design contexts in which optimization of materials and the way they are put together is of issue, the use of AI can identify superior designs to those based on legacy strategies [20]. This theme of harnessing AI to identify ways of optimizing the assembly of materials, or the manner in which an objective function of whatever sort is optimized given some starting materials and appropriate yet basic principles for assembling them, was leveraged in the recent description of the system for playing the age-old game of GO developed by Google's DeepMind group [24]. Essentially, the system developed at DeepMind was not only able to easily beat all human experts as well as other GO-playing systems, but was able to do this by identifying strategies and moves that were completely beyond those which humans had used to play and try to master the game for centuries. Thus, there is the possibility that AI could help identify materials and structures to be used in constructing drugs and interventions that are beyond those in current drug and intervention development processes.

As noted previously, if a therapeutic target has been identified, then one could potentially pursue compound screening studies to identify compounds that modulate that target. Such studies often require a knowledge or use of a particular output or phenotype (e.g., the expression level of a target gene) that reflects what the drug is to modulate. In the absence of such a phenotype, high-content screens can be pursued, in which many different phenotypes are evaluated to see if any of the compounds, often numbering in the thousands or tens of thousands, affect any one or some subset of these phenotypes as this can be taken as a sign of its activity. AI techniques have been used to identify potential compounds impacting a target in high content screening settings [25–27].

Once a therapeutic concept or prototype drug has been defined, relevant and deployable versions of the drug, or an intervention apparatus, embodying the concept must be manufactured at scale for distribution. In this light, the manufacture of drugs and interventions of all sorts has been greatly facilitated by robotics and AI [28]. In the context of personalized medicines, it may be that the manufacture of drugs and interventions will require nuanced features based on patients' profiles and therefore have to be designed and crafted *in real time* as opposed to be created at scale, stored and distributed when needed—a topic to be discussed in a later section of this chapter, Sect. 11.8 [29, 30].

11.4 First-in-Human (T1) and Pathology (P1) Studies

Once an intervention or drug had been created, it must be shown to safe through phase I clinical trials and studies that are often referred to as 'first-in-human-studies' (T1 in the left panel of Fig. 11.2). Such studies focus on the safety of a proposed intervention and are typically pursued on a small number of individuals in case there are problems with the intervention. To minimize the risk of exposing individuals to a new intervention that might cause them harm, insights into the likelihood that individuals with a certain profile will have an adverse response are required. Studies that consider genetic factors that predispose to responses to drugs (good or bad) have revealed many compelling and clinically useful connections between genetic variants and drug responses. Discovering such 'pharmacogenetic' insights has been greatly enhanced through the use of AI tools applied to very large databases with relevant genetic and drug response information [31, 32].

The actual design of phase I clinical trials is an ongoing area of research. The fact that only a few individuals are enrolled in such trials, and a great sensitivity to the detection of the effects of the proposed drug or intervention are of focus, suggests that careful monitoring of the subjects enrolled in the trial is required. Extensions of N-of-1 and aggregated N-of-1 trial designs could be appropriate for phase I trials [33]. Although discussed in greater detail in the context of vetting the efficacy of a personalized medicine in Sect. 11.6 below, such studies can leverage massive amounts of data and AI techniques to identify patterns in a patient's data that might be indicative of response to the intervention (see, e.g., Serhani et al. [34]). Table 11.1 lists examples of studies that have focused on monitoring a single individual over time to explore how they responded to a particular intervention, or how their health status may have changed over that time, using various data collection schemes.

In the context of personalized medicine studies, once an individual is found to possess a certain pathology, a need to identify how that pathology can be corrected arises (P1 in the right-hand panel of Fig. 11.2). For many common chronic diseases, this is obvious (e.g., for someone diagnosed with high blood pressure, providing blood pressure lowering medications makes sense). However, nuanced features of the patient that could effect an intervention response, and the optimal way to correct the pathology given those nuances, are not often clear. AI-based strategies similar to those used for making diagnoses can be exploited to identify potentially correctable pathologies (P0 and P1 in the right panel of Fig. 11.2). For example, the company Arterys recently announced the first FDA-approved AI-based application to be used in facilitating clinical diagnoses. The Arterys system used deep learning applied to a medical imaging platform to help diagnose heart problems [35]. Other systems have been developed that consider more comprehensive approaches to understanding a patient's profiles in a way that could facilitate the choice of an intervention [36].

To assess and identify pathologies in the first place, biomaterial, usually in the form of biopsies, is needed from patients, and there is growing sophistication in the way that biopsied material or patient biosamples can be studied in a laboratory to identify targets for intervention. For example, emerging induced pluripotent stem cell (iPSC) and organoid technologies have shown great promise in yielding insights into patient-specific pathologies that could be overcome with specific interventions (see Table 2 of Schork and Nazor [6] as well as Rossi et al. [37]). When recently developed single cell assays are combined with the use of organoids, even greater resolution concerning pathologies and drug targets can be revealed, and AI-based analyses have been shown to be effective in this area [38].

Table 11.1 Single patient-oriented studies leveraging intensive monitoring to identify either health status changes or the effects of an intervention

Authors	Reference	Study elements	Comments
David et al. (2014) [93]	PMID: 25146375	Diet and microbiome	Two individuals fecal microbiome tracked for a year
Chen et al. (2012) [94]	PMID: 22424236	Multiomics profiling	Individual tracked over a year (the 'Snyderome' study)
Magnuson et al. (2016) [95]	PMID: 28781744	Sleep treatment study	Patient with multiple treatments for compromised sleep
Zeevi et al. (2015) [96]	PMID: 26590418	Glycemic responses to diet	800 people studied to develop *personalized* diets
Smarr et al. (2017) [97]	PMID: 29582916	Colonoscopy effects	Gut microbiome changes post colonoscopy
Trammell et al. (2016) [98]	PMID: 27721479	NAD dose response	Single individual dosing study + study of others
Forsdyke (2015) [99]	PMID: 26055103	Response to antihypertensives	Decade of seasonal variation in response to Losartan
O'Rawe et al. (2013) [100]	PMID: 24109560	Deep brain stimulation (DBS)	Two-year study of a man with OCD treated with DBS
Li et al. (2016) [101]	PMID: 27140603	Parkinson's cell replacement	Single individual traced for 24 years post cell transplant
Bloss et al. (2015) [102]	PMID: 25790160	Idiopathic neurologic disease	Severely disabled individual treated for sleep tremors
Piening et al. (2018) [103]	PMID: 29361466	Multiomics weight loss study	23 individuals observed over time
Zalusky and Herbert (1961) [104]	PMID: 14009735	Folate supplementation	Study of an individual with severe dietary constraints
Herbert (1962) [105]	PMID: 13953904	Folate supplementation	Study on the researcher himself; dietary restriction
Golding (2014) [106]	PMID: 25332850	Folate supplementation	Study on the researcher himself; dietary restriction

11.5 Late Human (T2) and Intervention Choice (P2) Studies

If a drug, intervention or health product has been shown to be safe and likely to be efficacious in early phase trials, then it must be tested for its general utility in the population at large. AI can be exploited in relevant large-scale population trials that seek to minimize the deployment and use of inappropriate drugs or interventions for participants in the trial, as described recently by Yauney and Shah [39]. Of great interest in this context are the design and conduct of bucket (or variations termed 'basket'), umbrella, and adaptive trial designs [40]. Although each has unique features, a simple description of bucket trials can provide the general strategy behind each of these trial designs and also points out where AI can be exploited. Essentially bucket trials enroll eligible patients, profile them to identify nuanced pathophysiologic profiles they possess (e.g., sequencing their tumor DNA in the context of a cancer clinical trial), and then assign each of them one of possibly many treatments based on the mechanisms of action of the treatments and their biologic connections to the patient pathophysiologic profiles (i.e., put each patient into one of many treatment 'buckets'). If the patients provided with treatments dictated by their pathophysiologic profiles (i.e., assigned to the different baskets) have better outcomes than those provided treatments without recourse to the profiling and treatment matching scheme, then one could infer that the strategy or 'algorithm' for matching the treatments to the patients has merit. AI could be of great use in not only identifying treatment targets in the patient profiles, but also aid in determining the strategy for matching the treatments to the patient profiles. This would especially be the case if one could envision the use of many different treatment buckets (e.g., due to the use of many treatment combinations or complicated temporal treatment schemes).

In the context of choosing an intervention for a particular individual via the personalized medicine paradigm (P2 in the right panel of Fig. 11.2), if available drugs and interventions exist, then the choice could be based on simply matching the patient's pathophysiologic profile to the mechanisms of action of the drugs, consistent with the underlying theme governing bucket trials. If the choice is not obvious, then one could leverage personalized drug screening strategies using biopsies or biomaterials obtained from the patient, as suggested by Kodack et al. in the context of cancer [41]. These, and more general, personalized drug screening strategies have been developed and could benefit from AI techniques to find patterns of relevance in the data that could indicate which drug or intervention is the most optimal for a given patient [42, 43].

11.6 Implementation (T3) and Clinical Assessment (P3) Studies

Once a drug, intervention or health product has been shown to benefit individuals in the general population, then considerations about the routine implementation and/or use of the product arise (T3 in the left side of Fig. 11.2). Implementation can come in many forms. For example, if clinical trials focusing on a specific drug provide sufficient evidence that the drug is safe and efficacious, it can be approved for use by regulatory agencies such as the FDA and become adopted in clinical practice. Of greater relevance to AI is the implementation of insights that might benefit physicians with respect to intervention choices when confronted with patients with unique profiles (e.g., implementing a treatment strategy of the type tested in a bucket trial). Implementing such insights requires codifying them and then providing them to physicians through, e.g., electronic medical record (EMR) systems typically used to convey patient information to physicians [44]. Implementation of AI-based insights is a major topic of discussion among pathologists since they are typically responsible for evaluating evidence that a patient has particular condition, as well as pointing out nuances associated with that condition that may require special attention when intervention decisions are made [45]. The provision of 'decision support' information of this type to physicians and healthcare workers—especially information derived from AI-based analyses—opens up a number of thorny ethical issues, however, such as who to blame if the use of the decision support leads to poorer outcomes (i.e., the algorithm and its developers or the users who may be using it inappropriately) [46].

One important element of the implementation of AI-based decision support tools in EMR systems is that as new patient data are collected, the prediction models they are based on can be improved. Thus, 'Learning Systems' can be created that continually evolve and improve based on the accrual of more patient information and outcomes [47–49]. Sophisticated AI techniques can be used to enhance this learning, including aggregating data from multiple EMRs or sources [50].

To vet the utility of an intervention for an individual patient (P3 in the right side of Fig. 11.2), N-of-1 trials can be pursued [33, 51]. AI techniques can be used to identify patterns in data collected on the patient—say through wireless sensors—that might be indicative of that patient's response (or lack thereof) to the intervention [34]. The studies listed in Table 11.1 provide example published N-of-1 studies focusing on an individual's response to a treatment or an individual undergoing monitoring for health status changes.

11.7 Post-deployment Evaluation (T4) Studies and Warehousing (P4)

After the implementation and adoption of a new drug, treatment intervention, or health product, continuous monitoring of that product must occur in order to determine if either unanticipated side effects are occurring or the product can be improved or replaced for various reasons (T4 in the left side of Fig. 11.2). AI-based learning systems of the type mentioned in the previous section provide an excellent foundation for such monitoring, and early experiences with such systems bear this out [52–54]. In addition to the creation of learning systems, there are many initiatives to aggregate data on patients and patient materials to enable data mining and AI-based analyses, for example in cancer contexts [55], but also for more general settings as well [56, 57].

The implementation of AI-based products, such as EMR decision support tools and learning systems, will also affect doctor/patient relationships in profound ways. This is especially likely with respect to the justification of intervention choices for an individual patient [58], but also with respect to predictions concerning future healthcare needs of that patient where the initiation of interventions might be appropriate [59]. In this light, large, government-sponsored national initiatives are being pursued to identify patterns among individuals tracked for healthcare-related phenomena that might be useful in clinical and public health practices in the future, such as the UK Biobank initiative in the United Kingdom and the 'All-of-Us' study in the USA [60, 61]. These studies raise important questions about the ethical, legal, and social implications of aggregating data on many individuals for the purpose of benefitting a smaller number of individuals who may need focused care going forward [61].

11.8 Integration and the Personalized Medicine Workflow

The P0–P4 personalized medicine translational workflow has many common elements with the T0–T4 drug and health product development workflow (Fig. 11.2) as noted. One important common element is that the transitions from each stage of the workflow need to be seemless and efficient. This can be difficult since the expertise and technologies needed at each stage are very different, often leading to their independent pursuit. However, emerging strategies and concepts in the way personalized medicine is practiced, coupled with the use of AI techniques, could lead to more holistic and efficient ways of treating individual patients that run through the entire P0–P4 workflow [6].

Thus, the ideal setting for personalized medicine and health care is one in which the diagnoses, treatment, and follow-up monitoring of individual patients are streamlined into a single process with very smooth and coordinated transitions from one relevant activity or sub-process to another. A good paradigm for this involves the creation of cell replacement therapies for a wide variety of conditions [62, 63]. For example, in certain immunotherapeutic-oriented cell replacement therapies for cancer, a patient's tumor is profiled for the existence of unique 'neo-antigens' or mutations that might attract the host's own immune system to attack the cells harboring those mutations. If such neo-antigens are found, then cells from either a donor (allogeneic transplantation) or from the patient him or herself (autologous transplantation) are harvested and sensitized to recognize the neo-antigens. The basic idea is that these modified cells will attract the host's immune cells to the tumor cells harboring the neo-antigens when introduced into the patient's body [62, 63]. Since the creation and manufacture of the cells cannot be pursued in advance of knowing what neo-antigens are present in the patient's tumor, they must be created in near real time. The production of treatments for patients in real time based on the patient's unique and immediate needs is termed the 'magistral' production of treatments, as opposed to the traditional or 'officinal' production of treatments [29, 30]. Magistral production of treatments such as drugs is likely to be a reality for personalized medicine in many settings, even beyond cancer, since it would be too difficult to anticipate all the treatments (e.g., cells sensitive to every neo-antigen profile) and stockpile them for use in the future, as is assumed in the case with the officinal production of treatments.

To advance and generalize this concept of the magistral production of personalized medicine treatments, one could imagine leveraging AI-powered robotics technologies to enable the efficient and precise manufacture of relevant treatments [64]. 3D printing of treatments also has the potential to facilitate the realtime production of treatments, as the first US FDA-approval for a 3D printed drug was made in 2015 [65]. One could also envision the immediate conduct of N-of-1 trials involving AI-based pattern discovery with sophisticated treatment outcome monitoring devices after a treatment has been crafted to assess its impact on the patient [33, 51, 66]. Further, one could potentially exploit AI-based simulation studies to anticipate directions that a treatment strategy might take [67].

11.9 Limitations of AI in Advancing Personalized Medicine

There are many limitations to the use of AI in the development of personalized medicines. We briefly discuss some of the more salient issues below. First, there is an argument that many big data analyses that combine information on many individuals to identify patterns that reflect *population-level* relationships between data points do not get at important *individual-level* relationships [68]. This potential lack of 'ergodicity' could result in models that are not useful for making individual treatment decisions. It has been shown that, in terms of identifying trends in a target individual's health data that could indicate a health status change for that target individual based on data collected on a large number of individuals, as more data points are collected on each individual, any predictions of the target individual's heath trajectory will rely (in a statistical sense) more on the legacy data points on that target individual and less on the population-level data [69]. Sensitizing AI techniques to this fact is crucial for advancing personalized medicine.

Second, there is a need to vet or test the utility of healthcare products rooted in AI. This is motivated by the inconsistent results observed with the use of some AI or big data-based healthcare products, such as IBM's Watson treatment decision support system [70, 71]. Testing such systems via traditional randomized clinical trials has been discussed in the literature, and some AI-based decision support tools have in fact been shown evidence for efficacy in *bona fide* clinical trials [72]. A potential need for vetting AI-based decision support products, like IBM's Watson, is that if the underlying system's decision making capability is trained on an incomplete or biased data set, then the recommendations or predictions it provides are likely to be unreliable. A rather infamous case of this involves Google's system for predicting flu outbreaks [73]. In addition, in the context of bucket trials, in which the underlying scheme for matching drugs to patient profiles is being tested, if the scheme is shown not work better than standard of care or an alternative way of matching drugs to patient profiles, then a couple of questions could be raised. It could be that the drugs are ineffective, or some subset are ineffective, essentially negatively impacting the overall performance of the matching scheme. Alternatively, it could be that the drugs work, but simply are not matched properly to the patient profiles; i.e., the matching algorithm or scheme is simply wrong. These questions were raised in the context of the SHIVA trial—a bucket trail in which the drug matching scheme was shown not to benefit the patients any more than legacy ways of treating patients [74].

Third, it may be that the best way to vet at least decision support tools, is not to test them in randomized clinical trials, but rather to implement them in learning systems in which the decision support rules or algorithms are continuously updated [66, 75–78]. However, learning systems of this sort require a lack of bias in the initial data sets used to seed the system in order to ensure generalizable results. In addition, it could take a long time for the system to evolve into a one with an accurate and reliable decision scheme.

Fourth, many AI-based decision support products leverage deep learning and neural network-based algorithms. Such algorithms can produce very reliable predictions if a large enough training set is used, but the connections between the inputs (i.e., data) and the outputs (i.e., predictions) can be very hard to understand. Thus, the 'Black Box' problem associated with many AI-based tools can be problematic and lead to a lack of confidence or sense of trepidation about relying on the predictions in the real world where real lives are at stake [79]. In addition, not all AI techniques are designed to identify causal relationships between various inputs and outputs, but rather mere associations or predictions (i.e., they focus on correlation and not causation) [80]. This may suffice if the goal is to develop accurate predictions, but if the goal is to, e.g., identify a drug target that, when modulated, leads to a desired effect, then identifying causal relationships is crucial.

11.10 Future Directions and Concluding Remarks

The future contributions of AI in advancing personalized medicine are likely to be very pronounced, as this chapter makes clear. Not only will there be greater adoption of AI-based health products in the near term, but such products could be developed and exploit emerging and more long term computing capabilities such as quantum computing [81, 82] to achieve increased speed and an ability to handle larger and larger data sets. These larger data sets are likely to derive from better and more sophisticated monitoring health devices which can be used to gather data to seed and key off for the development of more reliable predictions [83].

In addition to exploiting greater speed and computational efficiency, AI-based health products and tools will likely incorporate greater understanding of biology in the future. For example, the discovery of simple input/output relationships among data points that has been focus of a great deal of AI, machine learning and statistical analysis research, could be pursued with constraints that are known to govern phenomena of relevance (e.g., known biophysical constraints involving the production of metabolites in a biochemical pathway, first principles having to do with Watson-Crick base pairing, etc.), leading to more biologically compelling models [84, 85].

Finally, as a closing note, much of the use of AI in the development of personalized medicines has focused on the treatment of individuals with overt disease: identifying the underlying pathology, determining which interventions might make most sense to provide given what is known about that pathology and the mechanisms of action of interventions, and testing to see if a chosen intervention works. Thus, the vast majority of AI-based products and tools used in advancing personalized medicine focus on the diagnosis, prognosis, and treatment of individuals. This makes sense as there is a great need for advances and efficiency gains in treating patients given the costs of current treatments, especially in the context of cancer. However, the application of AI to disease *prevention* is gaining a great deal of attention and traction. For example, AI and machine learning techniques have been shown to be useful in the development of 'polygenic risk scores' that can be used to identify individuals with an elevated genetic risk for disease who could be monitored more closely [86–88]. In addition, by combining insights into genetic predisposition to disease with continuous monitoring to identify early signs of disease, one could potentially stop diseases in their tracks before complicated treatments are needed [89, 90]. Such monitoring could be greatly enhanced by applying AI techniques to the data collected by novel sensors provided to patients [91, 92].

Ultimately, enthusiasm for leveraging AI techniques is not likely to slow down any time soon. AI is likely to impact virtually every industry, from manufacturing, to sales and marketing, to banking, to transportation. In fact, many of these industries have already experienced changes with the introduction of AI. The healthcare industry is no less likely to benefit from AI, as this chapter has made clear, as long as appropriate integration and vetting occurs.

References

1. Russell S, Norvig P (2009) Artificial intelligence: a modern approach, 3rd edn. Pearson, Carmel, IN
2. Mahmud M et al (2018) Applications of deep learning and reinforcement learning to biological data. IEEE Trans Neural Netw Learn Syst 29(6):2063–2079
3. Webb S (2018) Deep learning for biology. Nature 554(7693):555–557
4. Fleming N (2018) How artificial intelligence is changing drug discovery. Nature 557(7707): S55–S57
5. Committee to Review the Clinical and Translational Science Awards Program at the National Center for Advancing Translational Sciences, Board on Health Sciences Policy, Institute of Medicine, Leshner AI, Terry S (eds) (2013) The CTSA program at NIH: opportunities for advancing clinical and translational research. The national academies collection: reports funded by National Institutes of Health. National Academies Press, Washington, DC
6. Schork NJ, Nazor K (2017) Integrated genomic medicine: a paradigm for rare diseases and beyond. Adv Genet 97:81–113
7. Telenti A et al (2018) Deep learning of genomic variation and regulatory network data. Hum Mol Genet 27(R1):R63–R71
8. Esteva A et al (2017) Dermatologist-level classification of skin cancer with deep neural networks. Nature 542(7639):115–118

9. Gerstung M et al (2017) Precision oncology for acute myeloid leukemia using a knowledge bank approach. Nat Genet 49(3):332–340
10. Gulshan V et al (2016) Development and validation of a deep learning algorithm for detection of diabetic retinopathy in retinal fundus photographs. JAMA 316(22):2402–2410
11. Cohen JD et al (2018) Detection and localization of surgically resectable cancers with a multi-analyte blood test. Science 359(6378):926–930
12. Bray MA et al (2017) A dataset of images and morphological profiles of 30 000 small-molecule treatments using the Cell Painting assay. Gigascience 6(12):1–5
13. Ma J et al (2018) Using deep learning to model the hierarchical structure and function of a cell. Nat Methods 15(4):290–298
14. Ideker T et al (2001) Integrated genomic and proteomic analyses of a systematically perturbed metabolic network. Science 292(5518):929–934
15. Bohannon J (2017) The cyberscientist. Science 357(6346):18–21
16. King RD et al (2009) The automation of science. Science 324(5923):85–89
17. Sparkes A, Clare A (2012) AutoLabDB: a substantial open source database schema to support a high-throughput automated laboratory. Bioinformatics 28(10):1390–1397
18. Butler KT et al (2018) Machine learning for molecular and materials science. Nature 559(7715):547–555
19. Sanchez-Lengeling B, Aspuru-Guzik A (2018) Inverse molecular design using machine learning: generative models for matter engineering. Science 361(6400):360–365
20. Aage N et al (2017) Giga-voxel computational morphogenesis for structural design. Nature 550(7674):84–86
21. Segler MHS, Preuss M, Waller MP (2018) Planning chemical syntheses with deep neural networks and symbolic AI. Nature 555(7698):604–610
22. Ahneman DT et al (2018) Predicting reaction performance in C-N cross-coupling using machine learning. Science 360(6385):186–190
23. Radovic A et al (2018) Machine learning at the energy and intensity frontiers of particle physics. Nature 560(7716):41–48
24. Silver D et al (2017) Mastering the game of Go without human knowledge. Nature 550(7676):354–359
25. Madhukar NS et al (2018) A new big-data paradigm for target identification and drug discovery. BioRxiv. https://doi.org/10.1101/134973
26. Chen B, Butte AJ (2016) Leveraging big data to transform target selection and drug discovery. Clin Pharmacol Ther 99(3):285–297
27. Hu Y, Bajorath J (2017) Entering the 'big data' era in medicinal chemistry: molecular promiscuity analysis revisited. Future Sci OA 3(2):FSO179
28. Hernandez D (2018) How robots are making better drugs, faster. In: Wall Street Journal. Dow Jones & Company, New York, NY
29. Patient-centered drug manufacture (2017) Nat Biotechnol 35(6):485
30. Schellekens H et al (2017) Making individualized drugs a reality. Nat Biotechnol 35(6): 507–513
31. Lavertu A et al (2018) Pharmacogenomics and big genomic data: from lab to clinic and back again. Hum Mol Genet 27(R1):R72–R78
32. Kalinin AA et al (2018) Deep learning in pharmacogenomics: from gene regulation to patient stratification. Pharmacogenomics 19(7):629–650
33. Schork NJ (2015) Personalized medicine: time for one-person trials. Nature 520(7549): 609–611
34. Serhani MA et al (2017) New algorithms for processing time-series big EEG data within mobile health monitoring systems. Comput Methods Programs Biomed 149:79–94
35. Marr B (2017) First FDA approval for clinical cloud-based deep learning in healthcare. In: Forbes. Forbes Publishing Company, New York City
36. Miotto R et al (2016) Deep patient: an unsupervised representation to predict the future of patients from the electronic health records. Sci Rep 6:26094

37. Rossi G, Manfrin A, Lutolf MP (2018) Progress and potential in organoid research. Nat Rev Genet
38. Deng Y et al (2018) Massive single-cell RNA-seq analysis and imputation via deep learning. BioRxiv. https://t.co/EGBwlYFLLK
39. Yauney G, Shah P (2018) Reinforcement learning with action-derived rewards for chemotherapy and clinical trial dosing regimen selection. In: Proceedings of machine learning research, vol 85
40. Biankin AV, Piantadosi S, Hollingsworth SJ (2015) Patient-centric trials for therapeutic development in precision oncology. Nature 526(7573):361–370
41. Kodack DP et al (2017) Primary patient-derived cancer cells and their potential for personalized cancer patient care. Cell Rep 21(11):3298–3309
42. Gorshkov K et al (2018) Advancing precision medicine with personalized drug screening. Drug Discov Today
43. Miranda CC et al (2018) Towards multi-organoid systems for drug screening applications. Bioengineering (Basel) 5(3)
44. Scott IA et al (2018) Using EMR-enabled computerized decision support systems to reduce prescribing of potentially inappropriate medications: a narrative review. Ther Adv Drug Saf 9(9):559–573
45. Dreyer KJ, Geis JR (2017) When machines think: radiology's next frontier. Radiology 285(3): 713–718
46. Nabi J (2018) How bioethics can shape artificial intelligence and machine learning. Hastings Cent Rep 48(5):10–13
47. Etheredge LM (2007) A rapid-learning health system. Health Aff (Millwood) 26(2): w107–w118
48. Shrager J, Tenenbaum JM (2014) Rapid learning for precision oncology. Nat Rev Clin Oncol 11(2):109–118
49. Shah A et al (2016) Building a rapid learning health care system for oncology: why CancerLinQ collects identifiable health information to achieve its vision. J Clin Oncol 34(7): 756–763
50. Hastie T, Tibshirani R, Friedman J (2009) The elements of statistical learning: data mining, inference, and prediction, 2nd edn. Springer, New York
51. Schork NJ, Goetz LH (2017) Single-subject studies in translational nutrition research. Annu Rev Nutr 37:395–422
52. Agarwala V et al (2018) Real-world evidence in support of precision medicine: clinico-genomic cancer data as a case study. Health Aff (Millwood) 37(5):765–772
53. Williams MS et al (2018) Patient-centered precision health in a learning health care system: Geisinger's genomic medicine experience. Health Aff (Millwood) 37(5):757–764
54. Rajkomar A et al (2018) Scalable and accurate deep learning with electronic health records. NPJ Digit Med 1(18)
55. Ali M, Aittokallio T (2018) Machine learning and feature selection for drug response prediction in precision oncology applications. Biophys Rev
56. Mathe E et al (2018) The omics revolution continues: the maturation of high-throughput biological data sources. Yearb Med Inform 27(1):211–222
57. Varghese J et al (2018) CDEGenerator: an online platform to learn from existing data models to build model registries. Clin Epidemiol 10:961–970
58. Lerner I et al (2018) Revolution in health care: how will data science impact doctor-patient relationships? Front Public Health 6:99
59. Savage N (2017) Machine learning: calculating disease. Nature 550(7676):S115–S117
60. Bycroft C et al (2018) The UK Biobank resource with deep phenotyping and genomic data. Nature 562:203–209
61. Sankar PL, Parker LS (2017) The Precision Medicine Initiative's All of Us Research Program: an agenda for research on its ethical, legal, and social issues. Genet Med 19(7): 743–750

62. Li C et al (2018) Application of induced pluripotent stem cell transplants: autologous or allogeneic? Life Sci
63. Graham C et al (2018) Allogeneic CAR-T cells: more than ease of access? Cells 7(10)
64. Tan R, Yang X, Shen Y (2017) Robot-aided electrospinning toward intelligent biomedical engineering. Robotics Biomim 4(1):17
65. Osouli-Bostanabad K, Adibkia K (2018) Made-on-demand, complex and personalized 3D-printed drug products. Bioimpacts 8(2):77–79
66. Schork NJ (2018) Randomized clinical trials and personalized medicine: a commentary on deaton and cartwright. Soc Sci Med 210:71–73
67. Shamsuddin R et al (2018) Virtual patient model: an approach for generating synthetic healthcare time series data. In: IEEE international conference on healthcare informatics. IEEE Computer Society
68. Fisher AJ, Medaglia JD, Jeronimus BF (2018) Lack of group-to-individual generalizability is a threat to human subjects research. Proc Natl Acad Sci U S A 115(27):E6106–E6115
69. Drescher CW et al (2013) Longitudinal screening algorithm that incorporates change over time in CA125 levels identifies ovarian cancer earlier than a single-threshold rule. J Clin Oncol 31(3):387–392
70. Zhou N et al (2018) Concordance study between IBM Watson for Oncology and clinical practice for patients with cancer in China. Oncologist
71. Schmidt C (2017) M. D. Anderson breaks with IBM Watson, raising questions about artificial intelligence in oncology. J Natl Cancer Inst 109(5):4–5
72. Abramoff MD et al (2018) Pivotal trial of an autonomous AI-based diagnostic system for detection of diabetic retinopathy in primary care offices. NPJ Digit Med 1(39)
73. Lazer D et al (2014) Big data. The parable of Google Flu: traps in big data analysis. Science 343(6176):1203–1205
74. Le Tourneau C et al (2015) Molecularly targeted therapy based on tumour molecular profiling versus conventional therapy for advanced cancer (SHIVA): a multicentre, open-label, proof-of-concept, randomised, controlled phase 2 trial. Lancet Oncol 16(13): 1324–1334
75. Ioannidis JPA, Khoury MJ (2018) Evidence-based medicine and big genomic data. Hum Mol Genet 27(R1):R2–R7
76. AI diagnostics need attention (2018) Nature 555(7696):285
77. Frieden TR (2017) Evidence for health decision making—beyond randomized, controlled trials. N Engl J Med 377(5):465–475
78. Abernethy A, Khozin S (2017) Clinical drug trials may be coming to your doctor's office. In: Wall Street Journal. Dow Jones & Company, New York, NY
79. Voosen P (2017) The AI detectives. Science 357(6346):22–27
80. Marwala T (2015) Causality, correlation and artificial intelligence for rational decision making. World Scientific, New Jersey
81. Ciliberto C et al (2018) Quantum machine learning: a classical perspective. Proc Math Phys Eng Sci 474(2209):20170551
82. Li RY et al (2018) Quantum annealing versus classical machine learning applied to a simplified computational biology problem. npj Quantum Inf 4
83. Vashistha R et al (2018) Futuristic biosensors for cardiac health care: an artificial intelligence approach. 3 Biotech 8(8):358
84. Palsson B (2015) Systems biology: constraint-based reconstruction and analysis, 2nd edn. Cambridge University Press, Boston, MA
85. Ideker T, Dutkowski J, Hood L (2011) Boosting signal-to-noise in complex biology: prior knowledge is power. Cell 144(6):860–863
86. Khera AV et al (2018) Genome-wide polygenic scores for common diseases identify individuals with risk equivalent to monogenic mutations. Nat Genet 50(9):1219–1224
87. Warren M (2018) The approach to predictive medicine that is taking genomics research by storm. Nature 562(7726):181–183

88. Schork AJ, Schork MA, Schork NJ (2018) Genetic risks and clinical rewards. Nat Genet 50(9):1210–1211
89. Patel CJ et al (2013) Whole genome sequencing in support of wellness and health maintenance. Genome Med 5(6):58
90. Schork NJ (2013) Genetic parts to a preventive medicine whole. Genome Med 5(6):54
91. Mapara SS, Patravale VB (2017) Medical capsule robots: a renaissance for diagnostics, drug delivery and surgical treatment. J Control Release 261:337–351
92. Topol EJ (2019) Deep medicine: how artificial intelligence can make healthcare human again. Basic Books, New York
93. David LA et al (2014) Host lifestyle affects human microbiota on daily timescales. Genome Biol 15(7):R89
94. Chen R et al (2012) Personal omics profiling reveals dynamic molecular and medical phenotypes. Cell 148(6):1293–1307
95. Magnuson V, Wang Y, Schork N (2016) Normalizing sleep quality disturbed by psychiatric polypharmacy: a single patient open trial (SPOT). F1000Research 5:132
96. Zeevi D et al (2015) Personalized nutrition by prediction of glycemic responses. Cell 163(5): 1079–1094
97. Smarr L et al (2017) Tracking human gut microbiome changes resulting from a colonoscopy. Methods Inf Med 56(6):442–447
98. Trammell SA et al (2016) Nicotinamide riboside is uniquely and orally bioavailable in mice and humans. Nat Commun 7:12948
99. Forsdyke DR (2015) Summertime dosage-dependent hypersensitivity to an angiotensin II receptor blocker. BMC Res Notes 8:227
100. O'Rawe JA et al (2013) Integrating precision medicine in the study and clinical treatment of a severely mentally ill person. PeerJ 1:e177
101. Li W et al (2016) Extensive graft-derived dopaminergic innervation is maintained 24 years after transplantation in the degenerating parkinsonian brain. Proc Natl Acad Sci U S A 113(23): 6544–6549
102. Bloss CS et al (2015) A genome sequencing program for novel undiagnosed diseases. Genet Med 17(12):995–1001
103. Piening BD et al (2018) Integrative personal omics profiles during periods of weight gain and loss. Cell Syst 6(2):157–170 e8
104. Zalusky R, Herbert V (1961) Megaloblastic anemia in scurvy with response to 50 microgm. of folic acid daily. N Engl J Med 265:1033–1038
105. Herbert V (1962) Experimental nutritional folate deficiency in man. Trans Assoc Am Physicians 75:307–320
106. Golding PH (2014) Severe experimental folate deficiency in a human subject—a longitudinal study of biochemical and haematological responses as megaloblastic anaemia develops. Springerplus 3:442

MIX
Papier aus verantwortungsvollen Quellen
Paper from responsible sources
FSC® C105338

If you have any concerns about our products,
you can contact us on
ProductSafety@springernature.com

In case Publisher is established outside the EU,
the EU authorized representative is:
Springer Nature Customer Service Center GmbH
Europaplatz 3, 69115 Heidelberg, Germany

Printed by Libri Plureos GmbH
in Hamburg, Germany